Topics in Palliative Care
Volume 3

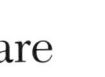

Series Editors
Russell K. Portenoy, M.D.
Eduardo Bruera, M.D.

TOPICS IN PALLIATIVE CARE

Volume 3

Edited by

Russell K. Portenoy
Beth Israel Medical Center
New York, New York

Eduardo Bruera
Grey Nuns Community Health Centre
University of Alberta
Edmonton, Alberta

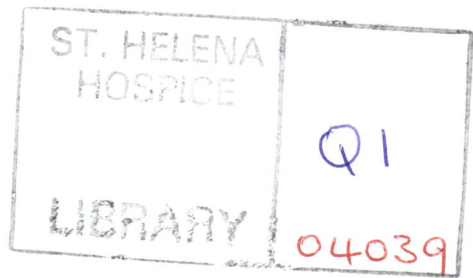
New York   Oxford
OXFORD UNIVERSITY PRESS
1998

Oxford University Press

Oxford New York
Athens Auckland Bangkok Bogotá Buenos Aires Calcutta
Cape Town Chennai Dar es Salaam Delhi Florence Hong Kong Istanbul
Karachi Kuala Lumpur Madrid Melbourne Mexico City Mumbai
Nairobi Paris São Paulo Singapore Taipei Tokyo Toronto Warsaw

and associated companies in
Berlin Ibadan

Published by Oxford University Press Inc.,
198 Madison Avenue, New York, New York 10016

Library of Congress Cataloging-in-Publication Data
Topics in palliative care / edited by Russell K. Portenoy, Eduardo Bruera.
p. cm.—(Topics in palliative care : v. 3)
Includes bibliographical references and index.
ISBN 0-19-510246-0
1. Cancer—Palliative treatment.
I. Portenoy, Russell K.
II. Bruera, Eduardo.
III. Series.
[DNLM: 1. Palliative Care. 2. Neoplasms—drug therapy.
Pain—drug therapy.]
WB 310 T674 1997] RC271.P33T664 1997
616.99'406—dc20 DNLM/DLC for Library of Congress 96-22250

9 8 7 6 5 4 3 2 1
Printed in the United States of America
on acid-free paper.

04039
Q1

AUTHOR PORTENOY

TITLE Topics in palliative care Vol. 3.

No Date	NAME	Name DATE
Temp Mem	J Baston	15 NOV 2001
1295	KL Wesson	19 NOV ???
. . . .		. . . .
. . . .		. . . .
. . . .		. . . .
. . . .		. . . .
. . . .		. . . .
. . . .		. . . .
. . . .		. . . .
. . . .		. . . .
. . . .		. . . .
. . . .		. . . .
. . . .		. . . .

DG 1301

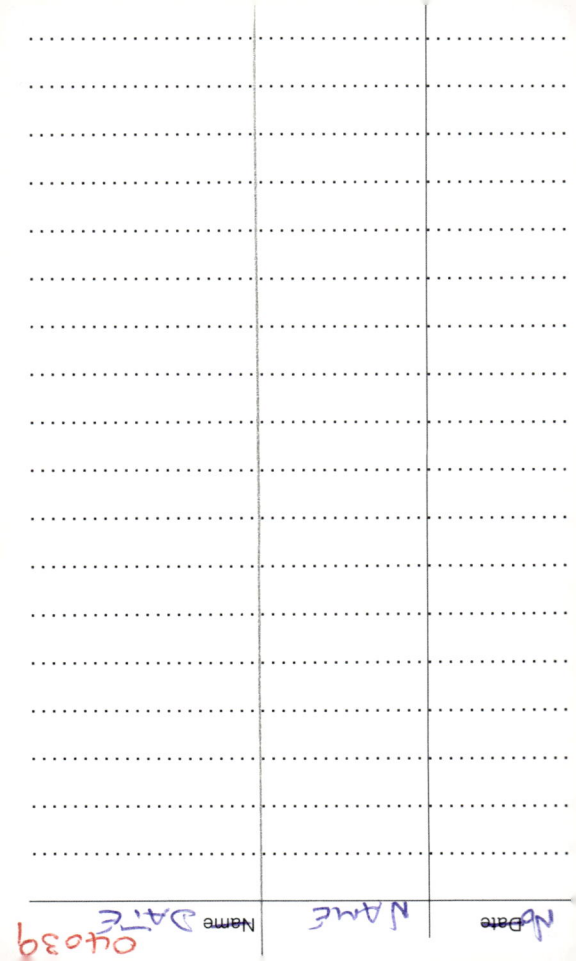

To our wives,
Susan and Maria,
whose love and support
make our work possible.

Preface to the Series

Palliative Care, a series devoted to research and practice in palliative care, was created to address the growing need to disseminate new information about this rapidly evolving field.

Palliative care is an interdisciplinary therapeutic model for the management of patients with incurable, progressive illness. In this model, the family is considered the unit of care. The clinical purview includes those factors—physical, psychological, social, and spiritual—that contribute to suffering, undermine quality of life, and prevent a death with comfort and dignity. The definition promulgated by the World Health Organization exemplifies this perspective.°

> Palliative care is the active total care of patients whose disease is not responsive to curative treatment. Control of pain, of other symptoms, and of psychological, social and spiritual problems is paramount. The goal of palliative care is the achievement of the best possible quality of life for patients and their families.

Palliative care is a fundamental part of clinical practice, the "parallel universe" to therapies directed at cure or prolongation of life. All clinicians who treat patients with chronic life-threatening diseases are engaged in palliative care, continually attempting to manage complex symptomatology and functional disturbances.

The need for specialized palliative care services may arise at any point during the illness. Symptom control and psychological adaptation are the usual concerns during the period of active disease-oriented therapies. Toward the end of life, however, needs intensify and broaden. Psychosocial distress or family distress, spiritual or existential concerns, advance care planning, and ethical concerns, among many other issues, may be considered by the various disciplines that coalesce in the delivery of optimal care. Clinicians who specialize in palliative care perceive their role as similar to those of specialists in other disciplines of medicine: referring patients to other primary caregivers when appropriate, acting as primary caregivers (as members of the team) when the challenges of the case warrant this involvement, and teaching and conducting research in the field of palliative care.

With recognition of palliative care as an essential element in medical care and as an area of specialization, there is a need for information about the approaches used by specialists from many disciplines in managing the varied problems that

---

°World Health Organization. Technical Report Series 804, Cancer Pain and Palliative Care. Geneva: World Health Organization, 1990:11.

fall under the purview of this model. The scientific foundation of palliative care is also advancing, and similarly, methods are needed to highlight for practitioners at the bedside the findings of empirical research. Topics in Palliative Care has been designed to meet the need for enhanced communication in this changing field.

To highlight the diversity of concerns in palliative care, each volume of Topics in Palliative Care is divided into sections that address a range of issues. Various sections address aspects of symptom control, psychosocial functioning, spiritual or existential concerns, ethics, and other topics. The chapters in each section review the area and focus on a small number of salient issues for analysis. The authors present and evaluate existing data, provide a context drawn from both the clinic and research, and integrate knowledge in a manner that is both practical and readable.

We are grateful to the many contributors for their excellent work and their timeliness. We also thank our publisher, who has expressed great faith in the project. Such strong support has buttressed our desire to create an educational forum that may enhance palliative care in the clinical setting and drive its growth as a discipline.

New York, N.Y.   R.K.P.
Edmonton, Alberta   E.B.

Contents

IV   Skin Disorders and Their Management

Introduction: Medical and Psychosocial
Implications of Skin Disorders, 231
Eduardo Bruera

Contributors

WILLIAM BREITBART, MD
Cornell University Medical College
    and Psychiatry Service
Department of Psychiatry and Behavioral
    Sciences
Memorial Sloan-Kettering Cancer Center
New York, New York, USA

EDUARDO BRUERA, MD
Palliative Care Program
Grey Nuns Community Health Centre
Edmonton, Alberta, Canada

EDMUND Y.S. CHAO, PhD
Department of Orthopedic Surgery
The Johns Hopkins Hospital
Baltimore, Maryland, USA

JOHN J. COLLINS, MB, BS, FRACP
Pain and Palliative Care Service
The New Children's Hospital
Parramatta, New South Wales, Australia

BETTY DAVIES, RN, PhD
School of Nursing, University of British
    Columbia
and British Columbia Research Institute
    for Child and Family Health
Vancouver, British Columbia, Canada

D. SCOTT ERNST, MD, FRCP(C)
Department of Oncology
University of Calgary
Calgary, Alberta, Canada

DEBORAH ANNE FRASSICA, MD
Department of Radiation Oncology
Uniformed Services University of the
    Health Sciences
Bethesda, Maryland, USA

FRANK J. FRASSICA, MD
Department of Orthopedic Surgery
The Johns Hopkins Hospital
Baltimore, Maryland, USA

PATRICE GUEX, MD
Service de Psychiatrie de Liaison
Centre Hospitalier Universitaire Vaudois
Lausanne, Switzerland

LLOYD R. HALE, FRACGP
Dermatology Department
The Oxford Radcliffe Hospital
Oxford, United Kingdom

JENNIFER L. HAY, PhD
Department of Psychiatry and Behavioral
    Sciences
Memorial Sloan-Kettering Cancer Center
New York, New York, USA

CAMERON A. HUCKELL, MD
Department of Orthopedic Surgery
The Johns Hopkins Hospital
Baltimore, Maryland, USA

JOHN P. KOSTUIK, MD
Department of Orthopedic Surgery
The Johns Hopkins Hospital
Baltimore, Maryland, USA

MARCIA LEVETOWN, MD, FAAP
Departments of Pediatrics and Internal
    Medicine
University of Texas Medical Branch at
    Galveston
Galveston, Texas, USA

STEVEN A. LIETMAN, MD
Department of Orthopedic Surgery
The Johns Hopkins Hospital
Baltimore, Maryland, USA

J. STEPHEN McDANIEL, MD
Department of Psychiatry and Behavioral
  Sciences
Emory University School of
  Medicine
Atlanta, Georgia, USA

DOMINIQUE L. MUSSELMAN, MD
Department of Psychiatry and Behavioral
  Sciences
Emory University School of Medicine
Atlanta, Georgia, USA

CHARLES B. NEMEROFF, MD, PhD
Department of Psychiatry and Behavioral
  Sciences
Emory University School of Medicine
Atlanta, Georgia, USA

STEVEN D. PASSIK, PhD
Oncology Symptom Control
  Research
Community Cancer Care, Inc.
Indianapolis, Indiana, USA

JOSE PEREIRA, MD
Palliative Care Program
Grey Nuns Community Hospital
Edmonton, Alberta, Canada

RUSSELL K. PORTENOY, MD
Department of Pain Medicine and
  Palliative Care
Beth Israel Medical Center
New York, New York, USA

MARYFRANCES R. PORTER, BA
Department of Psychiatry and Behavioral
  Sciences
Emory University School of Medicine
Atlanta, Georgia, USA

PHYLLIS RAMPULLA, PT
Rehabilitation Service
Department of Neurology
Memorial Sloan-Kettering Cancer Center
New York, New York, USA

OLIVIER REAL DEL SARTE, PhD
Service de Psychiatrie de Liaison
Centre Hospitalier Universitaire Vaudois
Lausanne, Switzerland

TERENCE J. RYAN, MB BS
Dermatology Department
The Oxford Radcliffe Hospital
Oxford, United Kingdom

FRANKLIN H. SIM, MD
Department of Orthopedic Surgery
Mayo Clinic
Rochester, Minnesota, USA

ROSE STEELE, RN, MSc
School of Nursing
University of British Columbia
Vancouver, British Columbia, Canada

FRITZ STIEFEL, MD
Service de Psychiatrie de Liaison
Centre Hospitalier Universitaire Vaudois
Lausanne, Switzerland

RICHARD S. TUNKEL, MD
Rehabilitation Service
Department of Neurology
Memorial Sloan-Kettering Cancer Center
New York, New York, USA

PAUL WALKER, MD
Palliative Care Program
Grey Nuns Community Hospital
Edmonton, Alberta, Canada

STEVEN J. WEISMAN, MD
Pediatric Pain Service
Departments of Anesthesiology and
  Pediatrics
Yale University School of Medicine
New Haven, Connecticut, USA

I

Pediatric Palliative Care

Introduction

Pediatric Palliative Care: A Field in Evolution

STEVEN J. WEISMAN

Led by pediatric oncologists, pain specialists, nurses, social workers, and mental health professionals, the palliative care team has become an increasingly visible service in the pediatric tertiary care hospital. As a pediatric hematologist/oncologist, I became interested in some of the issues related to palliative care so that I might lessen the suffering of children dying of cancer. Children with cancer endured much suffering in the 1970s and early 1980s. Treatment modalities had progressed at a remarkable rate and most children with newly diagnosed malignancies could expect to achieve long-term survival. There was, however, the most rudimentary understanding of the means available to support these children through increasingly intensive treatment regimens, or to provide the help they and their families needed as death approached. In addition, I saw only the most elementary understanding of the techniques with which to treat the pain of the child's primary disease, the pain caused by the intensive multimodality treatment programs, or the pain caused by the frequent invasive procedures needed to monitor the progress of these new therapies.

In this same era, the American hospice movement began, and children with cancer were offered new programs of support, such as home care for the dying child. Unfortunately, progress in the universalization of these programs has been slow. I would argue that there may even be a regression in the use and availability of some "traditional" palliative care services, such as home hospice care for children. Further, even with the addition of the burgeoning population of ill children infected with the human immunodeficiency virus (HIV), hospice facilities designed specifically for children remain scarce.

These deficiencies notwithstanding, there has been a relative explosion of supportive care information, which is begging for application to children in need of palliative care. New drugs and therapeutic interventions have brought us to a point where much symptom management can be accomplished with minimal adverse effects. Pain management teams; often multidisciplinary, provide a broad range of services to children requiring supportive care, both in and out of the hospital. In fact, these pain management teams including pediatricians, nurses, anesthesiologists, physical therapists, psychologists, social workers, and child life specialists, I feel, have been the leading force in the organization and delivery of palliative care to children.

Several national and international organizations have developed and disseminated guidelines for pain management in children and adults, and in both groups of patients with cancer.[1-4] Unfortunately, these guidelines have not received wide dissemination beyond the realm of pain and cancer specialties. There remains an enormous lack of widely available published information in general and specialty pediatric textbooks to help guide caretakers in the business of either pain management or palliative care. Therefore, even simple symptom control can be quite challenging for the general pediatrician or pediatric resident providing primary care to the patient.

In institutions with palliative care teams or pain management teams, symptom control and both the organization and administration of care for the dying child should be available. Traditionally, these services have been provided largely to pediatric oncology patients. It is unfortunate when services that provide care to complex and desperately ill children with HIV disease, cystic fibrosis, sickle cell anemia, large surface area burns, etc. fail to enlist the support and opinions of the palliative care teams. Often, consultation is requested only when the child has entered or is well into the terminal phase of illness. Clearly, palliative care teams should be involved well before these milestones have been reached.

Ideally, palliative care should be part of the broad range of services provided to every patient with a significant medical or surgical illness. The palliative care team should be composed of a diverse group of caretakers, including the primary nurse, physician, appropriate specialty-prepared physicians, rehabilitative medicine specialists, social workers, psychologists/psychiatrists, and chaplains. Often, these services are headed by an oncologist, anesthesiologist, or less commonly, by a pediatrician with a special interest or training in the area.

The fundamental responsibility of the pediatric palliative care team should be to minimize and relieve suffering in children with complex illnesses. The team should be able to provide both inpatient and outpatient consultation. Palliative care teams should provide careful assessment of symptoms, especially pain.[5,6] Pain management should include management of the side effects of opioid therapy, coordination of therapies for procedural pain, and the planning of the transition to home therapy. To accomplish these goals, and provide other palliative care services, a trusting and supportive relationship with the various pediatric care providers is essential for all the members of the team.

If the speciality of pediatric palliative care is to continue to develop, financial support must be maintained for these services. It is not unusual for reimbursement for palliative care to be denied, yet the very same patient may receive compensated care from a variety of pediatric specialists, such as those from infectious diseases, cardiology, and pulmonary medicine. If, as compassionate health care providers, we maintain our commitment to alleviate the suffering of ill children, we must enlist the support of our medical colleagues, as well as patients and families, to emphasize the crucial role of the palliative care teams. At the same time, palliative care teams must evolve systems that assess and measure their successes and failures by implementing quality assurance and improvement programs.

Some of the potential regression in the evolution of the palliative care team may be a result of the institutionalization of serious illness and death in children. This trend may lead caretakers to remain focused on a variety of diagnostic, interventional, and therapeutic life-saving measures, while giving inadequate attention to supportive care. Home care for the child with medically complex needs is now often dictated by health maintenance organizations. Many of these organizations have various "preferred provider" contracts with home health agencies. Unfortunately, the agencies are often unable to organize a critical mass of professionals dedicated to the palliative care of children. Thus, it has become all too common once again to witness the death of children in the hospital instead of in the home environment. When the palliative care team is brought into the care plan of these children early in their hospital stay, it becomes possible to coordinate the provision of a home care plan of therapy. This might mean a shift back to the model of home care developed several years ago by clinicians such as Ida Martinson.[7,8] The guiding principle of this model is that the parent or equivalent is defined as the primary caretaker. A home care coordinator, who is available 24 hours per day, is identified. The coordinator visits the home periodically and as the family deems necessary. A supervising physician also helps coordinate care. Ultimately, this small team can follow the child until death.

The current widespread public debate about the ethical and legal implications of euthanasia and assisted suicide in our society[9] should not avoid a discussion of children. In my opinion, the thrust of palliative care medicine precisely avoids the need to argue in favor of either euthanasia or assisted suicide in children.

Complete pain management and other palliative care should always be provided to the critically ill child. Particularly for children with potentially terminal diseases (cancers, cystic fibrosis, HIV), pain management should not be sacrificed because of fear of respiratory depression. Other supportive interventions such as nutrition, oxygen delivery, and use of blood products or antibiotics may be considered if they can provide symptom control or relief. Careful analysis and discussions with the family and the patient will usually provide insight into the appropriateness of using or withholding a specific therapy. The palliative care team does not allocate health care resources based upon financial considerations, such as in-hospital costs or home health costs. Instead, the palliative care team must remain focused on the relief of suffering in all children.

References

1. Acute Pain Management Guideline Panel. *Acute Pain Management: Operative or Medical Procedures and Trauma.* Clinical Practice Guideline. AHCPR Publication No. 92-0032. Rockville, MD: Agency for Health Care Policy and Research, U.S. Department of Health and Human Resources, Public Health Service, 1992.
2. Jacox A, Carr DB, Payne R, et al. *Management of Cancer Pain.* Clinical Practice Guideline No. 9. AHPCR Publication No. 94-0592. Rockville, MD: Agency for Health Care Policy and Research, U.S. Department of Health and Human Resources, Public Health Service, 1994.
3. World Health Organization. *Cancer Pain Relief.* Geneva: Switzerland, 1986.
4. World Health Organization. *Cancer Pain Relief and Palliative Care.* Geneva: Switzerland, 1994.
5. Schechter NL, Altman A, Weisman S. Report of the consensus conference on the management of pain in childhood cancer. *Pediatrics* 1990; 86:813–834.
6. Schechter NL, Berde CB, Yaster M (eds). Pain In Infants, Children and Adolescents. Baltimore: Williams and Wilkins, 1993.
7. Martinson IM, Henry WF. Some possible societal consequences of changing the way in which we care for dying children. *Hastings Center Report* 1980; 10:5–8.
8. Martinson IM, Birenbaum L, Martin B, Lauer M, Ing B. Hospice/Home Care: A Nurses Manual for Management for Children. Alexandria, VA: Children's Hospice International, 1991.
9. Foley KM. Pain, physcian-assisted suicide, and euthanasia. *Pain Forum* 1995; 4:163–178.

1

Pharmacologic Management of Pediatric Cancer Pain

JOHN J. COLLINS

The Report of the Consensus Conference on the Management of Pain in Childhood Cancer[1] established guidelines in the United States for the assessment and management of disease-related and treatment-related cancer pain. More recently, the World Health Organization (WHO) initiated the global application of the principles of pain management and palliative care for children with cancer.[2] In so doing, WHO established these principles as a required standard of care. The pharmacologic approach to the management of pediatric cancer pain is an important modality of pain control that is often used in conjunction with therapies directed at the control of the underlying cancer (e.g., surgery, radiation therapy, and chemotherapy) and with non-pharmacological approaches to pain management (e.g., relaxation exercises, guided imagery, and hypnotherapy).

The Epidemiology of Cancer Pain in Children

The improvement in survival rates of children with cancer is due to the evolution of multimodality treatment protocols. This improvement has changed the epidemiology of pain associated with childhood cancer from a predominantly tumor-related epidemiology to one predominantly treatment-related. Tumor-related pain predominates at diagnosis and during the early treatment phase of childhood cancer. A study of children with non-central nervous system (CNS) malignancies at the National Cancer Institute[3] found that 62% presented to their practitioners with complaints of pain prior to the diagnosis of cancer. Pain was present for a median of 74 days before treatment was begun; the duration of pain experienced by patients with metastatic disease was not longer than that for patients without metastases. After the initiation of therapy directed at their cancer, the majority of children had resolution of pain. Children with hematological malignancy had a shorter duration of pain after the institution of treatment than those with solid tumors.[3]

Children with brain tumors present to their practitioners either with symptoms consistent with raised intracranial pressure, including headache, or abnormal neurological signs.[4] A retrospective review of children with spinal cord tumors showed that most of them present with a complaint of pain.[5] Metastatic spinal cord compression is unusual at diagnosis and is more likely to occur later in the course of the illness.[6] Back pain is more common than abnormal neurological signs or symptoms as a sign of spinal cord compression in children.[6]

As multimodality treatment protocols evolve for each disease, treatment-related, causes of pain predominate.[7,8] Causes of treatment-related pain include mucositis, phantom limb pain, infection, antineoplastic therapy–related pain, postoperative pain, and procedure–related pain (e.g., needle puncture, bone marrow aspiration, lumbar puncture, removal of central venous line). Tumor–related pain frequently recurs in patients at the time of relapse and during the terminal phase of an illness. Palliative chemotherapy and radiation therapy, depending on tumor type and sensitivity, are sometimes instituted as modalities of pain control in terminal pediatric malignancy. Severe pain in terminal pediatric malignancy occurs more commonly in patients with solid tumors metastatic to spinal nerve roots, nerve plexus, large peripheral nerve, or spinal cord compression.[9]

Analgesic Studies in Children with Cancer

The need to improve pain management in children with cancer is demonstrated by recent data which indicate that pain is often not adequately assessed and effectively treated in this population.[10] Improvement in pain management will be dependent not only on advances in pediatric analgesic therapeutics but also on strategies to correct the barriers to the adequate treatment of pain in these children.

Although the difficulties encountered in performing analgesic trials in children (Table 1.1) can be overcome, few studies have been performed in children with cancer (Table 1.2). For example, the ethical issue of performing novel drug trials in pediatrics is somewhat mitigated by delaying such studies until safety, efficacy, and tolerability data are available from adult studies. Similarly, obtaining the assent of a child for a drug trial, using age-appropriate explanations, mitigates the issue of obtaining an informed consent only from a proxy (usually a parent). The compromise to the unacceptable problem of repeated venipuncture in children for drug assays is using intravenous cannulae inserted at the time of anesthesia or blood collection from a central venous line.

The major difficulty in performing analgesic studies in children with cancer pertains to the heterogeneous nature of pain in this population. Other difficulties

Table 1.1. Analgesic study issues in children with cancer

General Issues
Ethics of performing drug trials in children

Consent/assent issues

Practical problem of blood sampling in this population

Specific Issues
The heterogeneity of pain in children with cancer

Epidemiological differences in cancer diagnosis compared with the adult population

Lack of validated instruments to measure pain and other symptoms in children with cancer, particularly younger children

Differences in response to and attitude towards anti-neoplastic therapy in children compared with the adult population

Lack of a relatively stable pattern of pain

The difficulties of performing drug trials in medically ill children

Lack of an appropriate analgesic study design which accounts for the difficulties

relate in part to the epidemiology of childhood cancer. Solid tumors are less common than in the adult population and it is less likely that children will have chronic cancer pain from their tumors. Children, particularly adolescent patients, tend to receive therapies directed at control of tumors growth until very late in the course of their illness and are frequently very ill and highly symptomatic. These epidemiological and treatment variables make it less likely that a sub-population of children with cancer exists that has a stable, chronic pattern of pain amenable to evaluation in a trial. The lack of validated measures of pain and other symptoms, and the lack of analgesic study designs based on appropriate pain models but allowing for small numbers of subjects, are further impediments to progress in pain management for children with cancer.

Given the difficulties of performing analgesic studies in children with cancer (Table 1.1), such studies in the pediatric age group have usually been based on other pain models (e.g., postoperative, musculoskeletal). Although the pharmacokinetic and major pharmacodynamic properties (analgesia and sedation) of most opioids have been studied in pediatrics, little information is available about oral bioavailability, potency ratios, and other pharmacodynamic properties in this population.

The few analgesic studies performed in the setting of pediatric cancer pain (Table 1.2) have conformed to one of the following indications: *(1)* the evaluation of a drug proven efficacious in other pain models but now targeted to the pediatric cancer pain population or *(2)* the evaluation of treatments for pain that is more or less specific to pediatric cancer patients. Most of these studies had small numbers of subjects, few were controlled studies, and only recently has

Table 1.2. Analgesic studies in children with cancer

Analgesic study design	Indication for study	Sample Age of subjects Study duration	Analgesic outcome measures	Analgesic outcome results	Major findings
Survey (Miser, 1980)[11]	To test the safety, efficacy of continuous iv morphine infusions in a heterogeneous group of terminally ill patients	n = 8 3–16 years 1–16 days	Composite impression from investigator, parents and patients	Adequate to complete pain control	Intravenous morphine infusions were effective, with minor side effects recorded.
Survey (Miser, 1983)[12]	To test the safety, efficacy of continuous sc morphine infusions in a heterogeneous group of terminally ill patients	n = 17 2–22 years 0.25–30 days	Adequate analgesia defined as freedom from pain + absence of complaints of pain >95% of the time	Satisfactory pain control	Subcutaneous morphine infusions were effective, with mild side effects recorded.
Open trial (Miser, 1986)[13]	To test the safety, efficacy of po methadone in a heterogeneous cancer population	n = 19 (22 courses of methadone in toto) 4–23 years 2–267 days (median 24 days)	Investigator's assessment using a visual analog scale	"Good" or "excellent" analgesia in 18 courses of methadone	"Adequate" pain control in 21 courses.
Prospective survey (Miser, 1986)[14]	To test the efficacy of iv/sc morphine infusions in a heterogeneous pediatric cancer population	n = 26 (30 infusions in toto) 0.75–154 days	Investigator's assessment using a visual analog scale	"Good" or "excellent" analgesia in 20 courses of iv/sc morphine	"Adequate" pain control in 29 courses.
Survey (Miser, 1987)[15]	To test the safety, efficacy tolerability of iv fentanyl infusion in children and young adults with cancer	n = 15 (20 fentanyl infusions) median age = 22 years (range 10–29) 0.5–33 days	Patient and investigator visual analog assessment of pain severity	Adequate analgesia in the majority of cases	Major toxicities included respiratory depression, acute aphonia, CNS toxicity.

Study type (reference)	Objective	Sample	Observers' assessment	Results	Comments
Pharmacokinetic study (Greene, 1987)[16]	To define the relationships between morphine pharmacokinetics in plasma and CSF in cancer patients receiving long-term iv infusions of morphine	Morphine infusions: n = 17 (21 infusions in toto) CSF specimens: n = 5	Not recorded	Not recorded	Variable linear relationship between morphine infusion rate and plasma concentration.
(i) Double-blind placebo controlled study (ii) Open cross-over study (Kapdushnik, 1990)[17]	To define the potential benefit of topical EMLA prior to lumbar puncture in children with cancer	(i) n = 10 Mean age 9.2 ± 3.9 (range 5–15) (ii) n = 18 Mean age 6.1 ± 2.1 years (range 4.5–11)	(i) Patient rated visual analog scale (ii) Patient rated visual analog scale or faces scale	(i) Favorable effect of EMLA (ii) Generally favorable effect of EMLA. EMLA inferior to placebo in 2 cases	Although the 2 studies suggested the favorable effects of EMLA the need for placebo, randomized controlled studies in children was emphasized.
Randomized controlled trial (Mackie, 1991)[18]	To compare patient-controlled analgesia (PCA) with continuous infusions for adolescents with prolonged oropharyngeal mucositis pain	n = 20 12–18 years	Daily morphine intake Self-report of pain intensity using visual analog scale	No difference in pain intensity scores between the 2 groups	PCA group reported less sedation and less difficulty concentrating. Less morphine intake in PCA group.
Randomized, placebo controlled double-blind cross-over study (Miser, 1994)[19]	To test the safety, efficacy of EMLA for pain relief during central venous port access in children with cancer	n = 47 3–21 years	Self-report of pain intensity using a faces and visual analog scale	EMLA superior to placebo	EMLA provides effective superficial anesthesia.
Randomized, double-blind 3 period cross-over study (Collins, 1996)[20]	To compare the efficacy, side effect profile, and potency ratio of morphine to hydromorphone, and to obtain pharmacokinetic data on these drugs in children with cancer	n = 10 8–19 years 10 days	Self-report of pain intensity using visual analog scale	No difference in analgesic and side effect profile between the 2 drugs. A 5.1:1 hydromorphone: morphine ratio may be a more appropriate estimate	The clearance of hydromorphone and morphine was greater than in previous studies. Morphine pharmacokinetics were similar to previous studies.

self-report been used to measure the effectiveness of analgesia. There have been no controlled clinical trials of adjuvant analgesic agents in pediatrics.

Analgesic Medications

Analgesic drugs can be divided into three groups: *(1)* non-opioid analgesics, *(2)* opioid analgesics, and *(3)* adjuvant analgesics. The prescription of these drugs for children with cancer pain is based on the WHO analgesic ladder, which endorses the prescription of analgesics according to pain severity, ranging from acetaminophen and nonsteroidal anti-inflammatory drugs (NSAIDs) for mild pain to opioids for moderate to severe pain (Fig. 1.1). This approach, thought to be effective for children as well as adults with cancer,[21–23] emphasizes pain intensity rather than etiologic factors as the guide to choice of analgesic. In children the choice of analgesics must be individualized to achieve an optimum balance between analgesia and side effects.

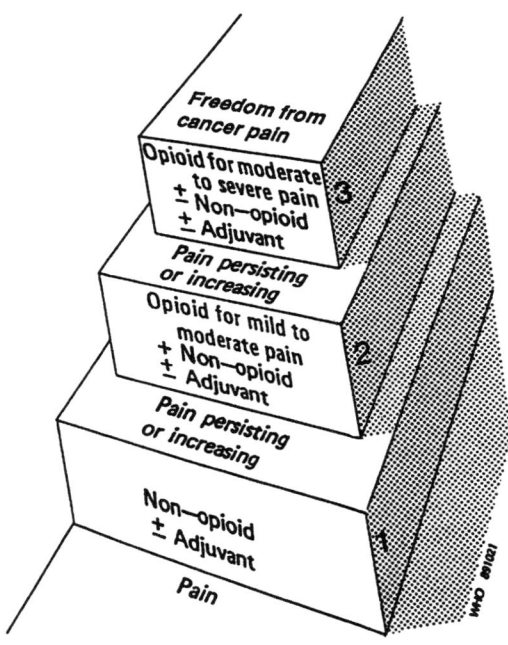

Figure 1.1. The World Health Organization (WHO) analgesic ladder. (Reproduced with permission from *Cancer Pain Relief and Palliative Care: Report of a WHO Expert Committee.* Technical Report series, No. 804. Geneva: World Health Organization, 1990.)

Non-opioid Analgesics

Acetaminophen

Acetaminophen is the most commonly used non-opioid analgesic in children. It inhibits prostaglandin synthesis primarily in the central nervous system. The elimination rate of unchanged acetaminophen is similar in neonates, children, and adults.[24] Pediatric dosing of acetaminophen is based on the dose-response for antipyretic effect, because pediatric dose-response studies for analgesia are unavailable. Oral dosing of 15 mg/kg every 4 hrs appears to be safe. Acetaminophen lacks the side effects of gastritis and inhibition of platelet function found with aspirin and NSAIDs. It has a potential for hepatic and renal injury,[25] but this is uncommon in therapeutic doses. Unlike aspirin, acetaminophen does not have the association with Reye's syndrome. The antipyretic action of acetaminophen may be contraindicated in neutropenic patients in whom it is important to monitor fever.

Aspirin and nonsteroidal anti-inflammatory drugs (NSAIDs)

Aspirin and NSAIDs are frequently contraindicated in pediatric oncology patients who are at risk for bleeding due to thrombocytopenia. Aspirin's effects are a greater concern because of its irreversible inhibition of platelet function; the reversible inhibition caused by NSAIDs terminates as the drug is cleared. In a comparative study of aspirin and ibuprofen in children with juvenile rheumatoid arthritis, the drugs were equally efficacious, but the drop-out rate caused by side effects was significantly higher in the aspirin group.[26] In selected children with adequate platelet number and function, NSAIDs may be extremely helpful analgesics, both alone and in combination with opioids.

Choline magnesium trisalicylate (Trilisate) has been widely recommended because of reports in adults of minimal effects on platelet function in vitro and experimental studies showing minimal gastric irritation in rats, in contrast to aspirin.[27] NSAIDs such as nabumetone and ibuprofen are generally considered to be relatively less likely than other NSAIDs to produce serious toxicity. Clinicians should view all such data with some caution, because the studies do not include medically frail patients with severe thrombocytopenia or other morbidities.

Opioid Analgesics

Codeine

Codeine is a phenanthrene alkaloid derived from morphine. In pediatrics it is most commonly administered via the oral route. It is often administered in combination with acetaminophen and is prescribed for mild to moderate pain. In equipotent doses, codeine has an analgesic and side-effect profile similar to morphine. Codeine is typically administered in pediatrics in oral doses of 0.5–1 mg/kg every 4 hr for children over 6 months of age.

Oxycodone

Oxycodone is a semi-synthetic opioid used for moderate to severe pain in children with cancer. In some countries oxycodone is available only as an oral preparation in combination with acetaminophen. The total daily acetaminophen dose may be the limiting factor in dose escalation of these products. In children aged 2–10 years, oxycodone has a higher clearance value and a shorter elimination half life ($t_{1/2}$) than in adults.[28,29] The oral pharmacokinetics of oxycodone have not been studied in children.

Morphine

Morphine is the most widely used opioid for moderate to severe cancer pain. The binding of morphine to plasma protein is age-dependent. In premature infants less than 20% is bound to plasma proteins.[30,31] Within the neonatal period for term infants, the volume of distribution is linearly related to age and body surface area,[32] but after the neonatal period the values are approximately the same as for adults.[33,34]

Morphine is metabolized by the liver. Neonates appear to produce morphine metabolites less effectively than do older children.[31,35–40] The major metabolite of morphine, morphine-6-glucuronide, produces analgesia and side effects comparable to morphine with chronic dosing. Morphine-6-glucuronide may accumulate and exacerbate sedation in patients with renal insufficiency.

Morphine clearance is delayed in the first 1–3 months of life. Primarily due to changes in clearance, the $t_{1/2}$ changes from values of 10–20 hr in preterm infants to values of 1–2 hr in pre-school children.[33] Starting doses in very young infants should be reduced by approximately 25%–30% on a per kg basis relative to dosing recommended for older children.

Morphine has significant first pass metabolism in the liver following oral dosing, so that an oral to parenteral potency ratio of approximately 3:1 is common during chronic administration. A typical starting dose for immediate release oral morphine in opioid-naive subjects is 0.3 mg/kg every 4 hr. If the oral route is not available, intermittent parenteral or continuous intravenous or subcutaneous morphine infusions are effective methods of pain control. Typical starting infusion rates are 0.02–0.03 mg/kg/hr beyond the first 3 months of life, and 0.015 mg/kg/hr in younger infants.

The intramuscular route is discouraged in children in general, not only because of the pain induced by a needle puncture, but also because this adverse experience may lead to the under-reporting of pain. Rectal administration is discouraged in the pediatric cancer population, not only because of the great variability of rectal absorption of morphine[41] but also because of concern regarding infection. Sustained-release preparations of morphine and oxycodone permit oral dosing either twice or three times daily. Crushing these tablets produces immediate release of morphine, which limits their use in children unable to tolerate the oral route.

Hydromorphone

Hydromorphone is commonly used as an alternative opioid in adults when dose escalation of morphine is limited by side effects. Hydromorphone is available for oral, intravenous, subcutaneous, epidural, and intrathecal dosing. Adults studies indicate that intravenous hydromorphone is 5–8 times as potent as morphine, although a recent pediatric study indicated that a potency ratio of 5.1:1 may be more likely in these patients.[20]

Fentanyl

Fentanyl is a synthetic opioid which is approximately 50–100 times as potent as morphine during acute intravenous administration. It is probably the most widely used intraoperative analgesic in pediatrics. Fentanyl is eliminated almost entirely by hepatic metabolism. The half-life of this opioid is prolonged in preterm infants undergoing patent ductus arteriosus ligation,[42] but values comparable with those of adults are reached within the first months of life.[43–46] The clearance of fentanyl appears to be higher in infants and young children than in adults.[43,44]

The effect of fentanyl is very rapid following intravenous administration because of its high lipid solubility and rapid entry into the brain. Its duration of action following intravenous bolus administration is much shorter than that of morphine. These features make fentanyl especially useful for brief noxious procedures, where rapid onset and short duration are useful. Fentanyl may also be used for continuous infusion for selected patients with dose-limiting side effects from morphine. Rapid administration of high doses of IV fentanyl may result in chest wall rigidity and severe ventilatory difficulty. Oral transmucosal fentanyl produces a rapid onset of effect and bypasses first-pass hepatic clearance. Schechter and colleagues[47] described the use of oral transmucosal fentanyl for sedation/analgesia during bone marrow biopsy/aspiration and lumbar puncture: this formulation was safe and effective, although the frequency of vomiting may be a limiting factor in its tolerability. The safety, efficacy, and tolerability of transdermal fentanyl in children is not known.

Meperidine

Meperidine is a short-acting synthetic opioid agonist that has been used for procedural and postoperative pain in children. Neonates have a slower elimination of meperidine than children and young infants, and are subject to great individual variation.[48–52] The major metabolite of meperidine is normeperidine, which can cause CNS excitatory effects including tremors and convulsions,[53] particularly in patients with impaired renal clearance. Meperidine is not recommended for children with chronic pain unless there is no alternative available. Meperidine may be an acceptable alternative to fentanyl for short painful procedures; its duration of action is shorter than morphine. Meperidine in low doses (0.25–0.5 mg/kg IV) is uniquely effective among the opioids for prophylaxis and treatment of rigors following the infusion of amphotericin.

Methadone

Methadone is a synthetic opioid that has a long through variable half-life (Table 1.3). Following single parenteral doses, its potency is similar to that of morphine. It is absorbed efficiently following oral administration. The oral:parenteral potency ratio is approximately 2:1. In children undergoing surgery, methadone produced more prolonged analgesia than morphine.[54,55] The prolonged half-life of methadone has an associated risk of delayed sedation and overdosage occurring several days after initiating treatment. Therefore, frequent patient assessment is key to safe and effective use of methadone. If a patient becomes comfortable after initial doses, the dose should be reduced or the interval extended to reduce the

Table 1.3. Opioid agonist drugs

Drug	IM°	PO°	Half-life (hs)	Duration of action (h)
Codeine	130	200	2–3	2–4
Dihydrocodeine		200	2–3	2–4
Oxycodone	15	30	2–3	2–4
Morphine	10	30 (repeated dose)	2–3	3–4
		60 (single dose)		
Hydromorphone	1.5	7.5	2–3	2–4
Methadone	10	20	15–190	4–8
Meperidine	75	300	2–3	2–4
Oxymorphone	1	10 (PR)	2–3	3–4
Levorphanol	2	4	12–15	4–8
Fentanyl (parenteral)	0.1	—	1–2	1–3
Fentanyl transdermal system†				48–72

°Dose (mg) Equianalgesic to 10 mg I.M. morphine; IM = intramuscularly; PO = by mouth; PR = per rectum.
†Transdermal fentanyl 100 µ/h ~ 4 mg/h.
Source: Reproduced with permission from Cherny and Foley.[60]

Table 1.4. Starting Drug Doses of Opioids Commonly Used in Pediatrics

Drug	Usual IV starting dose (<50kg)	Usual IV starting dose (>50kg)	Usual PO starting dose (<50kg)	Usual PO starting dose (>50kg)
Morphine	0.1 mg/kg q3–4h	5–10 mg q3–4h	0.3 mg/kg q3–4h	15–30 mg q3–4h
Hydromorphone	0.015 mg/kg q3–4h	1–1.5 mg q3–4h	0.06 mg/kg q3–4h	4–6 mg q3–4h
Oxycodone	N/A	N/A	0.3 mg/kg q3–4h†	10 mg q3–4h
Meperidine°	0.75 mg/kg q2–3h	75–100 mg q3h	N/R	N/R
Fentanyl	0.5–1.5 µ/kg q1–2h	25–75 µg/kg q1–2h	N/A	N/A

°Meperidine is not recommended for chronic use because of the accumulation of the toxic metabolite nor-meperidine.
†Smallest tablet size is 5 mg.
N/A = not available; N/R = not recommended.
Source: Reproduced with permission from Collins JJ, Berde CB. Management of cancer pain in children. In: Pizzo PA, Poplack DG, eds. *Principles and Practice of Pediatric Oncology*, 3rd Ed. New York: Lippincott-Raven, 1997.

likelihood of subsequent somnolence. If a patient becomes oversedated early in dose escalation, it is recommended to stop dosing, not just reduce the dose, and to observe the patient until there is increased alertness. Although "as needed" dosing is discouraged for most patients with cancer pain, some clinicians find this approach a useful way to establish a dosing schedule for methadone.[54,55] Methadone remains a long-acting agent when administered either as an elixir or as crushed tablets.

The starting dosage schedule for the commonly used opioids in pediatrics is shown in Table 1.4. The initial opioid dosing on a milligram per kilogram basis in infants less than 6 months of age should be one-quarter to one-third the comparable dose for older children. Infants receiving opioids should be supervised where continuous observation and immediate intervention are possible.

Routes and Methods of Analgesic Administration

Oral

Analgesics should be administered to children by the simplest, safest, most effective, and least painful route. Oral administration is the first choice for most patients. Oral dosing is generally predictable, inexpensive, and does not require invasive procedures or technologies. Oral dosing is not feasible in some children with severe nausea, ileus, mucositis, or in the occasional child who is rendered uncooperative by fear, delirium, or respiratory distress.

Topical

The eutectic mixture of local anesthetics, EMLA, is a topical preparation that provides localized anesthesia to the skin, dermis, and subcutaneous tissues if applied under an occlusive dressing for at least one hour. It has been shown to be useful for procedural pain, including lumbar puncture[17] and central venous port access[19] in children with cancer.

Intravenous

Intravenous administration has the advantage of rapid onset, relative easy dose titration, complete bioavailability, and constant effect when infusions are used. Typical starting intravenous morphine infusion rates are 0.03–0.04 mg/kg/hr beyond the first 3 months of life, and 0.015 mg/kg/hr in younger infants.[11,56]

Subcutaneous

A convenient alternative for children with poor intravenous access who require parenteral opioids is continuous subcutaneous infusions[12] of morphine or hydromorphone. A small catheter or butterfly needle (27 gauge) may be placed under the skin of the thorax, abdomen, or thigh, with sites changed every 3–5 days as needed. Solutions are generally concentrated so that infusion rates do not exceed 1–3 cc/hr.[57] Needle placement can be made less noxious by prior use of EMLA cream.

Intramuscular

Intramuscular dosing should be avoided in most circumstances. It is painful and may lead to the under-reporting of pain. It does not permit easy dose titration or infusion.

Patient-controlled analgesia

Patient-controlled analgesia (PCA) is a method of opioid administration that uses a device, usually computer-controlled, that permits the patient to self-administer small bolus doses within set time limits. PCA allows titrated dosing of opioid to compensate for individual variation in pharmacokinetics, pharmacodynamics, and pain intensity.

PCA has been used successfully for the management of prolonged oropharyngeal mucositis pain in children and adolescents.[18,20,58] A controlled comparison of PCA and staff-controlled continuous infusion (CI) of morphine in adolescents with oropharyngeal mucositis pain after bone marrow transplantation found that the PCA group had equivalent analgesia but had less sedation and less difficulty concentrating.[18]

PCA allows appropriately selected children control over their analgesia. In patients with painful mucositis, for example, opioid dosing can be timed with routine mouth care and other causes of incidental mouth pain. It also allows children to find a balance between the benefits of analgesia and the side effects of opioids. In postoperative use, PCA is widely used successfully by children aged 6–7 and above. Although anecdotal experience suggests that some children aged 4–6 can use PCA successfully, there is a higher chance of inadequate analgesia due to failure to associate pain relief with pressing the button device on the PCA pump.

Opioid Dose Titration, "By the Clock" Dose Administration, and "Rescues"

Opioid dose escalation in the absence of a progressive physical or psychological disorder is an uncommon event during the long-term treatment of adult patients with pain.[59] The analgesic effects of opioids increase in a log–linear function, until either analgesia is achieved or somnolence occurs.[60] An analgesic regimen is typically created for children whereby stable analgesia is achieved using "by the clock administration." This means that unless a child's episodes of pain are truly incidental and unpredictable, analgesics should be administered at regular times, by the clock, to prevent breakthrough pain. "Rescues" are supplemental "as needed"-doses of opioid incorporated into the analgesic regimen to allow a patient to have additional analgesia if required. Rescue doses of opioid may be calculated as approximately 5%–10% of the total daily opioid requirement and may be administered every hour.[60]

Opioid dose escalation is usually required after opioid administration begins and periodically thereafter. The size of a dose increment may be calculated as follows: (1) If greater than approximately six rescue doses of opioid are given in a 24-hour period, then the total daily dose should be increased by the total quantity of rescue medication. For example, the hourly average of this rescue opioid should be added to the baseline opioid infusion. An alternative to this method would be to increase the baseline infusion by 50%.[60] (2) Rescue doses are kept as a proportion of the baseline opioid dose. As noted, this dose can be 5%–10% of the total daily dose. An alternative guideline during opioid infusion is 50%–200% of the hourly basal infusion rate.[60]

Opioid Switching for Dose-Limiting Side Effects

The usual indication for an opioid switch is dose-limiting toxicity. This approach is recommended by the observation that a switch from one opioid to another is often accompanied by change in the balance between analgesia and side effects.[61] A favorable change in opioid side effects will be experienced if there is less

Table 1.5. Management of opioid side effects

Side effect	Treatment
Constipation	1. Regular use of stimulant and stool softener laxatives (fiber, fruit juices are often insufficient). 2. Ensure adequate water intake.
Sedation	1. If analgesia is adequate, try dose reduction. 2. Unless contraindicated, add non-sedating analgesics, such as acetaminophen or NSAIDs, and reduce opioid dosing as tolerated. 3. If sedation persists, try methylphenidate or dextroamphetamine 0.05–0.2 mg/kg PO b.i.d. in early am & midday. 4. Consider an opioid switch.
Nausea	1. Exclude disease processes (e.g., bowel obstruction, increased intracranial pressure). 2. Anti-emetics (phenothiazines, ondansetron, hydroxyzine). 3. Consider an opioid switch.
Urinary Retention	1. Exclude disease processes (e.g., bladder neck obstruction by tumor, impending cord compression, hypovolemia, renal failure, etc.). 2. Avoid other drugs with anticholinergic effects (e.g., tricyclics, antihistamines). 3. Consider short-term use of bethanechol or Crede maneuver. 4. Consider short-term catheterization. 5. Consider opioid dose reduction if analgesia adequate or an opioid switch if analgesia inadequate.
Pruritus	1. Exclude other causes (e.g., drug allergy, cholestasis). 2. Antihistamines (e.g., diphenhydramine hydroxyzine). 3. Consider an opioid dose reduction if analgesia adequate, or an opioid switch. Fentanyl causes less histamine release.
Respiratory depression Mild-moderate	1. Awaken, encourage to breathe. 2. Apply oxygen. 3. Withhold opioid dosing until breathing improves, reduce subsequent dosing by at least 25%.
Severe	1. Awaken if possible, apply oxygen, assist respiration by bag and mask as needed. 2. Titrate small doses of naloxone (0.01 mg/kg increments as needed). Stop when respiratory rate increases to 8–10/min in older children or 12–16/min in infants; do not try to awaken fully with naloxone. DO NOT GIVE A BOLUS DOSE OF NALOXONE, AS SEVERE PAIN AND SYMPTOMS OF OPIOID WITHDRAWAL MAY ENSUE 3. Consider a low-dose naloxone infusion or repeated incremental dosing. 4. Consider short-term intubation in occasional cases where risk of aspiration is high.
Dysphoria/Confusion/ Hallucinations	1. Exclude other pathology as a cause for these symptoms before attributing them to opioids. 2. When other causes excluded, change to another opioid. 3. Consider adding a neuroleptic such as haloperidol (0.01–0.1 mg/kg po/iv every 8 hours to a maximum dose of 30 mg/day).
Myoclonus	1. Usually seen in the setting of high dose opioids, or alternatively, rapid dose escalation. 2. No treatment may be warranted, if this is infrequent and not distressing to the child. 3. Consider an opioid switch or treat with clonezepam (0.01 mg/kg PO every 12 hours to a maximum dose of 0.5 mg/dose) or a parenteral benzodiazepine (e.g., diazepam) if the oral route is not tolerated.

Source: Reproduced with permission from Collins JJ, Berde CB. Management of cancer pain in children. In: Pizzo PA, Poplack DG, eds. *Principles and Practice of Pediatric Oncology,* 3rd Ed. New York: Lippincott-Raven, 1997.

cross-tolerance at the opioid receptors mediating analgesia than at those mediating adverse effects.[59]

Following a prolonged period of regular dosing with one opioid, equivalent analgesia may be attained with a dose of a second opioid that is smaller than that calculated from an equianalgesic table, as shown in Table 1.3.[59] Thus, the opioid switch is usually accompanied by a reduction in the equianalgesic dose (approximately 50% for short half-life opioids).

This dose reduction may be smaller if the switch is made in the setting of grossly inadequate pain control; it may be greater in the medically fragile and those with severe opioid toxicity. In contrast to other opioids, the doses of methadone required for equivalent analgesia after switching may be of the order of 10%–20% of the equianalgesic dose of the previously used short half-life opioid. A protocol for the dose conversion and titration of methadone has been previously documented.[62]

The Treatment of Opioid Side Effects

The assessment of analgesic effectiveness includes an assessment of opioid side effects. Tolerance to sedation, nausea and vomiting, and pruritus often develop within the first week of opioid administration. All opioids can potentially cause the same constellation of side effects (Table 1.5). Those experienced by individual patients receiving different opioids may vary, and children do not necessarily report side effects voluntarily (e.g., constipation, pruritus) and should be asked specific questions about these problems.

Also, children often do not develop tolerance to constipation, so concurrent treatment with a stool softener and a stimulant should always be considered. If opioid side effects limit opioid dose escalation, then consideration should be given to an opioid switch.

Adjuvant Agents

Adjuvant analgesics are a heterogeneous group of drugs that have a primary indication other than pain but are analgesic in some painful conditions.[63] Common classes of these drugs are antidepressants, anticonvulsants, neuroleptics, psychostimulants, antihistamines, corticosteroids, and centrally acting skeletal muscle relaxants, among others. These agents are commonly, but not always, prescribed with primary analgesic drugs.

Antidepressants

Tricyclic antidepressants have been used for a variety of pain conditions in adults, including postherpetic neuralgia,[64] diabetic neuropathy,[65] tension headache,[66] migraine headache,[67] rheumatoid arthritis,[68] chronic low back pain,[69] and cancer pain.[70] In the absence of controlled trials in children, data from adult studies have guided use in pediatrics.

The choice of antidepressant is usually made on the basis of side-effect profile. For example, patients with insomnia and pain may benefit most from a sedating compound at bedtime. Prior to treatment with a tricyclic antidepressant, it is prudent to obtain baseline hematology and biochemistry tests (including liver function tests) and an electrocardiogram (ECG) to exclude Wolff-Parkinson-White syndrome or other cardiac conduction defects.[71] Measurement of antidepressant plasma concentration allows confirmation of compliance and ensures that optimization of dosage has occurred before discontinuing the antidepressant. An ECG is recommended periodically during long-term use, or if standard mg/kg dosages are exceeded.[72]

Psychostimulants

Psychostimulants have multiple potential benefits as adjuvant drugs in pain management. Dextroamphetamine potentiates opioid analgesia in postoperative adult patients.[73] Methylphenidate counteracts opioid-induced sedation[74] and cognitive dysfunction[75] in advanced cancer patients and may allow dose escalation of opioids in cancer patients who have somnolence as a dose-limiting side effect.[76]

The safety, efficacy, and tolerability of dextroamphetamine and methylphenidate was reported in a retrospective survey of eleven children receiving opioids for a variety of indications, including cancer pain.[77] Somnolence was reduced without significant adverse side effects. The potential side effects of methylphenidate include anorexia, insomnia, and dysphoria.

Corticosteroids

Corticosteroids may produce analgesia by a variety of mechanisms, including anti-inflammatory effects and reduction of tumor edema.[78] In adult studies, they have a role in bone pain from metastatic bone disease,[79] cerebral edema from either a primary or metastatic tumor,[80,81] epidural spinal cord compression,[82] and possibly neuropathic pain.[83] Dexamethasone tends to be used most frequently because of its high potency, long duration of action, and minimal mineralocorticoid effect.

Anticonvulsants

Lancinating neuropathic pain and other episodic neuropathic pains characterized by a paroxysmal onset are considered an indication for a trial of anticonvulsants.[76] The mechanism of action of anticonvulsants in controlling lancinating pain is not known but is probably related to reducing paroxysmal discharges of central and peripheral neurons. The use of phenytoin, carbamazepine, and valproate may be problematic in the pediatric cancer population because of their potential adverse effects on the hematologic profile. The novel anticonvulsant, gabapentin, is well tolerated and appears to have a benign efficacy-to-toxicity ratio in children.[84] There is anecdotal clinical evidence from the adult literature that gabapentin may be useful for the treatment of all types of neuropathic pain.[85] Controlled studies are awaited.

Radionuclides

One recent case report indicates the potential role of [^{131}I]iodine-meta-io-dobenylguanidine ([^{131}I]MIBG) for painful bone disease related to disseminated neuroblastoma.[86] Administration of [^{131}I]MIBG occurred on three separate occasions and allowed cessation of opioids subsequent to the administration of this agent. The side effects of [^{131}I]MIBG were thrombocytopenia and cystitis. The use of other radionuclides for painful metastatic bone disease has been reported in the adult literature.[87]

Neuroleptics

Methotrimeprazine, a phenothiazined, is analgesic in the setting of adult cancer pain.[88] It may be useful as an adjuvant analgesic in a patient with advanced cancer who experiences pain associated with anxiety, restlessness, or nausea.[76] Methotrimeprazine should not be considered a substitute for opioid analgesia. The mechanism by which methotrimeprazine produces analgesia and its role as an adjuvant agent in pediatric cancer pain is unclear.

Tolerance, Physical Dependence, Addiction

Analgesic tolerance refers to the progressive decline in potency of an opioid with continued use, so that increasingly higher doses are required to achieve the same analgesic effect. Tolerance also develops to nonanalgesic opioid effects, including side effects. When tolerance develops to a particular opioid, cross-tolerance to other opioids concomitantly develops, but the degree of cross-tolerance to the various effects is not complete. Patients and parents are often reluctant to increase dosing because of a fear that tolerance will make opioids ineffective at a later date. Parents should be reassured that tolerance in the majority of cases can be managed by simple dose escalation, use of adjunctive medications, or perhaps by opioid switching in the setting of dose-limiting side effects.

Physical dependence is a physiologic state characterized by withdrawal (abstinence syndrome) after dose reduction or discontinuation of the opioid, or administration of an opioid antagonist. Initial manifestations of withdrawal include yawning, diaphoresis, lacrimation, coryza, and tachycardia.

Addiction is a psychological and behavioral syndrome characterized by drug craving and aberrant drug use. Some parents may fear that exposure to opioids will lead to a drug addiction. The incidence of opioid addiction was examined prospectively in 12,000 hospitalized adult patients who received at least one dose of a strong opioid.[89] There were only four documented cases of subsequent addiction among patients without a prior history of drug abuse. These data suggest that iatrogenic opioid addiction is an exceedingly uncommon problem,[89] an observation consistent with a large worldwide experience with opioid treatment of cancer pain.

References

1. Report of the Consensus Conference on the Management of Pain in Childhood Cancer. *Pediatrics* 1990; 86:813–834.
2. *Cancer Pain Relief and Palliative Care in Children.* World Health Organization Monograph. Geneva: World Health Organization, in press.
3. Miser AW, McCalla J, Dothage JA, Wesley M, Miser JS. Pain as a presenting symptom in children and young adults with newly diagnosed malignancy. *Pain* 1987; 29:85–90.
4. Heideman RL, Packer RJ, Albright LA, et al. Tumors of the central nervous system. In: Pizzo PA, Poplack DG, eds. *Principles and Practice of Pediatric Oncology.* Philadelphia: Lippincott-Raven, 1997: 633–698.
5. Hahn YS, McLone DG. Pain in children with spinal cord tumors. *Childs Brain* 1984; 11:36–46.
6. Lewis DW, Packer RJ, Raney B, Rak IW, Belasco J, Lange B. Incidence, presentation, and outcome of spinal cord disease in children with systemic cancer. *Pediatrics* 1986; 78:438–443.
7. Miser AW, Dothage JA, Wesley RA, Miser JS. The prevalence of pain in a pediatric and young adult cancer population. *Pain* 1987; 29:73–83.
8. Elliott SC, Miser AW, Dose AM, et al. Epidemiologic features of pain in pediatric cancer patients: a co-operative community-based study. *Clin J Pain* 1991; 7:263–268.
9. Collins JJ, Grier HE, Kinney HC, Berde CB. Control of severe pain in children with terminal malignancy. *J Pediatr* 1995; 126:653–657.
10. Ljungman G, Kreuger A, Gordh T, Berg T, Sörensen S, Rawal N. Treatment of pain in pediatric oncology: a Swedish nationwide survey. *Pain* 1996; 68:385–394.
11. Miser AW, Miser JS, Clark BS, et al. Continuous intravenous infusion of morphine sulfate for control of severe pain in children with terminal malignancy. *J Pediatr* 1980; 96:930–933.
12. Miser AW, Davis DM, Hughes CS, et al. Continuous subcutaneous infusion of morphine in children with cancer. *Am J Dis Child* 1983; 137:383–385.
13. Miser AW, Miser JS. The use of oral methadone to control moderate and severe pain in children and young adults with malignancy. *Clin J Pain* 1986; 1:243–248.
14. Miser AW, Moore L, Greene R, et al. Prospective study of continuous intravenous and subcutaneous morphine infusions for therapy related or cancer related pain in children and young adults with cancer. *Clin J Pain* 1986; 2:101–106.

15. Miser AW, Dothage JA, Miser JS. Continuous intravenous fentanyl for pain control in children and young adults with cancer. *Clin J Pain* 1987; 3:152–157.
16. Greene RF, Miser AW, Lester CM, et al. Cerebrospinal fluid and plasma pharmacokinetics of morphine infusions in pediatric cancer patients and rhesus monkeys. *Pain* 1987; 30:339–348.
17. Kapelushnik J, Koren G, Solh H, et al. Evaluating the efficacy of EMLA in alleviating pain associated with lumbar puncture; comparison of open and double-blinded protocols in children. *Pain* 1990; 42:31–34.
18. Mackie AM, Coda BC, Hill HF. Adolescents use patient-controlled analgesia effectively for relief from prolonged oropharyngeal mucositis pain. *Pain* 1991; 46:265–269.
19. Miser AW, Goh TS, Dose AM. Trial of a topically administered local anesthetic (EMLA cream) for pain relief during central venous port accesses in children with cancer. *J Pain Symptom Manage* 1994; 9:259–264.
20. Collins JJ, Geake J, Grier HE, et al. Patient-controlled analgesia for mucositis pain in children: a three period cross-over study comparing morphine and hydromorphone. *J Pediatr* 1996; 29:722–728.
21. Berde C, Ablin A, Glazer J, et al. Report of the subcommittee on disease-related pain in childhood cancer. *Pediatrics* 1990; 86:818–825.
22. Miser AW. Management of pain associated with childhood cancer. In: Schecter NL, Berde CB, Yaster M, eds. *Pain in Infants, Children and Adolescents*. Baltimore: Williams and Wilkins, 1993:411–424.
23. McGrath PA. Pain control. In: Doyle D, Hanks GWC, MacDonald N, eds. *Oxford Textbook of Palliative Medicine*. London: Oxford University Press, 1993:685–689.
24. Miller RP, Roberts RJ, Fischer LJ. Acetaminophen elimination kinetics in neonates, children and adults. *Clin Pharmacol Ther* 1976; 19:284–294.
25. Sandler DP, Smit JC, Weinberg CR, et al. Analgesic use and chronic renal disease. *N Engl J Med* 1989; 320:1238–1243.
26. Giannini EH, Brewer EJ, Miller ML, et al. Ibuprofen suspension in the treatment of juvenile rheumatoid arthritis. *J Pediatr* 1990; 117:645–652.
27. Stuart JJ, Pisko EJ. Choline magnesium trisalicylate does not impair platelet aggregation. *Pharmatherapeutica* 1981; 2:547.
28. Pelkonen O, Kaltiala EH, Larmi TKL, et al. Comparison of activities of drug metabolizing enzymes in human fetal and adult liver. *Clin Pharmacol Ther* 1973; 14:840–846.
29. Poyhia R, Seppala T. Lipid solubility and protein binding of oxycodone in vitro. *Pharmacol Toxicol* 1994; 74:23–27.
30. Bhat R, Chari G, Gulati A, et al. Pharmacokinetics of a single dose of morphine in pre-term infants during the first week of life. *J Pediatrl* 1990; 117:477–81.
31. McRorie TI, Lynn A, Nespeca MK, et al. The maturation of morphine clearance and metabolism. *Am J Dis Child* 1992; 146:972–976.
32. Pokela ML, Olkkala KT, Seppala T, et al. Age-related morphine kinetics in infants. *Dev Pharm Ther* 1993; 20:26–34.
33. Stanski DR, Greenblatt DJ, Lowenstein E. Kinetics of intravenous and intramuscular morphine. *Clin Pharmacol Ther* 1978; 24:52–59.
34. Olkkola KT, Maunuksela EL, Korpela R, et al. Kinetics and dynamics of postoperative morphine in children. *Clin Pharmacol Ther* 1988; 44:128–136.

35. Chay PC, Duffy BJ, Walker JS. Pharmacokinetic–pharmacodynamic relationships of morphine in neonates. *Clin Pharmacol Ther* 1992; 51:334–342.
36. Choonara IA, McKay P, Hain R, et al. Morphine metabolism in children. *Br J Clin Pharm* 1989; 28:599–604.
37. Choonara I, Lawrence A, Michaelkiewicz A, et al. Morphine metabolism in infants and neonates. *Br J Clin Pharm* 1992; 34:434–437.
38. Bhat R, Abu-Harb M, Chari G, et al. Morphine metabolism in acutely ill pre-term newborn infants. *J Pediatr* 1992; 120:795–799.
39. Hartley R, Green M, Quinn M, et al. Pharmacokinetics of morphine infusion in premature neonates. *Arch Dis Child* 1993; 69:55–58.
40. Hartley R, Quinn M, Green M, et al. Morphine glucuronidation in premature infants. *Br J Clin Pharm* 1993; 35:314–317.
41. Gourlay GK, Boas RA. Fatal outcome with use of rectal morphine for postoperative pain control in an infant. *BMJ* 1992; 304:766–767.
42. Collins C, Koren G, Crean P, et al. Fentanyl pharmacokinetics and hemodynamic effects in preterm infants during ligation of patent ductus arteriosus. *Anesth Analg* 1985; 64:1078–1080.
43. Johnson KL, Erickson JP, Holley FO, et al. Fentanyl pharmacokinetics in the pediatric population [abstract]. *Anesthesiology* 1984; 61 (3A):A441.
44. Gauntlett IS, Fisher DM, Hertzka RE, et al. Pharmacokinetics of fentanyl in neonatal humans and lambs: effects of age. *Anesthesiology* 1988; 69:683–687.
45. Koren G, Goresky G, Crean P, et al. Pediatric fentanyl dosing based on pharmacokinetics during cardiac surgery. *Anesth Analg* 1984; 63:577–582.
46. Koren G, Goresky G, Crean P, et al. Unexpected alterations in fentanyl pharmacokinetics in children undergoing cardiac surgery: age related or disease related? *Dev Pharmacol Ther* 1986; 9:183–191.
47. Schechter NL, Weisman SJ, Rosenblum M, et al. The use of oral transmucosal fentanyl citrate for painful procedures in children. *Pediatrics* 1995; 95:335–339.
48. Pokela ML, Olkkola KT, Kovisto M, et al. Pharmacokinetics and pharmacodynamics of intravenous meperidine in neonates and infants. *Clin Pharmacol Ther* 1992; 52:342–349.
49. Hamunen K, Maunuksela EL, Seppala T, et al. Pharmacokinetics of iv and rectal pethidine in children undergoing ophthalmic surgery. *Br J Anesthesia* 1993; 71:823–826.
50. Koska AJ, Kramer WG, Romagnoli A, et al. Pharmacokinetics of high dose meperidine in surgical patients. *Anesth Analg* 1981; 60:8–11.
51. Mather LE, Tucker GT, Pflug AE, et al. Meperidine kinetics in man: intravenous injection in surgical patients and volunteers. *Clin Pharmacol Ther* 1975; 17:21–30.
52. Tamsen A, Hartvig P, Fagerlund C, et al. Patient-controlled analgesic therapy, part 1: pharmacokinetics of pethidine in the pre- and postoperative periods. *Clin Pharmacokinet* 1982; 7:149–163.
53. Kaiko RF, Foley KM, Grabinski PY, et al. Central nervous system excitatory effects of meperidine in cancer patients. *Ann Neurol* 1983; 13:180–185.
54. Berde CB, Sethna NF, Holzman R, et al. Pharmacokinetics of methadone in children and adolescents in the perioperative period. *Anesthesiology* 1987; 67:A519.

55. Berde CB, Beyer JE, Bournaki MC, et al. Comparison of morphine and methadone for prevention of postoperative pain in 3- to 7-year-old children. *J Pediatr* 1991; 119:131–141.

56. Koren G, Butt W, Chinyanga H, et al. Post-operative morphine infusion in newborn infants: assessment of disposition characteristics and safety. *J Pediatr* 1985; 107:963–967.

57. Bruera E, Brenneis C, Michaud M, et al. Use of the subcutaneous route for the administration of narcotics in patients with cancer pain. *Cancer* 1988; 62:407–411.

58. Dunbar PJ, Buckley P, Gavrin JR, Sanders JE, Chapman CR. Use of patient-controlled analgesia for pain control for children receiving bone marrow transplant. *J Pain Symptom Manage* 1995; 10:604–611.

59. Portenoy RK. Opioid tolerance and responsiveness: research findings and clinical observations. In: Gebhart GF, Hammond D1, Jensen TS, eds. *Progress in Pain Research and Management*. Seattle: IASP Press, 1994:615–619.

60. Cherny NI, Foley KM. Nonopioid and opioid analgesic pharmacotherapy of cancer pain. In: Cherny NI, Foley KM, eds. *Pain and Palliative Care*. Hematol Oncol Clin N Am 1996; 10(1):79–102.

61. Galer BS, Coyle N, Pasternak GW, Portenoy RK. Individual variability in the response to different opioids: report of five cases. *Pain* 1992; 49:87–91.

62. Inturrisi CE, Portenoy RK, Max M, Colburn WA, Foley KM. Pharmacokinetic–pharmacodynamic relationships of methadone infusions in patients with cancer pain. *Clin Pharmacol Ther* 1990; 47:565–577.

63. Portenoy RK, Waldman SD. Adjuvant analgesics in pain management: Part 1. *J Pain Symptom Manage* 1994; 9(6):390–391.

64. Watson CPN, Evans RJ, Reed K, Mersky H, Goldsmith L, Warsh J. Amitriptyline versus placebo in postherpetic neuralgia. *Neurology* 1982; 32:671–673.

65. Max MB, Culrare M, Schafer SC, et al. Amitriptyline relieves diabetic neuropathy pain in patients with normal or depressed mood. *Neurology* 1987; 37:589–596.

66. Diamond S, Baltes BJ. Chronic tension headache-treatment with amitriptyline—a double-blind study. *Headache* 1971; 11:110–116.

67. Couch JR, Ziegler DK, Hassanein R. Amitriptyline in the prophylaxis of migraine: effectiveness and relationship of antimigraine and antidepressant effects. *Neurology* 1976; 26:121–127.

68. Frank RG, Kashani JH, Parker JC, et al. Antidepressant analgesia in rheumatoid arthritis. *J Rheumatol* 1988; 15:1632–1638.

69. Ward NG. Tricyclic antidepressants for chronic low back pain: mechanism of action and predictors of response. *Spine* 1986; 11:661–665.

70. Magni G. The use of antidepressants in the treatments of chronic pain. *Drugs* 1991; 42(5):730–748.

71. Heiligenstein E, Gerrity S. Psychotropics as adjuvant analgesics. In: Schecter NL, Berde CB, Yaster M, eds. *Pain in Infants, Children, and Adolescents*. Baltimore: Williams and Wilkins, 1993:173–177.

72. Biederman J, Baldessarini RJ, Wright V, et al. A double-blind placebo controlled study of desipramine in the treatment of ADD: II. Serum drug levels and cardiovascular findings. *J Am Acad Child Adolesc Psychiatry* 1989; 28:903–911.

73. Forest WH, Brown BW, Brown CR, et al. Dextroamphetamine with morphine for the treatment of postoperative pain. *N Engl J Med* 1977; 296:712–715.

74. Bruera E, Miller MJ, Macmillan K, Kuehn N. Neuropsychological effects of methylphenidate in patients receiving a continuous infusion of narcotics for cancer pain. *Pain* 1992; 48:163–166.
75. Bruera E, Fainsinger R, MacEachern T, Hanson J. The use of methylphenidate in patients with incident pain receiving regular opiates: a preliminary report. *Pain* 1992; 50:75–77.
76. Portenoy RK: Adjuvant analgesics in pain management. In: Doyle D, Hanks GWC, MacDonald N, eds. *Oxford Textbook of Palliative Medicine*. Oxford: Oxford University Press, 1993:187–203.
77. Yee JD, Berde CB. Dextroamphetamine or methylphenidate as adjuvants to opioid analgesia for adolescents with cancer. *J Pain Symptom Manage* 1994; 9:122–125.
78. Watanabe S, Bruera E. Corticosteroids as adjuvant analgesics. *J Pain Symptom Manage* 1994; 9:442–445.
79. Tannock I, Gospodarowicz M, Meakin W, Panzarella T, Stewart L, Rider W. Treatment of metastatic prostatic cancer with low-dose prednisone: evaluation of pain and quality of life as pragmatic indices of response. *J Clin Oncol* 1989; 7:590–597.
80. Yamada K, Yukitaka U, Hayakawa T, Arita N, Yamada N, Mogami H. Effects of methylprednisolone on peritumoral brain edema. *J Neurosurgery* 1983; 59:612–619.
81. Weinstein JD, Toy FJ, Jaffe ME, Goldberg HI. The effect of dexamethasone on brain edema in patients with metastatic brain tumors. *Neurology* 1973; 23:121–129.
82. Greenberg HS, Kim J, Posner JB. Epidural spinal cord compression from metastatic tumor: results with a new treatment protocol. *Ann Neurol* 1980; 8:361–366.
83. Mullan S. Surgical management of pain in cancer of the head and neck. *Surg Clin North Am* 1973; 53:203–210.
84. Khurana DS, Riviello J, Helmers S, Holmes G, Anderson J, Mikati MA. Efficacy of gabapentin therapy in children with refractory partial seizures. *J Pediat* 1996; 128:829–833.
85. Mellick GA, Mellick LB. Letter. Pain Symptom Manage 1995; 10(4):265–266.
86. Westlin JE, Letocha H, Jakobson A, Strang P, Martinsson U, Nilsson S. Rapid, reproducible pain relief with [^{131}I]iodine-meta-iodobenzylguanidine in a boy with disseminated neuroblastoma. *Pain* 1995; 60:111–114.
87. Silberstein EB, Williams C. Strontium-89 therapy for the pain of osseous metastases. *J Nucl Med* 1985; 26:345–348.
88. Beaver WT, Wallenstein S, Houde RW, Rogers A. A comparison of the analgesic effects of methotrimeprazine and morphine in patients with cancer. *Clin Pharmacol Ther* 1966; 7:436–446.
89. Porter J, Jick J. Addiction is rare in patients treated with narcotics [letter]. *N Engl J Med* 1980; 302:123.

2

Families in Pediatric Palliative Care

BETTY DAVIES
AND ROSE STEELE

Family-centered care is a basic tenet of palliative care philosophy. Hospice care recognizes that terminally ill patients are not isolated, but exist within the family system. In pediatrics, the focus on families becomes even more critical. The child's illness affects the whole family, and in turn, the family's responses have their impact on the child. In addition, because of the child's dependency, the family becomes a partner in care more so than in adult palliative care—pediatric palliative care involves the child–family unit in all aspects of care and decision making.

Recognizing the importance of a family focus necessitates a clear definition of what is meant by "family". The family has usually been defined by bonds, such as biological or emotional connections, or by functions, such as fulfilling the physical and health needs of its members, or providing sociological and psychological roots.[1] Typically, a family shares values and rules, and members are joined emotionally, or legally, or both. When working with children, the family often encompasses more than the ill child, parents, and siblings; it may include grandparents, aunts, uncles, cousins, and even friends, neighbors, and schoolmates, because a child's illness and death affects all those who know the child. Although the focus here is on parents and siblings because they are usually the central players in the child's experience, any of these others may need attention in the clinical setting.

Scope of Pediatric Palliative Care

In adult palliative care, most of the patients have cancer and are expected to die relatively soon. This is not the case in pediatric palliative care, where children targeted for intensive palliative care are those who suffer from a wide variety of diseases and syndromes. Many will have progressive neuromuscular or neurodegenerative conditions that will eventually cause death, but in a time frame that may be prolonged. For many ill children, families provide care at home over a period that may be measured in years rather than in days, weeks, or months. Consequently, the scope of pediatric palliative care must always include respite care in addition to terminal care. Bereavement care is the third integral component.

Ideally, palliative care is introduced early in the child's illness, preferably at the time of diagnosis. This approach is recommended in the model developed by the Canadian Palliative Care Association.[2] Over time, attention shifts from curative treatments to palliative care, and then to bereavement care. As children and families progress through this continuum of care, they experience transitions from respite care to terminal care; and then to bereavement care. They also experience the transitions involved in moving between hospital and home, and possibly hospice, and the transitions associated with the normal growth and development of children and families. These transitions are identified as difficult periods by parents of children with chronic illnesses.[3,4]

Although families may require additional support during critical transition periods, their need for ongoing support continues regardless of the phase of illness or location of care. In this chapter, we do not differentiate care for each phase of illness, but believe that the elements of care apply throughout the continuum.

The Impact on Families When a Child Has a Progressive, Life-threatening Illness

A child's progressive, life-threatening illness has a profound impact on every dimension of family life. Not only are families affected emotionally, psychologically, and financially, but their very structures and ways of organization are forever altered.

Emotional and psychological impact

The health care system is often a major source of distress to parents who are frustrated with perceived inadequacies and fragmented care.[5] Parents view themselves as their child's case manager, yet health care professionals may fail to acknowledge parents' skills and knowledge. Thus, the parents' frustration is increased, and sometimes the child is inappropriately treated or is admitted to the hospital because physicians who are unfamiliar with the child overreact instead of listening to the parents. Sometimes communication is unclear between health care professionals about a child's change of status from active treatment to palliative care. This lack of communication may create gaps in the support services provided to patients and families.[6] Faulty communication may cause parental anxiety, which impedes satisfactory care. Feelings of frustration may arise as parents try unsuccessfully to get needed information or to acquire equipment for the home.[6,7]

High levels of internal distress are common in families. One source of distress is the discrepancy between the parents' need to talk about feelings related to their child's death and dying, or planning the funeral, and the unwillingness of family and friends to discuss these issues.[6] Parents worry about the child's symptoms and about the course of the illness, and they are anxious about caring for the child if their own health should fail. Worries about the eventual death, such as where it will take place, what it will be like, and how they will manage, also concern parents. Moreover, anxious parents may suffer from insomnia, and become socially dysfunctional; some may start to use or increase their use of tranquilizers, antidepressants, or cigarettes to relieve their anxiety.[8] Many parents also struggle with trying to balance the demands of their ill child with the needs of their healthy children.

In addition, ill children themselves may experience emotional problems, such as anxiety and unhappiness. They often are aware of their prognosis, and may worry about its effect on their parents. They may go to great lengths to protect their parents from further distress.

Siblings also experience distress when a brother or sister is dying. In fact, in some families, siblings have more problems than the dying child.[8] Siblings may experience both emotional and behavioral problems, such as difficulty in dealing with their school work, problems establishing and maintaining relationships with peers, ambivalent feelings about the ill child (such as envy because of the attention given to the ill child, or shame and embarrassment because of how the ill child looks), and increased aggression or withdrawal. However, many siblings are aware of their parents' heavy burden and will accommodate their own behavior to the parents' needs so as to not compound their parents' distress.

Lack of acceptance within the broader community adds to a family's stress.[5] Lack of appropriate facilities, rude comments, curious stares, or even overly sympathetic responses from people in public places such as restaurants may result in families' being unwilling to venture far from home. Families may also experience difficulty in trying to balance the child's educational and medical needs because of inadequate in-hospital schooling, nonexistent home-school programs, or inappropriate program placement in public schools.

Financial impact

The financial burden on families is significant, though not always recognized by professionals. Financial problems occur because of cumulative costs associated with expenses related to the needs of the ill child (e.g., diapers, special equipment, food for special diet, medications, special clothing, ancillary services); attending health care facilities (e.g., airfare, taxi, parking, gas, food for the family while staying at the hospital, telephone); and meeting the needs of other family members (e.g., baby-sitting costs for other children, long-distance phone calls to keep in touch with siblings and grandparents).

Indirect costs increase the financial burden for some families. Many mothers give up their jobs to care for the child, or reduce their hours, resulting in a loss of family income.[8] Some fathers may refuse promotions or transfers; others may become unemployed or bankrupt. Those parents with insurance may be unable to change jobs because new insurance companies will not cover them. Even when families have insurance coverage, either by private coverage as they do in the U.S. or through government health plans as they do in Canada, families still incur great financial costs when a child is ill. For many families, a high percentage of weekly income may be spent on non-medical out-of-pocket expenses, causing a drain on family resources.[9] Consideration of financial support is an integral part of family-focused palliative care. When finances become a problem, the entire family is affected. Early involvement of a social worker may be helpful in preventing financial problems from becoming overwhelming.

Impact on family structure and organization

A child's terminal illness disrupts family patterns of interaction, requires family re-organization, and poses shared adaptational challenges. Tangible and intangible resources may be reallocated from family members to the ill child. In a study of families whose children were cared for in Helen House, the world's first free-standing hospice for children established in Oxford, England in 1982, parents reported several changes in social routines and functioning.[8] There was not enough time for social and leisure activities, and restrictions imposed by the ill child's need for care meant that families rarely left the home together. In addition, families had less contact with members of the extended family than they might normally have had. Other parents of children with medically complex needs reported that members of the extended family were often afraid of the ill child.[5] This fear may help account for the decreased family contact reported by many parents. Those parents whose children had medically complex needs also described deterioration of the family structure due to lack of time to do things as a couple or as a family. Again, following the routines imposed by the child's complex medical needs and day-to-day personal care needs interfered with the daily routines of family life.

The family reorganizes in response to the numerous changes in roles needed to manage a child's illness. Mothers usually take on the primary caregiving role, often giving up outside employment to be with the child. Consequently, mothers may feel particularly housebound because of exhaustion, concern about leaving the child safely in someone else's care, and worry about finding a suitable babysitter. Fathers generally continue working, but often use vacation time or take time off from work to attend to the child's needs. Siblings are often expected to assume responsibilities beyond those normally expected, and these tasks and duties may be more than they are ready to handle. Siblings may also have less free time, and have fewer friends than their peers.[8] Frequently, siblings feel that they do not receive enough attention from their parents, though they understand that the ill child requires a disproportionate share of their parents' time.

Importance of Family Functioning

How families adapt to the changes imposed by the child's illness and impending death depends in large part upon their level of functioning. The concept of family functioning has received considerable attention from family theorists, family therapists, and others who focus on family-centered care. In a study by Davies and colleagues,[10] familial level of functioning was related to how families managed the transition associated with the dying of an adult family member with advanced cancer. Family functioning also characterized how grieving parents adapted to the death of their child.[11] The dimensions of functioning occur along a continuum of functionality; family interactions tend to vary along the continuum rather than being positive or negative, good or bad. Table 2.1 summarizes the dimensions of family functioning.[11]

Dimensions of family functioning

Integrating the past
Previous experience with illness, loss, and other adversity influences the current situation of family members. Some families are able to learn from previous painful experiences, particularly of loss, and to incorporate that learning into the present situation. They recall painful events of the past, while also reminiscing about happy times. They are able to see potential regrets for actions taken or not taken as part of a normal response in a stressful situation: "I could have taken him to the doctor sooner, but I did the best I could." Though not negating their pain, they are still able to see the lighter side of life, believing that incorporating some of the frivolous aspects of life is important to continuing on with life. They are able, though with great sadness, to accept the inevitability of their child's death, and to alter in realistic ways the focus of their hope as the child's condition deteriorates. In one family, for example, when the child relapsed for what was to be the final time, family members hoped he would go into remission as he had done before. As the child became weaker, they hoped he would be able to swallow even small amounts of fluids. At the very end, they hoped he would die peacefully. After the child's death, they recalled both the good and bad behaviors of the child.

Other families dwell only on the painful experiences of the past, not having learned or grown along the way. Such families seem guided more by illusion than reality—they may continue to expect miracle cures and never really expect the child to die. They may insist on active treatment until the very end. They regret what they had or had not done that might have contributed to their child's illness and death. "If only" is a common phrase in their conversation. "Regret-focused"

Table 2.1. Dimensions of family functioning

Integrating the past	Describes painful experiences as they relate to present experience	Describes past experiences repeatedly
	Describes positive and negative feelings concerning the past	Dwells on painful feelings associated with past experiences
	Incorporates learning from the past into subsequent experiences	Does not integrate learning from the past to the current situation
	Reminisces about pleasurable experiences in the past	Focuses on trying to "fix" the past to create happy memories of situations that were absent from family life
Dealing with feelings	Expresses a range of feelings including vulnerability, fear and uncertainty	Expresses predominately negative feelings, such as anger, hurt, bitterness, and fear
	Acknowledges paradoxical feelings	Acknowledges little uncertainty or few paradoxical feelings
Solving problems	Identifies problems as they occur	Focuses more on fault finding rather than on finding solutions
	Reaches consensus about a problem and possible courses of action	Dwells on the emotions associated with the problem
	Considers multiple options	Unable to clearly communicate needs and expectations
	Is open to suggestions	Feels powerless about influencing the care they are receiving
	Approaches problems as a team rather than as individuals	Approaches problems from an individual perspective rather than as a family
		Displays exaggerated responses to unexpected events
		Withholds or inaccurately shares information with other family members
Utilizing resources	Uses a wide range or resources	Utilizes few resources
	Is open to accepting support	Reluctant to seek help or accept offers of help
	Is open to suggestions regarding resources	Receives help mostly from formal sources rather than from informal support networks
	Takes the initiative in procuring additional resources	Describes fewer friends and acquaintances who offer help
	Expresses satisfaction with results obtained	Expresses dissatisfaction with help received

Table 2.1. *(Continued)*

	Describes the involvement of many friends acquaintances and support persons	
Considering others	Acknowledges multidimensional effect of situation on other family members	Individuals focus concern on own emotional needs
	Expresses concern for well-being of other family members	Minimizes or misinterprets how others might be affected emotionally by the situation
	Focuses concern on patient's well-being	Fails to acknowledge or minimizes extra tasks taken on by others
	Appreciates individualized attention from health care professionals, but does not express a strong need for such attention	Displays inordinate need for individualized attention
	Directs concerns about how other family members are managing rather than with themselves.	
Portraying family	Identifies characteristic coping styles of family unit and of individual members	Describes own characteristic coping styles rather than the characteristic way the family unit copes
	Demonstrates warmth and caring toward other family members	Allows one member to dominate group interaction
	Considers present situation as potential opportunity for family's growth and development	Lacks comfort with expressing true feelings in the family group
	Values contributions of all family members	Feigns group consensus where none exists
Fulfilling roles	Demonstrates flexibility in adapting to role changes	Demonstrates rigidity in adapting to role changes and responsibilities
	Shares extra responsibilities willingly	Demonstrates less sharing of responsibilities created by extra demands of patient care
	Adjusts priorities to incorporate extra demands of patient care and expresses satisfaction with this division	Expresses resentment over perceived lack of support in caregiving
		Refers to caregiving as a duty or obligation
		Criticizes or mistrusts caregiving provided by others

(continued)

Table 2.1. Dimensions of family functioning (*Continued*)

Tolerating differences	Allows differing opinions and beliefs within the family	Displays intolerance for differing opinions or approaches of caregiving
	Tolerates different views from people outside the family	Demonstrates critical views of friends who fail to respond as expected
	Willing to examine own belief and value systems	Adheres rigidly to beliefs and value system

families may maintain a somber attitude, dismissing what they perceive as "frivolous"—there is little room for fun. After the child's death, they remember only the child's good characteristics, forgetting that he or she had been a normal child who misbehaved as all children do sometimes.

Dealing with feelings

Some families express a range of feelings, from happiness and satisfaction, through uncertainty and dread, to sadness and sorrow. They describe these feelings, and express the associated vulnerabilities. They express their anger, most often directed at a particular event. They acknowledge the uncertainty of the situation. They supplement descriptions of their situation with accounts of the associated feelings. They seem more process-oriented, that is, they focus on their whole experience rather than fixing on tangible incidents. Other families do not have this freedom of expression. They describe a narrow range of feelings, most often concentrating on anger, hurt, and fear. Anger is pervasive rather than directed towards a particular event. They seldom acknowledge their uncertainty, nor talk about their ambivalence. They appear to avoid issues of turmoil surrounding the impending death, and instead appear to shield themselves from the pain. This may be apparent when such families are asked to talk about their situation; their responses focus primarily on the events, with little, if any, mention of the associated feelings. Such families are more content-oriented.

Solving problems

When families are more focused on feelings and process, this awareness leads to action. Such families, for example, can anticipate the sadness and sorrow that will accompany the child's death. Though they cannot avoid it, they will begin to plan for how to manage their lives during those especially difficult times, for example, by asking other family members or friends to stay with them. These families identify problems as they occur and openly exchange information. They participate in identifying solutions, share in implementing strategies, and openly acknowledge each other's contributions. Other families do not discuss problems in order to arrive at the best solution. Instead, each member has his or her own version of the problem. Although they may all seem to agree with one another in family interviews, each criticizes the others and blames them for inappropriate action when alone. Family members may feel persecuted, or singled out to receive poor treatment. They often seem unable to communicate what they expect from the health care system, and become angry when their expectations remain unfulfilled.

Using and reorganizing resources

Some families use a variety of resources, including friends, community agencies, health care personnel, and each other. They are able to ask for and graciously receive assistance, friendship, support, and empathy. They are open, flexible, and adaptive in their organization and mobilization of resources. Other families use few resources, appearing reluctant to seek or accept help. They describe few friends and acquaintances who offer assistance, and when they do receive assistance, they appear dissatisfied. "The home care nurse comes every morning, but is never here early enough." These families are more rigid in their reorganization, regretting and resenting the changes.

Considering others

In some families, members show concern for each other and acknowledge one another's responsibilities. Siblings are concerned about their parents' fatigue and worry; parents appreciate their children's concern. The family is focused on the ill child's comfort, with compassion for the sacrifices being made by everyone. In contrast, in other families members focus their concerns on themselves, seemingly unaware of the responsibilities and contributions of others. Each person in the family appears to be alone in the experience, or misunderstood by the others.

Portraying family identity

In families with a strong family identity, members share in the acknowledgement of their family's unique characteristics. Statements about the family are usually positive and expressive of warmth and caring. All members participate in discussions, correcting and clarifying one another amiably. Views expressed within the group correspond with views expressed individually. There is a focus on the family as a system. In more individual-focused families, however, family members tend to talk more about their own personal characteristics than how they see the family. There is often discrepancy between what is acknowledged as the truth when the family is together and what is expressed in individual conversations. One person may speak authoritatively on behalf of the others; there is little correcting or clarifying of one another.

Fulfilling roles

Some families are flexible in sharing and changing roles. A mother may continue to work outside the home, while the father adjusts his schedule to be with the ill child; or the well siblings may assume household responsibilities while their parents are busy with the ill child. After the death, grief is allowed free expression, regardless of gender or age. Other families rigidly maintain roles as, for example, in the reinforcing of traditional gender-related behavior exemplified by one father who did not allow his surviving son to cry over his sister's death. There is a sense that these families do not adjust easily to the new situation, and do not accept roles being taken over by others, particularly by "outsiders."

Tolerating differences
In some families, the expression of differing opinions and beliefs is encouraged. These families, for example, may question their religious beliefs or their values as a way of trying to understand the situation and their reactions. The family environment encourages expression of the struggle involved in trying to make sense of the world. In less tolerant families, differing viewpoints are not welcomed, and the world is seen mostly from a rigid point of view. Beliefs, particularly religious beliefs, are not openly questioned.

Implications of the continuum of family functioning

Some families will be easier to work with than others, depending on their level of functioning. Professionals must be aware that family interactions, based on the dimension of functioning, will contribute to their ease or difficulty in managing transitions. Consequently, a prerequisite for working with families in palliative care is an assessment of family functioning. Such an assessment provides practitioners with an accurate understanding of how a family normally functions, enables practitioners to be more effective in their interactions with families, and provides direction for developing interventions in conjunction with the family.

Interventions

In pediatric palliative care, interventions for family support are needed at three different levels: the program level, the family level, and the individual level. Interventions often occur simultaneously at all three levels. The two principles underlying interventions are open communication and treating parents as partners in care. At the time of diagnosis, open communication about all aspects of the child's illness sets the tone for ongoing interactions between parents and health care providers. Giving information directly and honestly, yet sensitively, with a tolerance for varied parental responses, creates a milieu which fosters trust and a feeling of safety for parents.[12] Parents who feel safe can cope more effectively with their child's illness.

Health professionals and parents must work in interdependent, rather than adversarial, roles. As the child's illness progresses, parents become experts in the care of their child, and health professionals should respect and acknowledge this expertise.[13] While parents are capable of providing most of the child's care, they will need support in varying degrees. Parents frequently emphasize the difficulty in identifying sources of help and in obtaining help in a way that lets them retain control of their lives.[14] They tire of repeating their story to new health care providers each time the child is admitted to the hospital, or of making repetitive phone calls to track down a needed piece of equipment for use at home. Parents need one identified person, someone who knows them and their child, and is familiar with the child's condition, to provide continuity of care and central place for information and consultation. They need someone who can help them negotiate the system. In short, they need a "cornerstone carer,"[14] a person who has a good relationship with the family be it a physician, nurse, social worker, or other professional.

Program level

There are palliative care services for children in a variety of programs. For most of the 20th century, dying children have been cared for in hospitals. Home care programs, however, are becoming the most common form of care delivery in North America. In addition, Helen House serves as a model for many similar free-standing hospice facilities which have been developed in the United Kingdom over the past 15 years. This same program is the model for North America's first free-standing hospice for children (Canuck Place in Vancouver, Canada), and for what will be Australia's first such facility (Bear Cottage in Sydney).

Although parents can provide much of the care for their children, they require assistance in doing so. The child's wishes should be taken into account when deciding on a program of care. Families must be able to choose from hospital, home, or hospice care, and should be able to change their options as desired. An integrated, coordinated program of palliative care should offer these options.

Hospital care
In the hospital, pediatric palliative care can be provided in several ways. Some children's hospitals are now developing specialized palliative care units for children. These units are rare, however; it is more common for a hospital to designate palliative care beds, particularly on oncology, neurology, or cardiac units. Other children's hospitals have palliative care teams comprising health professionals with expertise in palliative care. Palliative care teams are called upon for consultation by staff who are caring for children who are admitted to general hospitals for palliative care. It is important that hospital staff have access to experienced palliative care teams for consultation, either in the community or at children's hospitals.

Home care
Home is often perceived as the ideal location for care. Care at home supports the family by keeping all members together, and by allowing everyone to share in the child's care and provide mutual support.[14] The home provides a secure, familiar,

and comfortable environment for the child, resulting in increased happiness, security, and physical comfort.[15] The child can maintain regular patterns of everyday living. He or she can eat favorite foods, treasured toys are available, the dog can rest nearby, and friends can visit whenever they want without having to plan for transportation. Parents feel more in control, and there is less disruption of family life for all members. The child and family can enjoy more privacy and freedom than in the hospital. Siblings are more involved, and can see for themselves their brother's or sister's gradual deterioration, which can enable them to approach death more realistically. Family members tend to be present at the time of death, and can grieve afterwards in an unhurried manner. They can sit with the child for as long as they desire without having to accommodate to hospital routines, limited space, and lack of privacy; friends and family can share the experience and offer support without worrying about infringing upon other patients, families, and staff in the hospital setting.

Yet home care is not for every family. Some parents may find it too painful to continuously watch their child's physical decline, or they may feel inadequate in providing care. They may be anxious about the child dying at home, about what to expect at the time of death, about their ability to continue living in the home afterwards, and about the effect of a home death on siblings. Even for families who want to keep the child at home, it is not always possible to do so. Medical complications, such as hemorrhage or intractable pain, may necessitate hospitalization. Parental stress and exhaustion related to 24-hour care of the child and coping with domestic duties may signal a need for the respite provided by placing the child in a hospital or other facility.

Community support systems need to be in place for home care to work well for families. Professional support 24 hours a day, seven days a week, is critical.[15,16] Parents want to know that they can call for help as needed at any time of the day or night, on weekdays, weekends, and holidays. Experience has shown that the vast majority of families do not overuse services. Indeed, the more important issue is the assurance that help is only a phone call away should it be needed. Home care staff must be knowledgeable and experienced in pediatric palliative care and must be able to share knowledge with families in supportive ways. Again, parents and staff must be partners in care. Staff must also be aware of community resources which might enhance the family's quality of life. For example, specialized equipment is often important in maintaining a child at home, yet families may be unaware of how to access such resources. Professionals can assist families in "cutting through the red tape" to obtain necessary equipment and other services in a timely fashion.

Caring for a child at home drains energy and is time consuming, especially for mothers, who most often are the primary caregivers. Teaching parents how to use special equipment, how to carry out procedures, and how to manage potential problems may enable families to manage the care of their child at home. Practical support from homemaking services or volunteers provides relief from dealing with the daily difficulties of housework and grocery shopping. Nighttime relief to allow parents to sleep may be obtained from either volunteers or professionals, depending on the needs of the child. Without periodic relief, parents become exhausted. Although they may continue to care for their child at home, it is often at the cost of their own health and well-being. Support services not only free parents to spend time with their ill child, but may also allow them some time alone or with their other children.

Hospice programs

Increasingly, hospice programs have developed as a complement to home and hospital care. Some programs have a hospice facility with outreach programs extending into the community. Families may have specific reasons for seeking hospice care, but there are often common themes. Families usually want care in a non-hospital environment that emphasizes emotional support, time to talk in a relaxed and homey atmosphere, relief of symptoms rather than active interventions, and respite care.[8,12] Pediatric hospice programs coordinate the care required to keep children at home. In addition, they provide respite, terminal, and bereavement care. For many families, hospice care may provide the additional support they need to keep the ill child at home for as long as possible.

Parents of children in the Helen House hospice program felt very well supported by the program.[12] Families welcomed the opportunity to meet and receive support from other families in a hospice, and were relieved to know that there was a place where their child could go if an emergency arose or the parents took ill. Many parents commented that the entire family, including the siblings, was made to feel welcome at the hospice, in contrast to the hospital, where families were often not well received. Parents were reassured by the staff's experience with the children's illnesses, especially the rarer ones, and they felt confident that the staff could manage the medical problems. The flexibility of the ongoing support, the helpfulness of rituals surrounding the death, and the opportunity to spend time with the child's body in an unhurried manner were especially supportive to families after the child had died.

Family level

Family level interventions are those that focus on the family unit. These interventions are directed toward all members of the family, rather than one member (e.g., mother) or a subgroup (e.g., parents). The aims of these interventions are to optimize family functioning and to promote the integrity of the family unit, so that families can care for the ill child, for individual family members, and for the family itself. Family interventions seek to sustain and improve family cohesion, communication, and social support.

As noted previously, different levels of functioning in families should be considered when planning intervention strategies to facilitate the family's coping with a child's terminal illness and subsequent death. Caution must be advised, however, against labeling families as "functional" or "dysfunctional," because there is a continuum and all families demonstrate various degrees of functionality.

Despite the importance of the family in palliative care, approaches for care of the family tend to be described in a general way. Using the dimensions of family functioning to assess families is suggested as a practical way to enhance family-focused care. For example, in families characterized by open expression of feelings, thoughts, and concerns, flexibility toward change, and consideration for one another, practitioners can approach the family as a unit. Practitioners can feel confident giving information to or discussing sensitive issues with one parent, knowing that the conversation will be shared accurately with the other parent, or with the ill child's siblings. In contrast, in families with indirect communication, little agreement about the nature of the problem, rigidly entrenched roles, and little tolerance for differing opinions, practitioners must direct their conversations to the entire family group, as well as to each member individually.

Communication is basic to assessing family functioning in all families, but particularly those who lack trust or who are reluctant to speak openly. Information should be obtained from more than one family member, and gathered over time, as some families take longer to develop trust. Allowing family members to tell their story is a major part of understanding the family. Most of the time, family members simply want someone to listen; they are not requesting assistance in "fixing" their family. It is critical for practitioners to recognize this difference. The goal is to support the family in doing what they want, not to "fix" families perceived as functioning less than optimally.

The family's level of functioning affects how practitioners obtain and share information, offer resources, and determine particular approaches. The use of family conferences, though widely advocated, may not work well for families whose members have difficulty listening to one another. It may be better to meet individually with each person, or, at least, to expect to have to answer questions and restate the information to the individual members outside of the group.

Support groups are also often highly recommended for families in palliative care. These groups are especially helpful for families who may benefit from hearing about the experiences of others; however, it may be unwise to recommend them for those who require more individualized attention.

The way a family functions profoundly affects the way the family deals with a dying child. For some families, the stress of palliative care coupled with their decreased level of family functioning makes the situation almost overwhelming. It is unrealistic to expect that all families will "pull together" to cope with the situation. It is essential that practitioners not judge families, nor label them as "dysfunctional" or "pathological," but rather appreciate that the family is doing the best it can under the most trying circumstances.

A point to consider is that most families with a dying child are young families. They may be relatively "new" as a family, may not be enmeshed in long-held patterns of interaction, and may still be open to new ways of relating to one another. Because children with progressive, life-threatening illnesses are usually ill for long periods of time, families get to know their caregivers very well. Consequently, health care providers may have both the time and the opportunity to facilitate and encourage optimal ways of family interaction. However, new ways of interacting should be introduced through modeling rather than by imposing behaviors upon families.

Assessing families also includes paying attention to cultural and religious beliefs and practices. For example, in some cultures it is believed that having a person die in the home is bad luck. To encourage home care of the dying child in such situations would be inappropriate. Practitioners must determine each family's preferences, rather than making assumptions based on their own beliefs.

Providing family level interventions means that the needs of families must be taken into account when planning palliative care services for children. For example, when designing structural aspects of pediatric palliative care, space must be provided for family members to stay with the ill child. Family suites should be provided so that whole families can stay in the same facility as the child. Many times, health care professionals make it easier for family members to stay with children in the hospital by providing cots or reclining chairs. Measures such as these are appreciated by families, but they occur as an adaptation of a system focused on the individual (in this case the ill child), rather than one that creates structures to support family care. Often only one parent can stay with the child, and the other parent and siblings must remain at home, or in a nearby motel room or other facility. To fully involve families, visiting policies must have open hours and no restrictions on who can visit; such restrictions should be left to the discretion of the family.

Involvement of the family must expand beyond the traditional practice of focusing on the mother's involvement with the ill child. Specific tasks need to be assigned to other family members, such as asking a sibling to read a favorite book to the ill child. A concerted effort must be made to include the father, siblings, and even other family members, such as grandparents. All family members should be included in discussions about the situation, in team conferences, and in meetings about the plan of care.

Often, educational and general support functions of interventions are integrated. Information must be provided in ways that empower families rather than constrain them.[17] Practitioners should help families define what they need, then help them find support on their own terms and in their own way. In this way, families can retain control over their own lives. The goal is to provide them with an array of choices, rather than with directives for what they must do.

Information should be accessible to all family members. Clear, simple explanations should be given, and drawings, diagrams, and booklets should be available. Care providers must take into account the developmental level of each member of the family, particularly the children. Preschool children require very different forms of information than do adolescents. In working with families, one must also take into account the developmental level of the family, as well as of the individual members. When the ill member is a child, the family is usually in the early developmental stages of family life. Such families often have other children whose ages may range from infancy to adolescence. Therefore, the range of developmental abilities is much greater than in families where members are all adults. These different abilities must be recognized.

Practitioners should also provide opportunities for families to discuss issues with one another. In interviews with families after the death of a child, many indicate that the interview, sometimes as long as three years after the death, was the first time they had discussed the death as a family. They may also indicate that, before the death, they had not discussed the illness as a family, although when they finally did so, they found it helpful. Caregivers need to create opportunities for family members to meet together, to share information, and to ask questions. In this way, caregivers can model effective patterns of interaction.

Individual level

Although family-focused care often implies that health professionals must view the family as a unit, consideration must also be given to the individuals who make up the unit.

In interactions with family members, caregivers should refrain from taking control of the situation and imposing preconceived notions of what the family needs. Instead, clinicians should listen to what is being said, then reflect and validate these perceptions. This may sound like a simple suggestion, but it is very difficult to do and requires practice and continuous effort. Caregivers should listen to what each family member wants and needs rather than lecturing and giving advice and information. They should provide opportunities for individuals to talk about their experiences, without being judgmental or offering explanations or platitudes. Nonverbal communication speaks louder than words in most interactions, and nonverbal behavior must be consistent with spoken words.

Involving the family means giving each person useful, concrete things to do. Directions for various procedures, or ways of meeting the ill child's needs, should be shared with all members of the family, not just with the mother. Involving everyone in discussions, explanations, and plans for treatment or care is critical to fostering cohesiveness among family members. It also serves to make each person feel a part of what is happening. All who want to be included should be.

Children with chronic illnesses have the same emotional needs as healthy children, but stresses from illness-related events can interfere with or change a child's emotional development. Health care professionals can provide the support and guidance needed by the child and family to optimize the child's ability to attain appropriate developmental tasks. Interventions such as home visits, telephone consultations, pre-hospital visits to the pediatric unit, play and educational sessions during and after hospitalization, parent and family education, and post-hospital follow-up can assist the child in meeting developmental tasks.

Caregivers should consider the different ways that children (both the ill child and siblings) and their parents view the world. Children understand the world differently simply because of their level of cognitive development. They may have fears and anxieties that seem irrational from the adult's perspective, and their understanding of events and explanations may be literal. For example, a child who, in anger, yelled at a sibling, "Get lost," or "I wish you were dead," may feel responsible for the sibling's subsequent illness and death. Health care providers should use simple and concrete language, and should only use abstract concepts, similes, and analogies with discretion. It is not wise to make assumptions, but to check out the meanings that various concepts hold for children (and adults). This is particularly significant in discussions about philosophical, religious, or theological concepts.

Professionals also should be aware that some parents and children will try to protect one another. Parents may be unwilling to include their children in discussions about death and dying because of the fear and anxiety they believe may result. On the other hand, children are curious about their illness, their prognosis, and about dying. They may avoid talking about these issues with adults because they realize the adults are uncomfortable. While respecting this desire to protect, professionals should strive to promote open communication among family members. When there has been open communication, families manage their grief more easily. Guidelines for providing support to the ill child, parents, and siblings are offered in Tables 2.2–2.4.

Table 2.2. Suggestions for supporting the ill child

Listen to what the child needs and wants.

Children are capable of being in control of their dying process; support them in whatever ways they need.

Grief work can be facilitated by encouraging the child to participate in the funeral planning, burial arrangements, and other rituals.

Children are curious about their illness and its prognosis, and about dying; provide opportunities for the child to talk.

Be comfortable with your own beliefs about death and dying, so that you can approach a child with openness and honesty.

Let the child control the conversation and set the pace for questioning.

Look for cues to what the child really wants to talk about.

Do not just lecture or give information.

Be truthful.

Use simple, concrete language.

Use pictures and stories for both gaining and sharing information.

Be aware that simply giving children the "facts" can be inadequate because of their different sense of reality; always validate a child's understanding of your answers and explanations.

Be prepared to accept fears and anxieties in children that may seem irrational from an adult perspective.

Children often have fears related to separation and pain, such as separation from their mother, painful or traumatic procedures, and the deaths of other children. Anticipate these fears and provide opportunities for the child to voice such fears.

Table 2.3. Suggestions for supporting parents

Listen to parents' needs and wants.

Provide opportunities for parents to talk, both individually and as a couple.

Help parents identify and discuss sources of distress.

Introduce intervention services early on.

Provide information about the child's particular health problem, current condition, and prescribed treatment, both in writing and verbally.

Provide information about programs and services, financial planning for the future, financial aid, and insurance plans.

Give information about the behavioral and emotional changes that might occur in the dying child and siblings.

Suggest ways of conveying information to siblings.

Encourage and facilitate social and recreational opportunities through the use of volunteer, family, and professional support.

Arrange for transportation to medical services.

Help families create reminiscences such as scrapbooks, tape recordings, and videos.

Facilitate contact with another parent who has had a similar experience.

Parent support groups may be useful; recommend as appropriate.

Provide counseling to help the family reorganize disrupted activities.

Provide information about the physical changes that indicate impending death.

Provide anticipatory information about how the death will likely occur.

Discuss the practical implications of the child's death, such as funeral arrangements.

After death, the family may benefit from a quiet time with the child's body.

Encourage families to participate in death rituals; suggest ways of performing rituals or assist families in developing their own.

Educating Professionals in Pediatric Hospice Care

Pediatric hospice care requires knowledgeable, skilled, and expert professionals who can provide the support families need, while also working with families as equal partners in care. For example, some families may have difficulty identifying and understanding the changes in family dynamics caused by the illness, so they may need assistance in articulating and understanding these changes. However, this assistance cannot easily be provided by an inexperienced professional.[18] Working with families requires skill and experience. Unfortunately, there is a lack of educational and training programs to help professionals become skilled pediatric hospice caregivers.

Although courses and special training in palliative care are now increasing, there is relatively little emphasis on preparing health care professionals to work with dying children and their families. Effective practitioners must be knowledgeable about the underlying principles of palliative care as well as about child development, child psychology, cultural and religious influences, pathophysiology

Table 2.4. Suggestions for supporting siblings

It is important to remember that siblings are also children, so many of the suggestions for working with the ill child apply to siblings as well.

Provide opportunities for siblings to talk.

Listen to what siblings tell you, and address their wants and needs.

Siblings may have their own version of what caused the child's illness, or may have misconceptions about the nature of the illness. Give a clear, unambiguous explanation of the illness and its cause, and try to free siblings of any wrong ideas they may have.

Reassure siblings that they will not get the same illness, if you can do this honestly.

Determine the nature of the relationship between the sibling and the dying child.

Provide information, include siblings in discussions, and keep them informed.

A support group may be beneficial.

Ask siblings to help in home care tasks.

Since parents tend to focus on the dying child and may neglect the siblings to some extent, pay attention to siblings.

Encourage parents to treat the children equally and to take each one's special needs into account.

Arrange for siblings to spend time alone with their parents.

Assist parents in staying in touch with siblings during hospital stays.

Encourage parents to permit siblings to continue their own lives as normally as possible.

Establish contact with the sibling's school to keep teachers informed of the child's experiences.

Include siblings in the experience of loss.

Allow siblings to say good-bye to the dying child.

Allow siblings to attend the funeral if they want to.

of disease, therapeutics, and pain control. In addition, they must acquire the skills to put this knowledge into practice. Moreover, they must then integrate this learning and combine it with superior communication skills, to work effectively with children and families. Indeed, Doyle[19] stresses that the teaching of communication skills is even more crucial than the teaching of clinical therapeutics. Clearly, optimal family care is dependent upon excellent communication skills, and symptom assessment and treatment must not be overemphasized at the expense of the fundamentals of communication. The importance of effective communication was emphasized by parents who participated in a recent study in a regional children's hospital, in which they described the experience of having their child die.[20] These parents appreciated competent care, but also wanted care providers to "act human," to take time to talk, explain, and just be there.

Conclusion

The death of a child is one of the most traumatic events that families must endure. Death and serious illness profoundly affect the lives of those they touch. Professionals must therefore provide not only safe and competent care, but must also provide sensitive and supportive care so that they can do all that is possible to prevent a difficult experience from having a lasting negative influence.

References

1. Leahey M, Wright L. *Families and Life-threatening Illness*. Springhouse, Pa.: Springhouse Corporation, 1987.
2. Canadian Palliative Care Association. *Palliative Care: Towards a Consensus in Standardized Principles of Practice*. Ottawa, Canada: 1995.
3. Clements D, Copeland L, Loftus M. Critical times for families with a chronically ill child. *Pediatr Nurs* 1990; 16(2):161–187.
4. Gravelle AM. Caring for a child with a progressive illness during the complex chronic phase: Parents' experience of facing adversity. *Adv Nurs* 1997; 25:738–745.
5. Diehl S, Moffitt K, Wade S. Focus group interview with parents of children with medically complex needs: An intimate look at their perceptions and feelings. *Child Health Care* 1991; 20(3):170–178.
6. Singleton R. Palliative home care program for terminally ill children. *Leadership Health Serv* 1992; 1(1):21–27.
7. Davies H. Living with dying: Families coping with a child who has a neurodegenerative genetic disorder. *Axone* 1996; 18(20):38–44.
8. Stein A, Wooley H. An evaluation of hospice care for children. In: Baum J, Dominica Sr. F, Woodward R, eds. *Listen: My Child Has a Lot of Living to Do*. New York: Oxford University Press, 1990:66–90.
9. Walker D, Epstein S, Taylor A, Crocker A, Tuttle G. Perceived needs of families with children who have chronic health conditions. *Child Health Care* 1989; 18(4):196–201.
10. Davies B, Reimer J, Brown P, Martens N. *Fading Away: The Experience of Transition in Families with Terminal Illness*. Amityville, N.Y.: Baywood Publishing Company, Inc., 1995.
11. Davies B, Spinetta J, Martinson I, McClowry S, Kulenkamp E. Manifestations of levels of functioning in grieving families. *J Fam Issues* 1986; 7(3):297–313.
12. Stein A, Forrest G, Woolley H, Baum J. Life threatening illness and hospice care. *Arch Dis Child* 1989; 64:687–702.
13. Ray L, Ritchie J. Caring for chronically ill children at home: Factors that influence parents' coping. *J Pediatr Nurs*, 1993; 8(4):217–225.
14. Woolley H, Stein A, Forrest G, Baum J. Cornerstone care for families of children with life-threatening illness. *Dev Med Child Neurol* 1991; 33:216–224.
15. Martinson I. A home care program. In: Armstrong-Dailey A and Goltzer S, eds. *Hospice Care for Children*. New York: Oxford University Press, 1993: 231–247.
16. Duffy C, Pollock P, Levy P, Budd E, Caufield L, Koren G. Home based palliative care for children. Part 2: The benefits of an established program. *J Palliat Care* 1990; 6(2):8–14.
17. Bakke K, Pomietto M. Family care when a child has late stage cancer: A research review. *Oncol Nurs Forum* 1986; 13(6):71–76.

18. Jefidoff A, Gasner R. Helping the parents of a dying child: An Israeli experience. *J Pediatr Nurs* 1993; 8(6):413–415.
19. Doyle D. Education in palliative medicine and pain therapy: An overview. In: Twycross RG, ed. *Edinburgh Symposium of Pain Control and Medical Education.* Edinburgh, Scotland: The Royal Society of Medicine, 1989: 165–174.
20. Davies B, Connaughty S. Final Report: Bereavement Care at British Columbia's Children's Hospital. Submitted to the Medical Advisory Council, B.C. Children's Hospital, 1996.

3

Treatment of Symptoms Other Than Pain in Pediatric Palliative Care

MARCIA LEVETOWN

The frequency of various symptoms among pediatric palliative care patients largely depends on the site of the survey. If patients are assessed following admission to a specialized program, the philosophy of the program influences the mix of patients and, consequently, the prevalence of symptoms. In England, for example, where patients are qualified for admission early in the disease process, there is a very large proportion of patients with slowly degenerative disorders, such as Sanfilippo syndrome, a metabolic disorder. This disease causes thickened facial features, progressive loss of intellect and other central nervous system functions, and seizures. Accordingly, a high proportion of English patients have this type of symptomatology.

A survey of 30 inpatients who died between 1983 and 1987 at Helen House, the first pediatric hospice in England, documented that 11 suffered slowly progressive metabolic disorders leading to neurologic dysfunction.[1] Thirteen had neoplastic diseases: of these, seven had brain tumors, one had a static central nervous system (CNS) disorder, three had unspecified congenital anomalies, one had a respiratory disorder and one a neuromuscular disorder. The most frequent non-pain symptoms documented were dyspnea, excess secretions, seizures, oral symptoms, psychological distress, swallowing difficulties, cough, muscle spasms, and excess sweating.[1]

In the United States, many hospice programs follow the Medicare guidelines for hospice admission, regardless of whether or not the patient is a child. Thus, a predicted prognosis for survival of six months or less is required. The few pediatric patients in these programs are often admitted only in the last weeks or days of their lives. Pediatric physicians and families often cannot admit that the child is terminally ill until the active dying phase is reached. Programs following Medicare guidelines will therefore primarily admit patients with end-stage cancers and children with severe congenital malformations such as anencephaly and Trisomy 18. The type and distribution of non-pain symptoms is thus considerably different than in England, with vomiting and bleeding being more prevalent.

Most nontraumatic pediatric deaths occur in the first year of life, and a large number occur in the 1–4-year-old population. However, many of these patients are not given the choice of palliative care. In a recent article on the development of a pediatric hospice program in Vancouver,[2] Davies wrote that children with a prognosis of less than a few days should not be considered hospice eligible.

The Butterfly Program, a program of pediatric supportive and palliative care in Galveston, Texas, takes another approach, allowing for a new, more inclusive set of non-pain symptoms to be the domain of the palliative care professional. The sole criterion for admission is that the patient is not expected to live to adulthood (age 18). Concurrent curative care may be undertaken at the discretion of the patient and family. In this situation, members of the "curative" care team are the primary caretakers and the palliative care team is consultative, addressing psychosocial issues and maintaining the treatment team's focus on the effective amelioration of symptoms and side effects. Uniquely, patients in the intensive care unit (ICU) are also eligible for supportive emotional and psychosocial care, with the understanding that all ventilator and pressor therapy will be discontinued within 24 hours if the patient is admitted to the palliative care service. This allows families losing children to acute illnesses or conditions to have some time to be reunited as a family and to say goodbye in a peaceful and humane setting. ICU patients usually have only a short course of palliation, mostly for respiratory symptoms.

Very little information is available concerning symptomatic treatment of children with terminal illness. What exists is rarely supported by controlled research trials in pediatric populations. Most literature documents personal practice, usually derived from adult palliative care experience. The research-supported information on symptom control for pediatric patients is primarily based on treatment during acute care, such as antiemetic therapy during antineoplastic regimens. This information may not necessarily apply to the hospice patient. Further research is needed to determine the best approaches to symptom management in the palliative care setting.

Feeding and Gastrointestinal Symptoms

Swallowing dysfunction

For the patient with a slowly progressive neurodegenerative disorder or a static CNS injury who cannot swallow effectively, but who can still experience hunger, feeding is indicated. One paper focusing on the ongoing care of children with static encephalopathies suggests that feeding without aspiration may be encouraged by positioning the patient 30 degrees reclined with the neck flexed.[3] Circumventing aspiration risk by percutaneously placed gastrostomy may be a preferable option, particularly if the patient does not seem to derive pleasure from eating. The care of patients unable to experience hunger, including most anencephalic patients, does not require feeding.[4] Even with the knowledge of the lack of hunger or suffering, and of the very real risk of aspiration pneumonitis, however, the family may prefer to feed the child. Ice chips and moistened swabs can be of benefit, particularly in the final phases of the illness.

Mouth discomfort

Oral candidiasis, aphthous ulcers, herpes, and other oral infections afflict terminally ill, debilitated children. Patients with AIDS have a differential diagnosis that also includes cytomegalovirus (CMV) and tuberculosis (TB). The diagnosis dictates therapy.

Candida is a particularly common infection among immunologically compromised patients and is present in 60% of symptomatic children with HIV.[5] Symptoms associated with oral candidiasis can include alteration of taste, pain and inflammation in the mouth, and bleeding during oral hygiene.[6] Candida infection in the oropharynx can have four manifestations: pseudomembranous, with plaques overlying reddened, friable mucosa; atrophic, associated with loss of tongue papillae; chronic hyperplastic, with erythematous and white plaques in a symmetric distribution; and angular cheilitis, with fissuring and erythema at the angle of the mouth.[5] For mild to moderate candidal infections, four treatments daily, consisting of clotrimazole troches (which can be put in a pacifier) or nystatin 200,000–500,000 U painted on the buccal mucosa and then swallowed, are indicated. Candida esophagitis is associated with dysphagia, retrosternal chest pain (which may manifest as arching in infants and young children), and, in some cases, a feeling of obstruction after swallowing.[6] Ketoconazole (5–10 mg/kg/day as a single dose) or fluconazole (3–6 mg/kg/day orally as a single dose) are indicated for more invasive or intractable cases.[7]

Oral herpes is treated with acyclovir, 250–500 mg/m² orally or intravenously every 8 hr[5] to shorten the symptomatic course. Recurrences can be frequent; chronic acyclovir therapy may be required in some patients.[7] Foscarnet has been used for acyclovir-resistant cases, in a dose of 40 mg/kg intravenously once daily, despite little pediatric experience with this drug.[7]

Aphthous ulcers may be treated with topical steroids (0.1% dexamethasone). Systemic steroids (prednisone, 2–5 mg/kg/day orally) may be used if the condition is severe.[8]

For mouth pain, palliative anesthetic treatments often include idiosyncratic mixtures combining diphenhydramine, magnesium oxide, lidocaine, or sucralfate. Caution is required in administering viscous lidocaine as an anesthetic because toxic doses are rapidly reached in the pediatric population; the maximum recommended dosage is 3 mg/kg/day.[9] Severe mouth pain should be treated with systemic opioids.[10,11]

Anorexia

Anorexia in children may arise due to mouth discomfort, nausea, inability to swallow effectively, constipation, unrelieved pain, advanced disease, depression, or irreversible CNS dysfunction. The approach in children is the same as for adults. Correctable problems should be treated, if appropriate. In the terminal phase, anticipatory counseling for the child and family regarding end-stage anorexia should be offered while providing small amounts of attractively presented favorite foods (regardless of nutritional "wholesomeness"). In primary anorexia preceding the terminal phase, some clinicians use the same medications administered to adult patients with AIDS-associated wasting, despite the lack of substantiating studies. Theses medications include corticosteroids, anabolic steroids, cyproheptadine, and antidepressants in selected instances. Other than the anabolic steroids, these drugs have been used widely and safely in children for other indications, and an increase in appetite has routinely been observed.

Nausea and vomiting

As with the adult population, the etiology of nausea and vomiting must be determined for effective treatment. A thorough review of sites and mechanisms of action of various classes of antiemetic agents is available, and guides the rational use of combination drug approaches.[12]

Ondansetron, a highly selective serotonin antagonist, is extremely effective for the treatment of chemotherapy-induced nausea.[13] Experience suggests that it is less effective in the absence of chemotherapy.[10] Controlled studies of the use of antiemetics in the pediatric population in the absence of chemotherapy are lacking, but some practitioners recommend a phenothiazine, lorazepam, or a corticosteroid such as dexamethasone in selected cases.[10]

In the case of vomiting caused by severe constipation, a bowel cleansing regimen is needed (see following section). Partial mechanical obstruction caused by tumor or adhesions, or as seen in cystic fibrosis, may be treated with cisapride, a prokinetic drug lacking specific antiemetic action.[14] The pediatric dosage is 0.2–0.3 mg/kg/dose, taken 15 minutes before eating three or four times daily. The dosage should be reduced in the presence of diarrhea. Cisapride may also be effective for gastrointestinal reflux, frequently found in the severely mentally retarded patient.[15]

Prolonged nausea and vomiting are not often caused by opioids, though they may occur during the first few days of therapy. When persistent, the best strategy is to change drugs, as individuals often respond with different side effect profiles to different opioids.[16] Failing this, it may be helpful to add an anxiolytic or antiemetic, such as lorazepam[10] or haloperidol.[11]

Nausea and vomiting can also be caused by metabolic disturbances such as hypercalcemia and uremia. One pediatric practitioner recommends the use of phenothiazines and serotonin antagonists for children with this origin of symptoms.[17] Other metabolic causes in pediatric patients are the relatively rare organic acidemias, aminoacidopathies, hyperammonemias, and MELAS syndrome.[18] There are no specific treatment recommendations for these etiologies.

Intracranial pathology is common among pediatric patients. Twenty-five percent of children with cancer have brain tumors; success in treating these malignancies has, so far, been disappointing. Most of these children will qualify to be hospice patients, by any criteria. Nausea accompanying brain tumors is most often treated with a corticosteroid such as dexamethasone. One practitioner avoids this drug in progressive brain tumors, because of its propensity to cause mood swings and excessive weight gain, and suggests an H_1 antihistamine, cyclizine, in this situation.[17] External beam radiation can be considered for single intracranial lesions as well,[10] though this therapy may be inconvenient and inappropriate for many patients in the final phase of the illness.

Constipation

Constipation can have a variety of causes in the pediatric setting. The most common in the healthy population is functional. However, immobility, severe retardation, smooth muscle dysfunction as seen in muscular dystrophy,[19] myelomeningocoele, pseudo-obstruction syndromes, and other neuronal dysplasias, congenital or acquired anal stenosis or stricture, or medication and metabolic effects may each cause constipation.

Treatment of constipation in the absence of reversible metabolic disturbances consists primarily of lubricants, softeners, and bulking agents, as well as laxatives, if needed. Suppositories and enemas are often not accepted well by the pediatric patient. In addition, many enemas are toxic to small children. Tap water enemas have resulted in severe hyponatremia, seizures, and death. Hypertonic phosphate enemas have caused hyperphosphatemia and numerous other electrolyte imbalances. Soapsuds enemas can result in bowel necrosis, perforation, and death.[20]

One group of pediatric gastroenterologists suggests aggressive oral administration of mineral oil (15–30 ml/age (yr)/day, up to 240 cc/day) to evacuate an impaction.[21] They claim 98% success in 3–4 days and no problems with fat-soluble vitamins even with maintenance therapy (15 ml × age (yr); max 90 ml qhs). However, caregivers are cautioned not to use this regimen in infants or neurologically impaired patients due to the risk of aspiration. Some patients benefit from disimpaction using a balanced polyethylene glycol-electrolyte solution (Go-Lytely). The correct dose results in discharge of clear fluid from the anus, usually 14–40 cc/kg/hr and in one series of children > 12 yr old, an average of 12 L over 23 hr.[78] Metoclopramide 5–10 mg is recommended for the accompanying nausea 15 minutes prior to lavage.[22] Other regimens for disimpaction include judicious use of hypertonic phosphate enemas (30 cc/5 kg body wt to maximum volume of

135 cc for children > 20 kg; maximum dose $= 2$ enemas or hyperosmolar milk-of-molasses [1:1 milk and molasses] given orally or by nasogastric tube until the child indicates discomfort [usual dose is 200–600 cc].[20] The dose may be repeated.

Once disimpaction is accomplished (if necessary), maintenance therapy may consist of increased fluid and dietary fiber intake, mineral oil as above, and/or laxatives. Laxatives will probably be needed if the patient is taking large opioid doses. Suggested starting doses are shown in Table 3.1.[22]

Treatment with osmotic laxatives (e.g., milk of magnesia, mineral oil, phosphate enemas) is rarely successful with neuromuscular causes of constipation, such as myelomeningocoele and muscular dystrophies, as they increase fecal incontinence. Increased fiber intake, daily doses of senna, and routine daily stimulation to defecate with suppositories, enemas, or manual stimulation are effective in these conditions.[20]

Table 3.1 Suggested pediatric constipation protocol

Medication	Starting Dosage[†]	Frequency	Comments/ Side effects
Malt soup extract (maltsupex)	*Breast-fed infants*: 5–10 cc in juice or water *Bottle-fed infants*: 7.5–30 cc/day	*Breast-fed infants*: twice daily *Bottle fed infants*: divided in alternating feeds	
Docusate	*<3 yr*: 10 mg *3–6 yr*: 20–60 mg *>6 yr*: 40–150 mg	*<3 yr*: up to 4 times daily *3–6 yr*: divided into as many as 4 doses daily *>6 yr*: divided into as many as 4 doses daily	
Milk of magnesia	1–3 cc/kg	Once or twice daily	*>6 mo old children*: larger dose for hard stools
Lactulose° (10 g/15 cc) or Sorbitol 70%	1–2 cc/kg	Once or twice daily	*>6 mo old children*: cramping, flatulence
Senna syrup	*1–5 yr*: 5 cc *5–15 yr*: 10 cc	Once or twice daily	

°Lactulose is very expensive but is associated with fewer side effects than senna extracts in one report describing the comparative use in children.[23]

†These are starting dosages only. Titrate to effect. More will be needed with decreasing mobility or increasing opioid dosage.

Diarrhea

Chronic diarrhea is a common problem in patients with severe immunodeficiencies,[24] including AIDS. In one survey, diarrhea occurred in 31% of long-term survivors and 50% of short-term survivors (<5 years) of perinatally acquired HIV.[25] In a study of infants in Zaire, diarrheal illness accounted for up to 50% of deaths in a 6-month follow-up of infants with perinatally acquired HIV.[26]

Diarrhea may be due to pathologic infection with normal flora, common pathogens, opportunistic infection, or HIV enteropathy. The principal causes of chronic diarrhea in AIDS patients are protozoans in the genus *Coccidia*, particularly *Cryptosporidium*. Another cause of protozoal diarrhea in children is infection with *Isospora belli*, which is treated with trimethoprim-sulfamethoxsazole (10 mg TMP–50 mg SMX/kg/day divided into 4 doses for 10 days, followed by half that dose divided into 2 doses for at least 3 weeks).[7] Other causes in this patient population include other parasites (*Giardia lamblia*, *Entamoeba histolytica*); bacteria including *Salmonella* and *Mycobacterium avium intracellulare* (*MAIC*); viruses, including CMV and HIV, which may lead to a chronic, untreatable course; and fungi, particularly *Candida albicans*.[27]

HIV enteropathy may take the form of villus atrophy due to immune-mediated enteropathy or necrotizing enterocolitis. It may mimic other better-known gastrointestinal pathologic processes.[24] One group at Schneider Children's Hospital reported four infants in whom a regimen of oral gentamicin (50 mg/kg/day divided in 6 doses for 3 days) and cholestyramine (1 g orally every 6 hr for 5 days) resulted in a decrease of stool frequency from 10–15 per day to 8–12 per day, with a concomitant increase in stool bulk.[28]

Respiratory Symptoms

Chronic progressive respiratory failure

In muscular dystrophy and some metabolic disorders, such as mucopolysaccharidosis, progressive respiratory failure may occur in the weeks and months prior to death. Weakness leading to respiratory compromise can be exacerbated by skeletal abnormalities such as profound scoliosis, which may be related to the underlying disorder. Symptoms of respiratory failure include irritability, fear of sleep, daytime somnolence, morning headaches, palpitations, and nausea. In some instances, ventilatory support such as continuous positive airway pressure, bipap, or mechanical ventilation (portable negative pressure ventilation such as a curaiss, or positive pressure ventilation) may be employed.[19] In many instances, the child is capable of deciding which is the correct course to take, and should be consulted unless intellectual capacity prevents it.

As with other forms of respiratory distress, opioids and benzodiazepines are beneficial in managing the distressing symptom of dyspnea.

Cough

The literature regarding cough in children primarily addresses the overuse of over-the-counter drugs in the treatment of cough related to viral upper respiratory tract illness. One paper comparing the efficacy of placebo vs dextromethorphan and codeine for acute cough suppression in children age 18 months to 12 years concluded that the two drugs were not effective,[29] but the study was flawed by the subjective scoring system used for cough severity. Other sources cite codeine and hydrocodone as efficacious for non-productive and irritative cough.[12]

The differential diagnosis in the child with a chronic cough has been reviewed.[30–31] While not specifically addressing terminally ill patients, the paper provides a good review of potentially reversible etiologies of chronic cough in children, some of which apply to the palliative care population. These include reactive airways disease (RAD, often seen in recurrent aspiration), gastrointestinal reflux, anatomical aberrations including tracheoesophageal fistulae, laryngotracheomalacia, heart failure, cystic fibrosis, and recurrent pneumonia (particularly in association with immunodeficiencies). These papers also cite adult literature to recommend codeine, dextromethorphan, and diphenhydramine to suppress irritative cough. By extrapolation, these medications may also provide benefit for children in whom a potentially reversible etiology of cough is found, but in whom, given the patient's overall condition, correction of the underlying problem is not appropriate. Other authors[17] suggest the use of opioids and nebulized local anesthetics, again based on work in adults.[32,33] Bronchodilators and steroids may be useful for RAD.

Secretion control and death rattle

Severe neurologic disability often impairs the ability to swallow saliva. This leads to the uncomfortable sensation of choking in addition to cosmetically unappealing drooling. Anticholinergic medications are most frequently employed to combat these problems. One English group preferred hyoscine patches, placed behind the ear and changed every three days, or benztropine 0.25 mg twice daily orally, increasing to a maximum of 1.5 mg twice daily based on response.[34] No patient weight guidelines were recommended. Practitioners at Helen House also use hyoscine for this purpose, but caution that, in their experience, prolonged use often results in paralytic ileus.[1] Others similarly endorse the use of hyoscine or scopolamine, given as a patch or subcutaneously.[17] If the onset of effects is too slow with transdermal dosing, atropine and hyoscine may be given intravenously or subcutaneously, 0.1–0.5 mg every 15 minutes, for rapid control.[35] Benztropine, 1–6 mg/day orally or intravenously, is also effective for treatment of drooling.[36]

Unlike some other transdermal delivery systems, the scopolamine patch, when available, can be cut to provide the appropriate dose. Whole patches deliver 0.5 mg/day. Access to the scopolamine patches has been limited in the United States recently, however, due to problems with the adhesive. Our approach, based on standard pediatric drug formularies,[37–38] has been to use atropine, 0.01 mg/kg/dose subcutaneously or orally, or hyoscyamine, 0.06125–0.250 mg orally, up to every 4 hr, or amitriptyline, starting at 0.1 mg/kg orally or (rarely) intramuscularly.

Pneumonia and other infections

Pneumonia, "the old man's friend," is often the terminally ill child's friend as well. If the child is not expected to return to his or her baseline status after recovery from pneumonia, or if the child's baseline status is unacceptable to the child or appropriate surrogate (usually the parents), then symptomatic care alone may be the most appropriate course. This may consist of oxygen,[10] bronchodilators, and possibly morphine[10,17,33,35,37,38] or sedation to alleviate dyspnea. There are, however, no research reports supporting the efficacy of these interventions in children. Additionally, in the case of cystic fibrosis, Rh deoxyribonuclease is currently thought to be inappropriate in the terminal phase, as a recent review reports a lack of efficacy in patients with forced vital capacity (FVC) of 40% or less.[39]

In the experience of the Butterfly Program, it may take time for the family to be able to forgo curative therapy for pneumonia, particularly in the setting of chronic illness associated with recurrent pneumonias which have been treated in the past with the goal of cure. In addition, "curative" therapy may be employed until the end of life for the patient with end-stage cystic fibrosis, in the hopes of receiving a lung transplant.[40]

While pursuing these goals, compassionate care would dictate ascertaining the possibility of, and discussing how to handle, death. For some patients, curative interventions may have been undertaken against the better judgment of the parents, who may have been threatened with charges of medical neglect or who had never before been offered the option of palliation only. In addition, some families have been destroyed by the relentless deterioration of the patient; for others, letting the child die may represent the loss of the raison d-être for the caretaker. These psychosocial "symptoms" within the family framework need to be acknowledged and addressed.

Dyspnea

Dyspnea frequently occurs among dying children.[1] However, only anecdotal reports are available regarding the treatment of dyspnea in children. Empiric treatments are largely based on experience with and research on adult patients.[32,33,41–45]

Simple practical measures may be efficacious. Whatever the etiology of the dyspnea, elevating the head of the bed (or assisting the child to sit up), a fan, and the confidence of the medical team are beneficial. Guided imagery may also help.

Specific etiologies of the dyspnea must be considered, as some may be amenable to treatment. These include pleural effusions, anemia, abdominal distention from ascites or swallowed air, chest wall pain, and superior vena cava obstruction. Childhood cancers that cause chest metastases and/or malignant pleural effusions are osteogenic sarcoma, Ewing's sarcoma, Wilms' tumor, and neuroblastoma.[35] Palliative transfusions can be very effective in prolonged alleviation of anemia-related dyspnea. Drainage of ascites or use of diuretics usually provides only brief relief. Supplemental oxygen is rarely of benefit to the patient in the active phase of dying.

Many of the children served in the Butterfly Program are ventilator-dependent. These include newborns with hypoplastic left heart syndrome or hypoplastic lungs, and children of any age with multisystem organ dysfunction based on sepsis syndrome or other etiologies.

Morphine is routinely available for treatment of dyspnea, but has rarely been needed. Indications for use include tachypnea accompanied by facial expressions of discomfort or use of accessory muscles of respiration, as well as family assessment of patient discomfort. Some patients have required extremely large doses of morphine for the treatment of dyspnea. One 10 kg, 2-year-old girl with AIDS and related encephalopathy had evidence of pain (facial grimace and bruxism) and profound dyspnea. Her clinical diagnosis was sepsis and possibly pneumonia. She was started on 0.1 mg/kg of morphine intravenously per dose, and was rapidly titrated to symptom abatement, doubling the dose every 15 minutes until relief of pain and dyspnea were noted. The final regimen was 60 mg (6 mg/kg) of morphine every 30 minutes (the interval was determined by symptom recurrence). This case illustrates the fact that high-dose morphine, when given to alleviate symptoms, is not lethal, even in children.

Central Nervous System Symptoms

Sleep disturbances

Sleep disturbance is a frequent occurrence in early childhood, even in the absence of medical illness.[45–46] Medical illness causes increased anxiety, lapses in normal schedules, and sometimes suspension of the usual house rules.[46] Most of these problems are best treated with behavioral interventions, emotional support, and security.[10,47,49,50] However, inadequately treated pain may precipitate sleep disturbances[46] and some illnesses themselves, particularly metabolic and neurodegenerative disorders, can produce sleep disturbance.[49,50] For these problems, adjunctive pharmacologic intervention is warranted.

In neuronal ceroid lipofuscinoses, disorders resulting in low cerebrospinal fluid gamma amino butyric acid (GABA) levels, sleep disturbance is often the presenting symptom. Some authors[49] recommend GABAergic drugs such as baclofen (15–25 mg/day, increasing to as much as 200 mg/day) and/or tizanidine (1–9 mg/day, increasing to 20–60 mg/day). In severe cases, these authors use intrathecal baclofen. Alternatively, benzodiazepines may be effective.

Chloral hydrate has been used liberally in some cases.[34] It has a slow onset of action and a short half-life. Tolerance is reported to develop within five weeks. Diphenhydramine is also commonly used to facilitate sleep. Tricyclic antidepressants, benzodiazepines, and phenothiazines are useful, but tolerance is a problem, at least for benzodiazepines and tricyclic antidepressants, and rebound insomnia is also a significant problem.[45,51,52] Paradoxical stimulation can occur in children with use of benzodiazepines and, with chronic dosing, there is concern regarding cognitive deficits, particularly in visuospatial and learning abilities.[51]

Clonidine, an alpha$_2$ presynaptic receptor agonist that inhibits the release of norepinephrine into the synaptic space, is useful in the treatment of attention-deficit hyperactivity disorder (ADHD). A beneficial side effect, in some cases, is somnolence. This drug effect can combat the insomnia associated with psychostimulants.[53] It may also prove effective in the treatment of patients with insomnia caused by other etiologies, including neurodegenerative processes.

Mood disturbances (anxiety, aggression, and depression)

Much anxiety can be alleviated by providing support and companionship to the child, and particularly by allowing parents and siblings to have unfettered access. The child may also have developmentally appropriate irrational fears that, once discovered and talked through, will disappear. For example, children often fear "irrationally" that a parent may precede the ill child in death. Also, children may often fret about how their family will cope with their death.[53] Such issues can often be readily handled if at least one adult can allow the child to express his or her concerns.

In general, pharmacologic management of anxiety in children has been hampered by diagnostic ambiguities.[36] When pharmacologic treatment of anxiety is necessary, benzodiazepines, including oral diazepam or intravenous or subcutaneous midazolam, are most often used.[17] If the benzodiazepines are not successful, haloperidol or methotrimeprazine may be substituted; if they are moderately successful but insufficient, haloperidol or methotrimeprazine may be added. These agents are compatible with morphine and can be given subcutaneously.

Aggression and hyperactivity, as seen in the progressive metabolic and neurodegenerative disorders, are treated by creating a safe environment that reduces both the likelihood of injury and parental anxiety. When drug therapy is called for, the English palliative care experience supports the use of haloperidol (0.25 mg twice daily, slowly increasing to up to 10 mg/day) or thioridazine (2.5

mg/kg/day). A very thorough, scientifically based, recent review of pediatric psychopharmacology also supports the use of neuroleptics, particularly in mentally retarded and autistic children as well as in the conduct-disordered child, but cautions that aggressive behavior has been poorly defined by clinical scientists.[36] It is also of concern that 30%–40% of mentally retarded people have tardive dyskinesias related to prolonged neuroleptic treatment.[55,56]

Some limited data support the use of fenfluramine, a serotonin reuptake inhibitor used as an anorexiant, to manage hyperactivity and aggression in retarded children. Methylphenidate is also useful in aggressive behaviors, particularly in association with hyperactivity. Other agents for which there is only limited information in children with aggressive behaviors, independent of underlying medical illness, include lithium (target blood levels 0.32–1.51 mEq/L), propranolol (dose range 50–300 mg/kg/day), and carbamazepine.[36] Propranolol has been shown to be efficacious in a small double-blind crossover study of 10 patients (ages not specified),[57] as well as in at least 14 other less well-controlled studies. Carbamazepine for this indication is dosed as it would be for seizure management.[36,57,58] Hyperactivity alone can be managed with desipramine (up to 5 mg/kg/day; adolescent maximum is 100 mg) or clonidine.[36]

There is limited information regarding the pharmacologic treatment of depression in prepubertal children. There are no double-blind, controlled studies documenting the efficacy of tricyclic antidepressants in this population, though they are commonly used in clinical practice. A recent article documents the safety and effectiveness of amitriptyline in intravenous form for eight children, two of whom received it for depression.[59] Though sleep and neuropathic pain were improved, it is not clear that depression was improved. Lithium or monoamine oxidase inhibitors may help nonresponders.[36] There is a case report of the successful use of methylphenidate as an antidepressant in an adolescent with AIDS, in whom fatigue was a significant source of depression.[60]

Seizures

Seizures are often a long-standing problem for children affected by neurodegenerative disorders. These children can usually continue their routine anticonvulsant therapy. However, as the terminal phase approaches, seizure control may become more challenging. Most patients respond to diazepam. In the experience of Helen House, children with either late infantile Batten disease or subacute sclerosing panencephalitis have seizures which are particularly difficult to control, and may require paraldehyde (no longer available in the United States).[50]

Seizures may also arise from more subacute metabolic disturbances, such as sodium, calcium, and magnesium imbalances. Depending on the status of the child and preferences of the family, correction may be indicated. If not, anticonvulsants such as phenytoin, phenobarbital, lorazepam, or carbamazepine can be used as needed.

Increased intracranial pressure

Increased intracranial pressure (ICP) is usually caused by primary or metastatic brain tumors. It may also be caused by progressive hydrocephalus, as can be seen in children[59] born prematurely who suffered intraventricular hemorrhages or meningitis in the neonatal period. While most groups advocate the use of dexamethasone for tumor–related increased ICP, similar to the adult setting,[10,61] one practitioner avoids this drug because of the disfigurement associated with prolonged use and the mood swings it can cause.[17] Single metastatic neoplastic brain lesions may respond to external beam radiation. The decision to use radiation therapy may be difficult in the palliative care setting because it involves travel to the hospital, with a significant associated expense, as well as a delayed onset of clinical benefit.

Spasticity

Painful muscle spasms as well as movement disorders occur in a significant number of children with neurodegenerative disorders.[1] Hunt and Burne report an incidence of more than one in three at Helen House.[50] Spasticity can accompany brain tumors, is well known in cerebral palsy and other brain injuries, and is seen in AIDS–related encephalopathy. Diazepam and baclofen are first-line treatments. Baclofen, a GABA-B agonist, works by presynaptic inhibition of 1a and 1b afferents and has relatively poor CNS penetration. It has a short half-life (2–4 hr), but is effective for flexor spasms and clonus.[62,63] Side effects include fatigue, muscle weakness, somnolence, GI distress, dizziness, incoordination, imbalance, and bladder dysfunction. Tolerance builds to these adverse effects if the dose is slowly titrated up. Benzodiazepines facilitate GABA-mediated alpha motor neuron function and also produce the adverse effects of sedation, imbalance, incoordination, and muscle weakness. A recent review of benzodiazepines indicates that their prolonged use may induce tolerance to the muscle relaxant effect of these agents.[51] Another source[12] reiterates this point and notes that tolerance to the relaxant properties of baclofen also occurs. Clonidine is undergoing trials as an antispasmodic for spinal cord injuries. Dantrolene sodium has also proven useful in treating spasticity; it acts by dissociating muscular excitation contraction. Weakness is an obvious side effect. This drug is most often used when the patient does not respond to baclofen or benzodiazepines.[62] Dantrolene is associated with drowsiness, fatigue, malaise, diarrhea, and potential hepatic toxicity. Newer drugs being tested include gabapentin and tizanidine. The latter appears to have antinociceptive properties as well,[59] but has only been tested in adults with spinal cord injuries, strokes, and multiple sclerosis.[66] Chemical or surgical treatment of spasticity (e.g., posterior rhizotomy) may be indicated in patients with a prognosis for a long survival. Injection of botulinum toxin may also be useful.[62,63] Continuous intrathecal baclofen may be an attractive alternative for these patients.[67,68] Another modality recently reported to be useful is neuromuscular electrical stimulation (NMES).[69,70]

Somnolence associated with opioid therapy

Few studies address the use of psychostimulants for opioid–associated somnolence in the pediatric age group. Two citations were found on an intensive literature search. One was a case study in which methylphenidate was found to be an effective treatment.[71] The other was a retrospective review of 11 patients, aged 12 to 20 years, who had inadequate pain relief on opioid dosages that induced excessive somnolence. Regimens of methylphenidate or dextroamphetamine were used, with improvement noted in five patients. Adverse effects were mild and in no case required cessation of the psychostimulant.[72] No attempt was made to determine any synergistic antinociceptive effects that these agents might provide.

Despite the lack of randomized, controlled studies to assess the efficacy of psychostimulants in children, there is extensive experience with these agents in the pediatric population. Methylphenidate has been shown to produce increased concentration in children, adolescents, and adults with attention-deficit disorder, as well as in normal populations.[73] It has also been used in narcolepsy, with limited experience in children.[48] Additional benefits of methylphenidate include antidepressive and antifatigue effects,[60] as well as a reported improvement of attention, language skills, memory, behavior, and academic achievement in patients who have received cranial irradiation with or without intrathecal chemotherapy for the treatment of brain tumors or acute lymphocytic leukemia.[74]

The adverse effects in the terminally ill population include the well-known anorexic effects. There are also scattered reports of rare drug interactions, including an increased incidence of tics when given in combination with thioridazine[75] and severe cognitive and mood deterioration when given in combination with imipramine.[76]

Miscellaneous Systems

Bleeding

Bleeding is distressing to both child and family.[61] Infiltration of the bone marrow by the more common malignancies of childhood puts the pediatric patient with oncologic disease at particular risk for bleeding. One approach is to counsel the child and family about this possibility, and to do everything to prevent it. Scheduled platelet transfusions are probably unreasonable (except perhaps in promyelocytic leukemia), but transfusions for clinical bleeding can be appropriate. Localized mucosal bleeding can sometimes be controlled by topical thrombin or tranexamic acid (available as a tablet or a mouthwash).[17,61]

Bleeding may also be caused by conditions leading to liver failure. Supplemental vitamin K can be beneficial, and fresh-frozen plasma may help if clinical bleeding occurs. Patients with cirrhosis may bleed from esophageal varices. Sclerosing may be indicated, depending on the status and preferences of the child and family.[17]

Skin breakdown

Skin problems are common in chronically ill children who progress to the terminal phase and develop malnutrition, sensory loss, and immobility. Appropriate bed coverings such as sheepskin, "bunny boots," and elbow covers help to prevent bedsores. Smaller children rarely benefit from expensive inflator beds; gel mattresses, "egg-crate" mattresses, and frequent turning can benefit immobile patients. Topical antibiotics may be indicated if skin breakdown occurs.[10]

Diaper dermatitis may also occur and is often severe in AIDS patients. The most common causes are Candida or chemical irritation from urine or frequent soiling. Antifungal ointments are helpful for fungal infections. In the author's own practice, chemical dermatitis is treated with keeping the diaper off as much as possible, using a heat lamp for 20 minutes every 4 hours, and, in the case of diarrhea-associated skin breakdown, using 10%–20% cholestyramine in aquaphor with each diaper change. This regimen has produced dramatic changes, even in severe cases. One author suggests Critic Aid by Sween for severely denuded skin.[77]

Itching

Itching can be associated with opioid therapy, skin afflictions, neuropathic injury, and dry skin. It is frequently treated with emollients and antihistamines such as hydroxyzine and diphenhydramine. Colloidal oatmeal baths can be effective. For neuropathic injury manifesting as itching, the usual regimens for neuropathic pain are used, including anticonvulsants and antidepressants. Itching associated with opioid therapy may necessitate switching to a different drug or, in the case of epidural opioids, the addition of low-dose naloxone.

Itching is also associated with jaundice and cholestasis, as may be seen in biliary atresia. Cholestyramine may be helpful in such cases. One author also has used rifampicin and ursodeoxycholic acid.[17]

Conclusion

In summary, there has been little research about the management of symptoms in children with terminal conditions. Even the definition of who these children are is a matter of contention.

Much work remains to be done to ensure that pediatric patients with terminal conditions receive sound, research-based therapy. The only way to accomplish this, given the relatively small number of patients as well as the diversity of ailments that afflict them, is to form collaborative research networks, such as has been done in pediatric oncology. Only then can we fulfill our mission to offer to children and their families relief from the suffering associated with life-threatening conditions.

References

1. Hunt AM. A survey of signs, symptoms and symptom control in 30 terminally ill children. *Dev Med Child Neurol* 1990; 32:347–355.
2. Davies B. Assessment of need for a children's hospice program. *Death Stud* 1996; 20:2347–2348.
3. Larnert G, Ekberg O. Positioning improves the oral and pharyngeal swallowing function in children with cerebral palsy. *Acta Paediatr* 1995; 84(6):689–692.
4. Nelson LJ, Rushton CH, Cranford RE, et al. Forgoing medically provided nutrition and hydration in pediatric patients. *J Law, Med Ethics* 1995; 23:33–46.
5. Prose NS. Mucocutaneous disease in pediatric human immunodeficiency virus. *Pediatr Clin North Am* 1991; 38(4):977–990.
6. Garber GE. Treatment of oral Candida infections. *Drugs* 1994; 47(5):734–740.
7. Brady MT. Treatment of human immunodeficiency virus infection and its associated complications in children. *J Clin Pharmacol* 1994; 34:17–29.
8. de Asis ML, Bernstein LJ, Scliozberg J. Treatment of resistant aphthous ulcers in children with acquired immunodeficiency syndrome. *J Pediatr* 1995; 127(4):663–665.
9. AIDS: The ultimate challenge for symptom management. *Syllabus for the Academy of Hospice Physicians Meeting.* American Academy of Hospice Physicians, Toronto, Ontario, 1996.
10. Miser JS, Miser AW. Pain and symptom control. In: Armstrong-Dailey A, Goltzer SZ, eds. *Hospice Care for Children.* New York: Oxford University Press, 1993:23–59.
11. Mackie AM, Coda BC, Hill HF. Adolescents use patient controlled analgesia effectively for relief from prolonged oropharyngeal mucositis pain. *Pain* 1991; 46:265–269.
12. Bennett DR, ed. *Drug Evaluations Annual 1995.* Chicago, Ill.: American Medical Association, 1995.
13. Plosker FL, Milne RJ. Ondansetron: A pharmacoeconomic and quality of life evaluation of its antiemetic activity in patients receiving anti-cancer therapy. *PharmacoEconomics* 1992; 2(4):285–304.
14. Barone JA, Jessen LM, Colaizzi JL, Bierman RH. Cisapride: A gastrointestinal prokinetic drug. *Ann Pharmacother* 1994; 28(4):488–500.
15. Staiano A, del Guidice E, Simeone D, et al. Cisapride in neurologically impaired children with chronic constipation. *Dig Dis Sci* 1996; 41(5):870–874.
16. Hanks G, Cherney N. Opioid analgesic therapy. In: Doyle D, Hanks GWC, MacDonald N, eds. *Oxford Textbook of Palliative Medicine.* 2nd ed. New York: Oxford University Press, 1998:331–355.

17. Goldman A, Byrne R. Symptom management. In Goldman A, ed. *Care of the Dying Child.* New York: Oxford University Press, 1994:52–75.

18. Gordon N. Recurrent vomiting in childhood, especially of neurologic origin. *Dev Med Child Neurol* 1994; 36(5):463–470.

19. Hilton T, Orr RD, Perkin RM, Ashwal S. End of life care in Duchenne muscular dystrophy. *Pediatr Neurol* 1993; 9(3):165–177.

20. Loening-Baucke V. Encopresis and soiling. *Pediatr Clin North Am Gastroenterology I.* 1996; 43(1):279–298.

21. Seth R, Heyman MB. Management of constipation and encopresis in infants and children. *Pediatr Gastroenterol* 1994; 23(4):621–636.

22. Loening-Bauke V. Chronic constipation in children. *Gastroenterol* 1993; 105:1557–1564.

23. Perkin JM. Constipation in childhood: A controlled comparison between lactulose and standardized senna. *Curr Med Res Opin* 1977; 4:540–543.

24. McLoughlin LC, Nord, KS, Joshi VV, Oleske JM, Connor EM. Severe gastrointestinal involvement in children with the acquired immunodeficiency syndrome. *J Pediatr Gastroenterol Nutr* 1987; 6:517–524.

25. Features of children perinatally infected with HIV surviving longer than five years. *Italian Register for HIV Infection in Children. Lancet* 1994; 343(8891):191–195.

26. Keusch GT, Thea DM, Kamenga M, Kakanda K, Mbalaa M, Brown C, Davachi F. Persistent diarrhea associated with AIDS. *Acta Paediatr Suppl* 1992; 381:45–48.

27. Arbo A, Santos JI. Diarrheal diseases in the immunocompromised host. *Pediatr Infect Dis J* 1987; 6:894–906.

28. Shapiro WL, Kain ZN. Diarrhea in infants with AIDS. *N Engl J Med* 1988; 319(8):517–518.

29. Taylor JA, Novack AH, Almquist JR, Rogers JE. Efficacy of cough suppressants in children. *J Pediatr* 1993; 122:799–802.

30. Hatch RT, Carpenter GB Smith LJ. Treatment options in the child with a chronic cough. *Drugs* 1993; 45(3):367–373.

31. Leung AKC, Robson WLM Tay-Uyboco J. Chronic cough in children. *Can Fam Physician* 1994; 40:531–537.

32. Cowcher K, Hanks G. Long-term management of respiratory symptoms in advanced cancer. *J Pain Symptom Manage* 1990; 5(5):320–330.

33. Bruera E, Macmillan K, Pither J, MacDonald RN. Effects of morphine on the dyspnea of terminal cancer patients. *J Pain Symptom Manage* 1990; 5(6):341–344.

34. Cleary MA, Wraith JE. Management of mucopolysaccharidosis type III. *Arch Dis Child* 1993; 69:403–406.

35. deVeber LL. Physiological differences between children and adults that affect physical findings and symptom development. In: Doyle D, Hanks GW, MacDonald N, eds. *Oxford Textbook of Palliative Medicine.* New York: Oxford University Press, 1993:694–695.

36. Gadow KD. Pediatric psychopharmacotherapy: A review of recent research. *J Child Psychol Psychiatry* 1992; 33(1):153–195.

37. Taketomo CK, Hodding JH, Kraus DM. *Pediatric Dosage Handbook.* 2nd ed. Hudson, OH: Lex-Comp, Inc., 1993–1994.

38. Binder RM, Howry LB. *Pediatric Drugs and Nursing Implications.* East Norwalk, Conn: Appleton and Lange, 1991.

39. Thompson AH. Human recombinant Dnase in cystic fibrosis. *Soc Med* 1995; 88(suppl 25):24–29.
40. Webb AK, David TJ. Clinical management of children and adults with cystic fibrosis. *BMJ* 1994; 308:459–462.
41. Ingeho KB, Heyman MD. Polyethylene glycol-electrolyte solution for intestinal clearance in children with refractory encopresis. *Am J Dis Child* 1988; 142:340–342.
42. Bruera E, Chadwick S, Brenneis C, Hanson J, MacDonald RN. Methylphenidate associated with narcotics for the treatment of cancer pain. *Cancer Treat Rep* 1987 70:67–70.
43. Bruera E, Brenneis, C, Paterson, AH, MacDonald RN. Use of methylphenidate as an adjuvant to narcotic analgesics in patients with advanced cancer. *J Pain Symptom Manage* 1989; 4(1):3–6.
44. Bruera E, Fainsinger R, MacEachern T, Hanson J. The use of methylphenidate in patients with incident cancer pain receiving regular opiates. A preliminary report. *Pain* 1992; 50:75–77.
45. Dahl RE. The pharmacologic treatment of sleep disorders. *Psychiatr Clin North Am* 1992; 15(1):161–178.
46. Horne J. Annotation: Sleep and its disorders in children. *J Child Psychol Psychiatry* 1992; 33(3):473–487.
47. Kerr S, Jowett S. Sleep problems in pre-school children: A review of the literature. *Child Care Health Dev* 1994; 20:379–391.
48. Mindell JA. Sleep disorders in children. *Health Pyschol* 1993; 12(2):151–162.
49. Santavuori P, Linnankivi T, Jaeken J, Vanhanen SL, Telakivi T, Heiskala H. Psychological symptoms and sleep disturbances in neuronal ceroid-lipofuscinoses (NCL). *J Inherit Metab Dis* 1993; 16:245–248.
50. Hunt A, Burne R. Medical and nursing problems of children with neurodegenerative disease. *Palliat Med* 1995; 9:19–26.
51. Ashton H. Guidelines for the rational use of benzodiazepines. *Drugs* 1994; 48(1):25–40.
52. Roth T, Roehrs TA. A review of the safety profiles of benzodiazepine hypnotics. *J Clin Psychiatry* 1991; 52(9 suppl):38–41.
53. Wilens TE, Biederman J, Spencer T. Clonidine for sleep disturbances associated with attention-deficit hyperactivity disorder. *J Am Acad Child Adolesc Psychiatry* 1994; 33(3):424–426.
54. Bluebond-Langner M. *Private Worlds of Dying Children*. Princeton, N.J.: Princeton University Press, 1978.
55. Gualtieri CT, Sprague RL, Cle JO. Tardive dyskinesia litigation and the dilemmas of neuroleptic treatment. *Psychiatry Law* 1986; 14:187–216.
56. Kalachnik JE, Harder SR, Kidd-Nielson P, Errickson E, Doebler M, Sprague RL. Persistent tardive dyskinesia in randomly assigned neuroleptic reduction, neuroleptic nonreduction and nonneuroleptic history groups: Preliminary results. *Psychopharmacol Bull* 1984; 20(1):27–32.
57. Sheard MH. Clinical pharmacology of aggressive behavior. *Clin Neuropharmacol* 1988; 11(6):483–492.
58. Campbell M, Gonzalez NM, Silva RR. The pharmacologic treatment of conduct disorders and rage outbursts. *Psychiatr Clin North Am* 1992; 15(1):69–85.

59. Collins JJ, Kerner J, Sentivany S, et al. Intravenous amitriptylene in pediatrics. *J Pain Symptom Manage* 1995; 10(6):471–475.
60. Walling VR, Pfefferbaum B. The use of methylphenidate in a depressed adolescent with AIDS. *Dev Behav Pediatr* 1990; 11(4):195–197.
61. Chambers EJ, Oakhill A, Cornish JM, Curnick S. Terminal care at home for children with cancer. *BMJ* 1989; 298(8):937–940.
62. Mitchell G. Update of multiple sclerosis therapy. *Med Clin North Am* 1993;77:231–249.
63. Andersson P-B, Goodkin DE. Current pharmacological treatment of multiple sclerosis symptoms. *West J Med* 1996; 165:313–317.
64. Cohen JA. Issues and challenges in the management of spasticity. In: Golanty SA, ed. *New Options for the Treatment of Spasticity*. Laguna Niguel, Calif.: Institute for Medical Studies, 1997:7–8.
65. Knobler RL. Conditions associated with painful muscle spasm. In: Golanty SA, ed. *New Options for the Treatment of Spasticity*. Laguna Niguel, Calif.: Institute for Medical Studies, 1997:14–16.
66. Jeffery DR. Patients with spinal cord injury and other neuromuscular disorders. In: Golanty SA, ed. *New Options for the Treatment of Spasticity*. Institute for Medical Studies, Laguna Niguel, Calif: 1997:12–13.
67. Albright AL, Cervi A, and Singletary J. Intrathecal baclofen for spasticity in cerebral palsy. *JAMA* 1991; 265(11):1418–1422.
68. Albright AL, Barron WB, Fasick P, Polinko P, Janosky J. Continuous intrathecal baclofen infusion for spasticity of cerebral origin. *JAMA* 1993; 270(20):2475–2477.
69. Carmack J. Clinical use of neuromuscular electrical stimulation for children with cerebral palsy. *Phys Ther* 1993; 73(8):505–527.
70. Zupan A, Gregoric M, Vandot S. Effects of electrical stimulation on muscles of children with Duchenne and Becker muscular dystrophy. *Neuropediatrics* 1993; 24:189–192.
71. McManus MJ, Panzarella C. The use of dextroamphetamine to counteract sedation for patients on a narcotic drip. *J Assoc Pediatr Oncol Nurs* 1986; 3:28–29.
72. Yee JD, Berde CB. Dextroamphetamine or methylphenidate as adjuvants to opioid analgesia for adolescents with cancer. *J Pain Symptom Manage* 1994; 9(2):122–125.
73. Peloquin LJ, Klorman R. Effects of methylphenidate on normal children's mood, event-related potentials and performance in memory scanning and vigilance. *J Abnorm Psychol* 1986; 95(1):88–98.
74. DeLong R, Friedman H, Friedman N, Gustafson K, Oakes J. Methylphenidate in neuropsychological sequelae of radiotherapy and chemotherapy of childhood brain tumors and leukemia. *J Child Neurol* 1992; 7:462–463.
75. Casat CD, Wilson DC. Tics with combined thioridazine–methylphenidate therapy: case report. *J Clin Psychiatry* 1986; 47(1):44–45.
76. Grob CS, Coyle JT. Suspected adverse methylphenidate–imipramine interactions in children. *Dev Behav Pediatr* 1986; 7(4):265–267.
77. Hagelgans NA. Pediatric skin care issues for the home care nurse. *Pediatr Nurs* 1993; 19(5):499–450.

II
Management of Bone Pain

Introduction

Bone Pain: Defining the Need for New Approaches

RUSSELL K. PORTENOY

Bone is the most common site of tumor metastasis, and bone pain is the most prevalent type of chronic pain reported by patients with metastatic solid tumors. There are numerous therapeutic options for bone pain, including primary treatments and diverse analgesic approaches. Together, these interventions offer the clinician and patient a varied menu from which to select treatments that may optimize comfort and function, and minimize patient burden and cost.

Unfortunately, very little is known about the development of pain in association with bone metastases, and the lack of empirical information constrains rational decision making. With limited data, it is difficult to develop therapeutic guidelines for available interventions, and even more difficult to identify the need for new approaches to manage refractory cases. The challenges inherent in this process become clear in highlighting some of the unresolved questions about the phenomenon of bone pain.

Bone Pain: Unresolved Questions

Much remains unknown about the pathogenesis, epidemiology, and treatment of malignant bone pain. Among the more salient issues are the following:

1. The pathophysiology of bone pain is not understood. Although it may be heuristic to speculate about the role of nociceptors that innervate periosteum or endosteum, tumor release of substances that can activate these nociceptors, release of cytokines or other factors from host tissues, or mechanical factors like intramedullary pressure, no specific process has been established as a cause of bone pain.[1] Accordingly, there is no

explanation for the remarkable observation that most bone metastases are not painful and most patients with painful sites of bone disease also have other non-painful ones. Clearly, the presence of a neoplasm in bone is necessary but not sufficient for the development of pain, and the mechanism or mechanisms that convert a painless lesion into a painful one are not known.

With such limited information about mechanisms, it is not possible to know if the pain associated with bone metastases represents a single disorder resulting from a specific pathologic response or multiple disorders. It is possible that pain is the final common outcome of many mechanisms. If this is true, the variability in the response to treatments may reflect differences in pathogenesis. For example, the utility of osteoclast inhibitors, such as the bisphosphonates, may be limited to those patients who have pain mediated by processes induced by these cells. Similarly, the efficacy of nonsteroidal anti-inflammatory drugs may be especially good only in a subgroup of patients whose pain is mediated by local release of prostaglandins. A nonpharmacologic approach, such as bracing, may only be helpful if pain is related to mechanical deformation of the bone. Additional research into the pathogenesis of bone pain may allow identification of subtypes relatively more likely to respond to one type of treatment than another. This information, in turn, will help clarify which patient subgroups respond poorly to current therapy. These subgroups are the most appropriate targets for the development of new treatments.

2. There are many relevant gaps in the known epidemiology of bone pain. Clinically, it is well recognized that bone pain often includes a breakthrough pain with movement, known as incident pain. Incident pain is associated with a relatively reduced responsiveness to optimal opioid therapy.[2,3] The proportion of patients with treatment-limiting incident pain is not known, however, and treatments for breakthrough pain are evolving.[4] The need for novel bone pain treatments may be decreased by the availability of specific therapies for incident pain. The extent to which this may occur, however, is difficult to know in the absence of epidemiologic data.

In a similar manner, little is known about the relationship between pain and other important complications of bone disease, such as fracture. These complications are not addressed by analgesic therapies, and their prevention may require the administration of primary therapy, such as radiation. Without information about the relationship between pain and other complications, it is difficult to rationalize the selection of primary treatments for analgesia vs. analgesic treatment alone in patients with bone pain. Certainly the relatively expensive alternative of radiation therapy should not be offered to every patient with focal pain related to a metastatic deposit in a long bone in lieu of potentially effective analgesic pharmacotherapy Some patients, however, such as those with evidence of imminent fracture on plain radiography, should receive radiation. Until better epidemiologic data are able to clarify the clinical predictors of fracture, clinicians must rely solely on the plain radiograph and clinical judgment to select those patients with focal bone pain who should receive primary therapy early.

3. There is also little known about the functional consequences of bone pain, another aspect of the epidemiology of this phenomenon. The effects on physical or psychosocial functioning of numerous pain characteristics, such as the number of sites of pain, the presence of incident pain, the development of pain at rest, and the response to analgesic therapy, are undetermined. Consequently, the efficacy of available therapies is understood only in very narrow terms. With such meager information about the impact of bone pain and its varied treatments on quality of life, the larger risks and benefits of available therapies are difficult to discern accurately and the need for new therapies remains poorly defined.

4. There have been important advances in the therapy of bone pain during the past two decades, but the available data are too limited to allow the development of evidence–based treatment guidelines. The efficacy of radiotherapy is well established, and there is some evidence that chemotherapy may be able to provide relief of bone pain associated with some tumor types.[5] Some patients benefit from surgery that resects or stabilizes a site of injured bone. There is widespread recognition that generally accepted guidelines for the pharmacotherapy of cancer pain[6] which emphasize the role of opioid therapy for all patients with moderate or more intense pain, apply to those with pain caused by metastatic bone disease. Based on clinical observations, nonsteroidal anti-inflammatory drugs and corticosteroids[7] are often added to the opioid regimen to enhance analgesia. Recent studies also have suggested that multifocal bone pain that has been refractory to routine drug therapies may be treated effectively with specific adjuvant analgesics. These drugs include bisphosphonate compounds such as pamidronate,[8] calcitonin,[9] gallium nitrate,[10] and bone-seeking radionuclides such as strontium-89 or samarium-153.[11]

Although the availability of these diverse therapies offers many options for therapy, the lack of comparative data is a significant concern. The use of the adjuvant drugs is usually based on clinician bias, patient preference, and the availability of insurance coverage for drug costs. Although it is possible that specific facets of the pain or the bone disease itself may predict a better response to one adjuvant drug than another, none of these potential relationships has been confirmed. Like radiotherapy, these adjuvants may be selected before the opioid regimen is optimized, difficult approach to justify in the absence of systematic data on cost–benefit.

Future research that evaluates the cost–benefit of these drugs must focus on the prevention of complications, as well as analgesia and functional outcomes, because a reduction in the morbidity of bone disease would strongly indicate early drug use. Evidence that the bisphosphonates may reduce fracture rate[12] while enhancing analgesia could justify earlier administration to patients with pain. Additional data of this type are needed to clarify the overall benefits and burdens associated with current and future therapies.

Conclusion: The Need for New Approaches

With these questions unresolved, it is difficult to optimize the use of the many available therapies for bone pain and determine the need for novel approaches. The proportion of patients with refractory pain is unknown and cannot be determined without information that rationalizes the use of radiotherapy and other primary approaches, and encourages the most appropriate selection and administration of analgesic drugs. More information about the pathogenesis and epidemiology of bone pain, and the risks, benefits, and costs of current therapies, would permit the development of novel therapies with an improved therapeutic index or cost–benefit. Until this information is acquired, clinicians should attempt to weigh carefully the advantages and disadvantages of each approach, and develop a therapeutic strategy based on a comprehensive assessment of the patient.

References

1. Healey J. The mechanism and treatment of bone pain. In: Arbit E, ed. *Management of Cancer-related Pain*. Mount Kisco, N.Y.: Futura Publications, 1993: 515–526.
2. Mercadante S, Maddaloni S, Roccella S, Salvaggio L. Predictive factors in advanced cancer pain treated only by analgesics. *Pain* 1992; 50:151–155.
3. Bruera E, Schoeller T, Wenk R, et al. A prospective multi-center assessment of the Edmonton staging system for cancer pain. *J Pain Symptom Manage* 1995; 10:348–355.
4. Portenoy RK. Managing the temporal aspects of cancer pain. *Semin Oncol*, 24(5) Suppl. 16, pp. S16–7 to S16–12 year
5. Tannock IF, Osoba D, Stockler MR, et al. Chemotherapy with mitoxantrone plus prednisone or prednisone alone for symptomatic hormone-resistant prostate cancer: a Canadian randomized trial with palliative endpoints. *J Clin Oncol* 1996; 14:1756–1764.
6. Jacox A, Carr DB, Payne R, et al. *Management of Cancer Pain*. Clinical Practice Guideline No. 9. AHCPR Publication No. 94-0592. Rockville, Md. Agency for Health Care Policy and Research, U.S. Department of Health and Human Services, Public Health Service, 1994.

7. Tannock I, Gospodarowicz M, Meakin W, et al. Treatment of metastatic prostatic cancer with low-dose prednisone: evaluation of pain and quality of life as pragmatic indices of response. *J Clin Oncol* 1989; 7:590–597.

8. Glover D, Lipton A, Keller A, et al. Intravenous pamidronate disodium treatment of bone metastases in patients with breast cancer. *Cancer* 1994; 74:2949–2955.

9. Roth A, Kolaric K. Analgetic activity of calcitonin in patients with painful osteolytic metastases of breast cancer: results of a controlled randomized study. *Oncology* 1986; 43:283–287.

10. Warrell RP, Lovett D, Dilmanian FA, et al. Low-dose gallium nitrate for prevention of osteolysis in myeloma: results of a pilot randomized study. *J Clin Oncol* 1993; 11:2443–2450.

11. Porter AT, McEwan AJ, Powe JE, et al. Results of a randomized phase-III trial to evaluate the efficacy of strontium-89 adjuvant to local field external beam irradiation in the management of endocrine resistant metastatic prostate cancer. *Int J Radiat Oncol Biol Phys* 1993; 25:805–813.

12. Hortobagyi GN, Theriault RL, Porter L, et al. Efficacy of pamidronate in reducing skeletal complications in patients with breast cancer and lytic bone mets. *N Engl J Med* 1996; 335:1836–1837.

4

Management of Bone Pain

JOSÉ PEREIRA

Pain is a common symptom in patients with cancer, occurring in 50%–85% of patients with advanced disease.[1,2] Metastatic cancer invades bone in 60%–84% of cases.[3] In several common cancers, such as breast and prostate cancers, the skeleton is the most common site of metastases. It is estimated that between 65% and 75% of patients with bone metastases present with bone pain,[4] and the high morbidity associated with bone metastases can be protracted. Although survival varies widely among patients with metastatic bone disease, patients suffering from metastatic breast disease survive on average 34 months after detection of the first metastasis, with a range of 1–90 months.[5] Survival with metastatic prostate cancer averages 24 months, and lung cancer patients have a poor prognosis of less than one year after bone metastases are first diagnosed.[6,7] Significant advances in our knowledge of the mechanisms of bone metastases and the pathophysiology of bone pain have prompted review of traditional treatment modalities and have offered new possibilities for managing malignant bone pain more effectively. This chapter reviews current knowledge regarding the pathophysiology and treatment of malignant bone pain.

Pathophysiology of Bone Metastases and Bone Pain

Cancer affects bone by three mechanisms: primary bone tumors, direct invasion from primary tumors, and hematogenous spread. The last is by far the most common. Hematogenous spread involves a cascade of linked steps which a neoplastic cell needs to traverse to successfully establish a secondary tumor in a distant bony site.[6] The mechanism whereby tumor cells are attracted to bone surfaces is complex but appears to involve various chemotactic factors such as type 1 collagen and osteocalcin.[8,9] Once the tumor cell adheres to the endosteum, factors within the bone matrix stimulate growth of the tumor (Fig. 4.1).

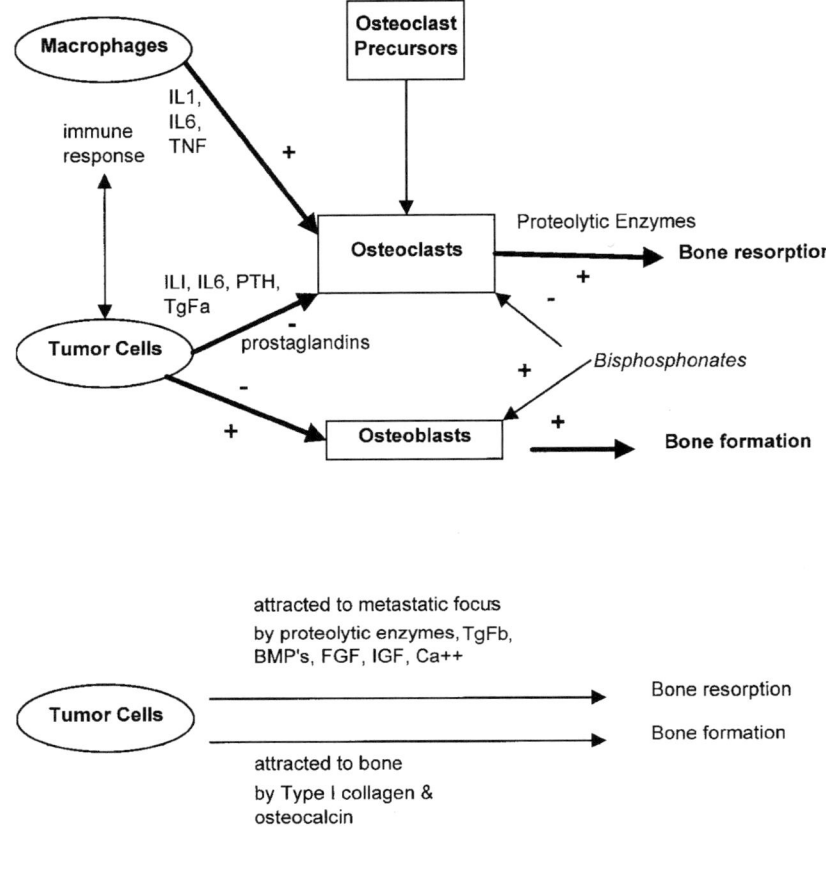

Figure 4.1. Metastatic osteolysis: the micromilieu. TgF = transforming growth factor; FGF = fibroblast-derived growth factors; TNF = tumor necrosis factor; BMP = bone morphogenic proteins; IL = interleukin; IGF = insulin-like growth factor.

The most important mechanism of bone destruction is the release of paracrine factors which stimulate osteoclasts to resorb bone.[8,9] It involves a chemical assault, in which various humoral mediators are produced by an interaction of tumor cells, neighboring osteoclasts, the immune system, and other systemic factors. The net result is an increase in osteoclast activity. Often a mixed activation of both osteoclasts and osteoblasts is evident. There is some recent evidence that bone itself is an important source of growth factors which are released during bone resorption and stimulate tumor growth.

The mechanism by which metastases cause bone pain is not well understood.[4] It is puzzling that not all bone metastases cause pain. Only 25%–32% of patients with skeletal metastases experience related pain.[10] Moreover, severe bone pain can result from the smallest of metastatic deposits.[11] Classically, the periosteum has been described as being richly innervated by free nerve endings; if true, this element would be the only part of bone that could generate pain when distended by tumor mass.[12] This traction theory, although plausible, does not explain why aneurysmal bone cysts are frequently painless. Traditionally, it has also been postulated that elevated bone marrow pressure (either as a result of tumor growth or inflammatory reactions) is in some way transduced to the periosteum, triggering the periosteal nerve endings.[13] This view, however, does not adequately explain why elevated hydrostatic pressure within the marrow, as occurs in bone infarctions, must be relieved by surgical decompression of the marrow compartment. This observation suggests that high pressure within bone compartments may cause pain via receptors distinct from those in the periosteum. In addition, various compounds known to mediate nociception have been found in the bone marrow and cortex of long bones.[12] Thus a combination of chemical and mechanical factors could be responsible for the nociceptive process in pain.

Clinical Features of Malignant Bone Involvement

The sites of pain are dependent on the pattern of metastasis. Some cancers exhibit osteotropism and predictably metastasize to bone.[14] For example, more than 50% of patients with breast, lung, or prostate cancer develop bone metastases.[15] Eighty percent of all bone metastases originate from tumors of the breasts, prostate, lungs, thyroid, and kidneys. The most common sites of bone metastasis are the spine, pelvis, ribs, femur, and skull.[4,15] There is an association between tumor type and the site of skeletal involvement. Prostate cancer, for example, shows predominant involvement of the pelvic bones.

Primary tumors of bone are for less common than metastatic neoplasms. They often present with persistent pain and some may grow rapidly. Osteosarcomas (18%) and chondrosarcomas (10%) are the more common primary bone malignancies.[15] Multiple myeloma, which arises in the marrow of bone, can also be the source of bone pain and other skeletal complications.

Bone metastases produce various complications, the most common being a somatic pain syndrome (bone pain) (Table 4.1). Continuous pain is the most frequent presentation of bone pain and is usually well localized to one or more specific bone areas. It usually develops gradually over a period of weeks or months, progressively becoming more severe in intensity. It is characteristically described as dull in character and constant in presentation. Bone pain often increases with pressure on the area. Continuous pain may be moderate during

Table 4.1. Clinical features associated with malignant bone involvement

---

Pain

    Continuous bone pain
    Breakthrough pain
    Incident pain
    Neuropathic pain
    Mixed bone and neuropathic pain

Impaired mobility and function

Pathological fractures

Hypercalcemia

Spinal cord and nerve root compression

Bone marrow infiltration and marrow depression

---

periods of rest but become more intense during periods of activity. The activity can include movements such as turning, standing, walking, or coughing. Even deep inspirations may worsen pain associated with rib metastases. Breakthrough pain, of which incident pain (pain with movement) is an example, is experienced by almost two-thirds of patients with cancer pain.[16] Depending on the associated activity, it can occur rarely or frequently in a given period and can be difficult to control. It is a poor prognostic indicator for adequate pain control.[17]

Neuropathic pain syndromes may complicate malignant bone involvement when bone destruction results in compression of adjacent neural structures. Radicular pain, for example, may occur if a vertebral tumor impinges on the adjacent nerve roots. A "burning" or "tingling" pain may be described, as well as occasional paroxysms of lancinating pain. The pain may be referred to other anatomical areas. Impingement of the first and third lumbar nerve roots, for example, may refer pain into the hip and knee, respectively. The presence of sensory or motor deficits is further indication of nerve involvement. Invasion of the epidural space and compression of the spinal cord may produce motor, sensory, and autonomic signs. Cord compression occurs in approximately 5% of cancer patients, and local or radicular pain may be the only sign of spinal cord compression before the development of paralysis.[18]

Metastases to the base of the skull region can cause headaches in that area, often with accompanying neck pain. Bone lesions in the proximity of cranial nerves, especially near their foramina, can result in specific cranial nerve dysfunction, such as trigeminal neuropathy, facial nerve palsy, glossopharyngeal neuropathy, or vagal nerve involvement.

Pathological fractures have been reported in 8%–30% of patients with bone metastases.[19,20] The proximal parts of long bones are more commonly involved. The bones fractured most often are the femur (50%) and humerus (15%).[4,20] A pathological fracture typically results in a sudden exacerbation of pain.

Hypercalcemia occurs in approximately 10%–40% of cancer patients during the course of their illness.[21] The underlying mechanism of hypercalcemia is osteolysis and calcium reabsorption from the kidney which, in 80% of cases, is caused by the release of a parathyroid hormone–related protein. The incidence of hypercalcemia does not, therefore, always correlate with the extent of metastatic bone disease, and hypercalcemia may be present even in the absence of extensive bone involvement.

Bone Pain Assessment

The diagnosis of malignant bone pain can usually be made by history and physical examination. The clinician should enquire about the quality, intensity, site, and radiation of the pain; factors that exacerbate or alleviate it; and other systemic symptoms. Simple pain measurement tools, such as visual analogue and numerical scales, should be used to document the intensity of pain on an ongoing basis, both before and after therapeutic interventions. The physical examination should include a general examination as well as a meticulous assessment of the musculo–skeletal and neurological systems. Signs such as tenderness over bony structures, crepitation, limb instability, and neurological deficits should be noted.

Close monitoring is necessary in patients with vertebral bone metastases, whether or not they have back pain. Although pain is usually the presenting feature of spinal cord compression, weakness, paresthesias, sensory deficits, or bladder and bowel impairment occasionally occur first.[18] The key to successful management of spinal cord compression is early diagnosis and prompt treatment. Neurological recovery is inversely related to the degree of pre-treatment neurological impairment. Approximately 80% of patients who are ambulatory at the initiation of treatment will remain ambulatory after treatment while only 50% of those who are paraparetic at the initiation of therapy will regain ambulation.[22] Only 10% of those who are already paraplegic when they first present will regain mobility after therapy.[22] The thoracic cord is at particularly high risk for compression because the vertebral canal is at its narrowest in that area. One study reported that 74% of patients presenting with the combination of back pain, a normal neurological examination, and vertebral body metastases had epidural disease documented by positive myelography.[23]

Plain radiographs of suspected involved bones and a bone scintigram may be useful in characterizing the extent of bone involvement.[24,25] Radiography is specific, but quite insensitive. At least 50% of the bone must be destroyed before involvement of the medulla can be seen radiographically; lesions that involve the cortex are detected when they are much smaller. Skeletal metastases generally develop in the medulla and cortical damage occurs later.[4]

Patients with a high risk for pathological fractures should be identified so that prophylactic management, either surgical or nonsurgical, can be implemented. Plain radiographs of painful upper extremity lesions and all lower extremity lesions may assist in determining fracture risk. Radiographic guidelines that identify a high risk for an impending fracture of the femur have been proposed[19,27,193] (Table 4.2). However, it has been reported that up to 40% of pathological fractures did not meet these criteria.[27] It is important to note that not all bone metastases are painful and that pathological fractures can occur without preceding pain.

Bone scintigrams, unlike radiographs, are highly sensitive for the detection of bone metastases. Bone scintigraphy can detect metastases as small as 2 mm; in contrast, radiography seldom detects metastases smaller than 1 cm.[28] Scintigraphy, however, lacks specificity.[28] The false negative rate for a bone scan is about 8%, while the false positive rate may be as high as 40%–50% when only a few positive lesions are observed.[29] Because bone scans commonly show abnormality where there is osteoblastic activity, it may be negative in purely lytic lesions, such as those that occur in multiple myeloma. Alternatively, it may be positive in such conditions as arthritis, infections, trauma, and Paget's disease.[28]

Computed tomography (CT) or magnetic resonance imaging (MRI) may give additional information, especially when spinal cord involvement is suspected.[25,30] Some suggest that all patients with vertebral column involvement be investigated by MRI; others suggest that CT and MRI of the spine should be reserved for patients who present with vertebral body compression of 50% or greater on plain radiograph and those who present with neurological involvement. In assessing patients with possible spinal cord compression, Portenoy et al. studied 43 cancer patients retrospectively to assess the risk of epidural disease associated with specific clinical, radiographic, and scintigraphic findings.[31] The study found that spinal radiography is predictive of epidural disease and the authors suggest that patients with pain and no neurological deficit should be considered for aggressive evaluation if spinal radiograph is abnormal. The need for aggressive evaluation is compelling if vertebral body collapse occurs, whereas greater flexibility is appropriate when the radiograph shows a small lesion limited to the body of the vertebra. Clinically "silent" areas of cord compression are not uncommon, and the poor correlation between

Table 4.2 Radiographic and clinical indications*
for prophylactic surgery or impending fractures

Cortical Lesions

  Destruction of > 50% of the cortical width
  Axial length of the lesion diameter of the bone
  > 2–3 cm lesion

Medullary Lesions

  Lesion that is > 50% of the medulla
  Lesions causing pain unrelieved by radiotherapy

*These apply specifically to large, weight-bearing bones.

site of vertebral body metastases and extent of epidural disease has been emphasized.[32] It is therefore suggested that the entire spine be imaged.

Occasionally, despite the presence of pain, no abnormalities are detected on plain radiography or bone scintigraphy.[33,34] MRI may have a role in this setting. These radiologically invisible lesions have been attributed to inter-trabecular infiltration by tumor cells. In contrast to the more typical osteolytic or osteoblastic patterns, this pattern does not result in marked alteration of the bony trabeculae and is therefore not easily identifiable on plain radiography.[35] A recent study found that, of 734 vertebral lesions, 255 were of an inter-trabecular pattern;[35] these inter-trabecular lesions were detected by only 7.1% of radiographs and 4.5% of bone scans, but were demonstrated in all of the MRI images. Bone scintigraphy therefore appears to demonstrate inter-trabecular lesions with great difficulty.

Patients with a polyostotic disease and a known primary neoplasm can usually be treated without obtaining a biopsy. Patients should be considered for biopsy when the response to treatment is atypical and when a metastatic bone lesion is suspected but no primary tumor is identified. Monostotic lesions, especially in patients younger than 40 years, may be a primary sarcoma and must be imaged before biopsy. To elucidate the full extent of the lesion for proper biopsy planning, CT or MRI is needed.[24] Almost all biopsy incisions need to be done with specific precautions.

Malignancy is not always the cause of bone–related pain in cancer patients. Spondylolisthesis, osteoporosis, osteoarthritis, osteomyelitis, prolapsed intervetebral discs, and other rheumatologic illnesses are benign causes of bone pain and need to be excluded.

Bone Pain Treatment

Malignant bone pain is best treated with a multimodality, interdisciplinary approach. For most patients, medical management plus radiotherapy generally suffice. Opioid analgesics remain the mainstay of symptom management, both for areas of isolated bone involvement and for diffuse bone pain (Table 4.3).

Opioid analgesics

Bone pain typically shows a good response to opioid analgesics.[36,37] A variety of strong agonist opioids are generally available, including morphine, hydromorphone, oxycodone, fentanyl, and methadone. The guidelines for the choice of drug, route, and dose of opioid are well described in many publications.[2,38] These include the use of fixed scheduled doses, of an agonist opioid for constant pain and so-called rescue doses on an as-needed basis for breakthrough pain. The dose is then titrated to achieve pain control. Care must be taken to manage common side effects, such as constipation and nausea.[39] The oral route is preferred, but

Table 4.3. Treatment modalities of malignant bone pain

	Focal bone pain	Multifocal bone pain
Mainstay Therapies	Analgesics	Analgesics
	Opioids	Opioids
	Non-opioids	Non-opioids
	External irradiation	External irradiation of localized areas
Additional Therapies	Adjuvant analgesics	Adjuvant analgesics
	NSAIDs	NSAIDs
	Corticosteroids	Corticosteroids
	Surgical reduction and	Bisphosphonates
	Internal fixation of	Bisphosphonates for
	pathological fractures	prevention of skeletal events
		Radioisotopes
Less Utilized Therapies	Anesthetic blocks	Hemibody irradiation
	Neurosurgical modalities	Anesthetic blocks
	Amputation	Neurosurgical modalities

occasionally an alternative route is required. The subcutaneous route has been shown to be as effective as the intravenous route, and is more convenient. Other options include rectal and transdermal formulations. To allow for rapid and safe titration, an immediate–release formulation is required when starting an opioid–naive patient on an opioid or when trying to control pain in an unstable situation such as uncontrolled pain or delirium. Once the pain is under control and stable, a controlled–release formulation may be introduced for convenience. Knowledge about neuropsychiatric side effects and their management strategies is essential.[40] When there are other complicating factors, such as incident pain, adequate titration of opioids may prove difficult. Severe sedation in such cases may become a dose-limiting toxicity of opioids during the intervals between incident pains. Addition of a psychostimulant may allow patients to tolerate a higher dose of opioids by reducing sedation, thereby improving analgesia.[40] The presence of factors such as severe psychological distress, neuropathic pain, incident pain, and a history of alcohol abuse (indicating maladaptive coping techniques) may complicate pain management.[17]

Adjuvant analgesics in bone pain

Occasionally, it may be necessary to add an adjuvant analgesic to the opioid regimen to effect better pain control. There have been no comparative trials of adjuvant analgesics for bone pain, and the selection of one over another is based on clinician preference, convenience, patient preference, and various clinical indicators such as localized pain versus multifocal pain.

Nonsteroidal anti-inflammatory drugs

Nonsteroidal anti-inflammatory drugs (NSAIDs) have been reported to be effective in managing cancer pain.[41,42] Various guidelines have advocated their use as single agents in the treatment of mild–to–moderate cancer pain, and in combination with opioids for moderate–to–severe pain.[2,43] Single-dose trials have suggested benefit from, among others, ibuprofen, naproxen, ketoprofen, zomepirac, diflusinal, and ketorolac.[44–51] Multiple dose studies have indicated benefit from aspirin, benzydamide, ibuprofen, diclofenac, ketorolac, indomethacin, sulindac, naproxen, piroxicam, and zomepirac.[52–59] Various routes, including the oral route, subcutaneous infusions (naproxen, diclofenac, and ketorolac), and intramuscular injections, have been used.[60–63]

A case is often made for a special role of NSAIDs in metastatic bone pain.[36,37,42] Although numerous studies have documented their effectiveness in the management of cancer pain in general, few randomized clinical studies have assessed their role specifically for metastatic bone pain.[41] This paucity of controlled studies is well illustrated in a recent meta-analysis of data from published randomized controlled trials of NSAIDs in cancer pain.[64] Of the 25 studies identified, a specific cancer diagnosis was reported for only 33% of all patients. Many of these studies had confounding factors and methodological difficulties. Thirteen of the studies tested a single dose effect, raising concern about the generalizability of the data to chronic dosing.[65] Only four studies[53,66–68] examined the analgesic efficacy of NSAIDs specifically for malignant bone pain.

In a randomized, double-blind trial, 83% of the patients analyzed had significant pain relief during the 6 hr following a loading dose of 550 mg of naproxen.[66] One-third of patients receiving a dose of 550 mg every 8 hr for 3 days experienced pain relief. Pain relief appeared to be better in patients receiving these higher doses than patients on a lower dose of naproxen (275 mg every 8 hr). In another study, patients whose pain was well controlled on an oxycodone/acetaminophen combination were randomized to receive either an additional 600 mg of ibuprofen 4 times a day over 7 days or no additional medications.[53] Those who received ibuprofen required significantly less oxycodone/acetaminophen combination than those who did not; the reduction in opioid use occurred within 24 hr and maximized at 5 days.[53] Daily pain intensity scores also improved. In a third study—a six-week, placebo-controlled, double-blind crossover study of flurbiprofen and placebo in patients with metastatic breast cancer to bone—the overall mean differences in pain scores showed better control of pain during treatment with flurbiprofen, but the difference was not statistically significant.[68] Patients in this study were also receiving a variety of other analgesics.

The effect of NSAIDs in cancer pain is neither predictable nor consistent. Although the various NSAIDs are often grouped by chemical structure into the fenamates, indoles, oxicams, propionates, and salicylates, there is substantial variation in the response to NSAIDs within the same chemical group. Possible reasons for this variability are differences in the ability of the various NSAIDs to block the prostaglandin pathway, intersubject pharmacokinetic differences,[37,69] inadequate trial designs, and insensitive measurements.

A few studies have attempted to compare the efficacy of various NSAIDs.[57] A double-blind study compared the efficacy and tolerability of acetylsalicylic acid, paracetamol, diclofenac, ibuprofen, indomethacin, pirprofen, sulindac, naproxen, and suprofen.[57] The most effective drugs appeared to be naproxen, diclofenac, and indomethacin.[57] However, no clinically noticeable superiority of an individual NSAID or class of NSAIDs over other NSAIDs has been clearly identified.[26] Furthermore, neither the percentage of responders nor the optimum doses or route of administration have been well established in prospective trials. Failure of one class does not exclude effectiveness of other NSAIDs. It is suggested that any particular NSAID be started at full anti-inflammatory dosage, and if adequate analgesia is not forthcoming, trial of another NSAID is warranted. For patient comfort, the oral route is preferred. Drugs that can be administered less frequently offer the potential advantage of increased convenience and compliance.

The analgesic effect of NSAIDs is presumed to result from inhibition of prostaglandin synthesis in the periphery.[70] This effect occurs via the inhibition of cyclo-oxygenase, an enzyme that catalyzes the conversion of arachidonic acid into endoperoxide (Fig. 4.2). Endoperoxide, in turn, serves as the substrate for the prostaglandins, thromboxanes, and prostacyclins, many of which are involved in inflammatory and nociceptive responses.[12] There is also increasing evidence that NSAIDs have central effects.[71] Recent basic research suggests that prostaglandins appear to have some role in modulating sensitization of the dorsal horn neurons of the spinal cord in response to repetitive stimuli.[41,71]

In clinical practice, the administration of NSAIDs as single analgesics in mild-to-moderate pain appears to be indicated for periods of less than 3–5 weeks because of long-term analgesic inefficacy, the presence of a ceiling effect, and the occurrence of adverse effects.[43,57,64] NSAIDs should, therefore, not be viewed as opioid substitutes for the management of moderate-to-severe cancer pain. Some authors have also suggested that NSAID may have an opioid-sparing effect,[56,72] and some trials have suggested that the combination of an opioid with an NSAID gives better analgesia than the opioid alone.[44,56,62,63] However, a recent small retrospective review did not confirm this.[73] It can be argued that a "narcotic–sparing effect" should not necessarily be an indication to add an NSAID to an opioid regimen. The same level of analgesia can be obtained by simply increasing the opioid dose by 20% to 40% without significant dose-limiting toxicity, rather than exposing the patient to polypharmacy and the potential NSAID-related adverse effects.

Toxicity remains the most significant factor limiting the long-term role of NSAID in the management of cancer pain.[36,37,41] There were 59 adverse events per 100 patients in the meta-analysis of pooled data from prospective, controlled

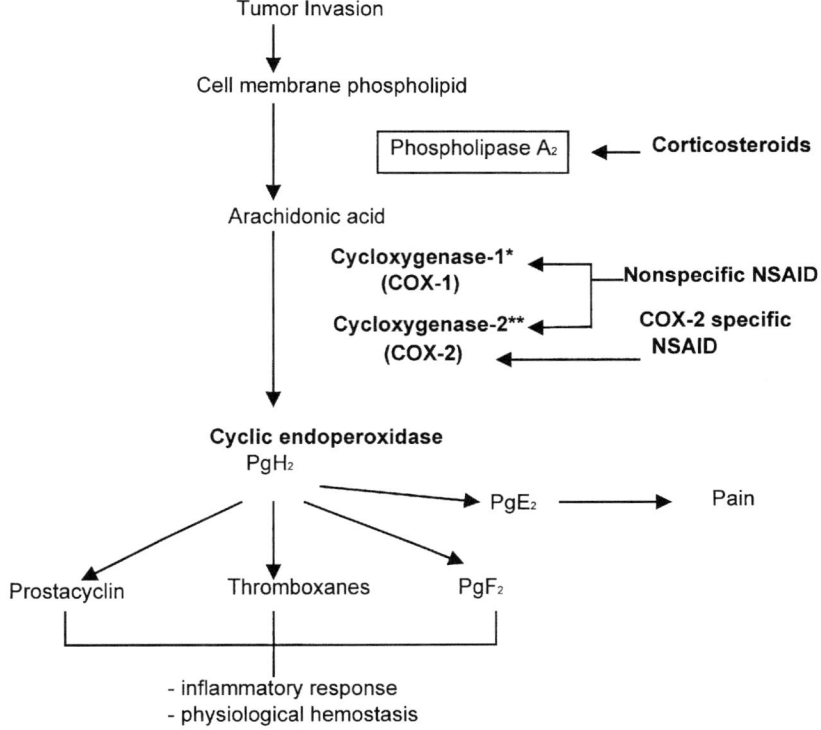

Figure 4.2. Mechanisms of corticosteroid and nonsteroidal anti-inflammatory drug action.

multiple-dose studies.[64] The most common of these adverse events involved the gastrointestinal tract, kidneys, and platelet functioning. Although the most common gastrointestinal effects are dyspepsia and nausea,[74,75] the potential for damage to the upper gastrointestinal tract is potentially the most hazardous complication of these drugs. The risk of gastric ulceration increases five-fold and the risk of duodenal ulceration appears to increase slightly during NSAID administration. Dyspepsia without mucosal damage is common, as is mucosal damage without any symptoms; 10–20% of patients on NSAIDs have an ulcer on endoscopy at any time.[76] Dyspeptic symptoms are therefore a poor guide to gastric mucosal damage in patients on NSAIDs. The risk of bleeding or perforation is increased substantially in patients with pre-existing gastric and duodenal ulcers. This risk also increases significantly with age, concomitant steroid use, past history of peptic ulceration, smoking, and possibly alcohol consumption.[74] The risk of ulcer formation is greatest within the first months of treatment and the degree of damage is dose–dependent. Other gastrointestinal adverse effects include hepatotoxicity, colitis, esophagitis, and proctitis.[75]

Both gastrointestinal and renal adverse effects are mediated by prostaglandin inhibition. NSAIDs may cause renal insufficiency by impairing intra-renal blood flow via the inhibition of prostacyclin, a renal vasodilator.[77] Patients with congestive heart failure, cirrhosis with ascites, nephrotic syndrome, or salt and water depletion are at higher risk for developing these adverse effects. Patients with advanced cancer may be at an increased risk of renal toxicity resulting from hypovolemia secondary to reduced fluid intake or prior therapy with nephrotoxic chemotherapy agents. In patients with advanced cancer, renal impairment can result in opioid metabolite accumulation, giving rise to various neuropsychiatric toxicities.[40]

Other less common adverse effects of the NSAIDs may affect the hematological, dermatological, pulmonary, and central nervous systems. It is difficult to obtain any clear data on the risks of individual NSAIDs.

Several strategies have been advocated in an attempt to improve the safety profile of NSAIDs. These include the use of non-oral routes of administration; the development of "enteric-coating," which limits local exposure of the gastric mucosa to the drug; co-administration of gastro–protective agents such as the histamine-2 receptor antagonists, sucralfate and misoprostol; and the use of drugs with unique kinetic properties.[78] The last approach involves the administration of a pro-drug, such as nabumetone, which is absorbed in the inactive form and then converted to its active form in the liver.[79] The effectiveness of this pro-drug strategy has not been confirmed in large studies. Misoprostol, a prostaglandin analogue, appears to be superior to either histamine-2 receptor antagonists or sucralfate in reducing the risk of gastric ulceration.[78] The evidence suggests that differences in the route of administration do not alter systemic inhibition of prostaglandin biosynthesis or change toxicity.

Recently two forms of the enzyme cyclo-oxygenase (COX), COX-1 and COX-2, have been identified.[80] Unlike COX-1, which is always present in the gastric mucosa and renal tubules, COX-2 is only induced as part of the inflammatory process at the site of inflammation. In theory therefore, if COX-2 is selectively inhibited over COX-1, fewer gastric and renal side effects should occur.[81] These selective NSAIDs hold promise, but their role remains to be clarified.

Corticosteroids
Corticosteroids have significant analgesic effects in a variety of cancer pain syndromes, including neuropathic, visceral, and bone pain.[82] They also may have other benefits for patients with very advanced disease, including improved appetite, decreased nausea, and an improvement in the sense of well-being.[83] When

used to reduce bone pain, short-term improvement can be dramatic, occurring within a day or two. The duration of pain relief appears to be shorter than 3–4 weeks.[84] The analgesic mechanism of action is probably similar to that of the NSAIDs, namely the inhibition of prostaglandin synthesis[85] (Fig. 4.2).

The ideal type of corticosteroid and the optimal dose have not been well established, and dose recommendations are based mainly on uncontrolled, anecdotal reports and clinical experience. Therapy is usually instituted with 4–8 mg of dexamethasone orally or subcutaneously 2–3 times per day, 16–32 mg of methylprednisolone orally 2–3 times a day, or 20–40 mg of prednisone orally 2–3 times per day.[86] Any clinical effect should be evident within 5 days, at which time a decision can be made to taper the drug either rapidly or gradually. Tapering is required to avoid adrenal insufficiency. If effectiveness is demonstrated, the dose should be gradually tapered to the lowest effective level or, if possible, be discontinued to avoid long-term adverse effects. If no benefits are noted after 5–7 days, the tapering can be more rapid, and the corticosteroids can be discontinued within a few days.

The special benefit of corticosteroids in spinal cord compression has been well demonstrated and they should be initiated early when spinal cord compression is suspected. The appropriate dose is controversial.[87,88] An uncontrolled study found that a high-dose regimen of 100 mg dexamethasone intravenously followed by 96 mg daily for 3 days, concurrent with radiotherapy, followed then by a tapering schedule over 2 weeks, yielded pain relief in 82% of patients; in some cases the relief preceded the radiotherapy.[88] An initial high dose of dexamethasone (100 mg) was compared with an initial low dose (10 mg) in a randomized double-blind study, and no significant difference in pain relief was observed; both groups received the same low-dose regimen after this initial dose.[87] The analgesia produced by these drugs may be due to the reduction in peri-tumoral edema; improvement in neurological dysfunction has been noted if therapy is started promptly.

The potential for toxicity from steroid administration, particularly with long-term administration, must be considered and monitored.[83,84] Toxic effects include edema, hyperglycemia, immunosuppression, osteoporosis, and proximal myopathy. In patients with a relatively long expected survival, maintenance therapy with corticosteroids should be carefully weighed against these potential side effects. In palliative care, the life expectancy of most patients is relatively short and these effects have limited relevance. During short-term treatment, however, side effects may occur, including infections, hyperglycemia, and psychiatric complications such as affective disorders, psychotic reactions, and cognitive impairment.[89] These adverse effects most commonly occur within the first two weeks of therapy and are largely reversible with rapid tapering and discontinuation of the drug. Although gastrointestinal damage is often feared, the ulcerogenic role of corticosteroids is controversial.[90,91] The available data suggest that these drugs are ulcerogenic only when used in combination with an NSAID.[91]

Inhibitors of Bone Resorption

The pathophysiology of metastatic bone destruction makes it logical to use inhibitors of osteoclast activity.[8,9,92,93] A variety of agents inhibit bone resorption, including plicamycin, calcitonin, gallium nitrate, and the bisphosphonates. Bisphosphonates are an extremely useful non-toxic modality for the treatment of bone pain, particularly where metastatic bone involvement is diffuse.

Bisphosphonates

Bisphosphonates are analogues of pyrophosphate, a natural inhibitor of the formation of calcium phosphate crystals. Following systemic administration, these compounds localize to bone and inhibit osteoclast activity.[93] Some bisphosphonates may also inhibit the maturation of mononuclear precursor cells into fully active osteoclasts. Clodronate and pamidronate have been studied the most extensively in malignant disease, particularly in multiple myeloma[94–96] and breast cancer.[97–104] Positive results have also been recorded with other adeno- and squamous carcinomas, including lung, gastrointestinal, and prostatic cancers.[97,105–107] Positive results in the presence of prostatic bone involvement stems from the fact that increased bone resorption may occur in the presence of osteoblastic metastases.[97,108–110] Etidronate is the weakest bisphosphonate in clinical use and is ineffective in malignant bone disease.[111] Newer, much more potent bisphosphonates include alendronate, risedronate, ibandronate and zolendronate.[92] These still need to be studied in the context of cancer.

As single intravenous infusions, both clodronate and pamidronate are useful for the relief of painful malignant bone disease.[105,106,112,113] In a randomized, double-blind, placebo-controlled study evaluating the analgesic benefit of intravenous clodronate in patients with metastatic bone disease of various primaries, a single, slow intravenous infusion of clodronate 600 mg was found to produce significant pain relief when compared with placebo.[105] Based on malignancy–induced hypercalcemia studies, a higher single infusion dose of 1500 mg of clodronate is now recommended.[99] Single intravenous infusions of pamidronate at doses of 60 mg to 120 mg are recommended. A single intravenous dose of 120 mg of pamidronate produced a significant subjective response in 58%–65% of patients.[106,112]

Numerous studies of multiple dosing regimens, using either oral or intravenous routes, have also been reported.[94,95,99–101,114–120] Most of these studies were relatively small and used open designs. In a large double-blind study which compared oral clodronate with a placebo, patients received 1600 mg of clodronate per day for 18 months.[98] There was a decreased need for palliative radiotherapy in the clodronate–treated group. In a randomized, double-blind study, patients received either 1600 mg per day of oral clodronate or a placebo.[121] Clodronate appeared to improve control of bone pain to a modest degree. In two other studies, intravenous pamidronate at doses of either 30 or 60 mg every 2 weeks showed relief of pain in 30%–60% of patients.[114,116] Regimens consisting of 60 mg or 90 mg every 4 weeks were found to be effective in both breast and prostate metastatic bone disease.[108] Rapid infusions of 45 mg over 1 hour have been well tolerated, provided renal function is not impaired.[117,118]

Onset of analgesia following bisphosphonate therapy usually occurs within the first two weeks. The duration of effect is variable. Pain relief was described by patients within the first few days of receiving an intravenous dose of clodronate 600 mg.[105] Hypercalcemia studies, as well as clinical experience, suggest an average duration of effect of 2 weeks for clodronate and 4 weeks for pamidronate. After a single intravenous infusion of 120 mg of pamidronate, the analgesic effect persisted for a median of 12 weeks.[112] The anti-osteolytic effect of a single dose of 120 mg of pamidronate persisted throughout the 8 weeks of observation in a recent study.[106]

Bisphosphonate analgesic effects appear to be dose-dependent. Pamidronate, at an intravenous dose of 90 mg every 3 weeks, had significantly more prolonged pain relief than doses of 60 mg every 3 weeks.[113] Some patients appear to require repeated infusions because of re-emergence of pain. More than one infusion may be needed if the initial one fails. One practical approach suggests a regimen of intravenous pamidronate 60 mg every 2 weeks for at least two or three treatments.[122] If there is no analgesic response, therapy can be discontinued; if pain declines, the biweekly scheduled can be continued until relief is optimal; the treatment interval can then be lengthened to the longest period possible without loss of effect. In certain settings, such as the home, intravenous administration may be difficult. Favorable results in the management of tumor-induced hypercalcemia with single subcutaneous infusions of 1500 mg of clodronate have been reported.[123] The clodronate is diluted in 1 liter of normal saline and infused over 12 hours. The effectiveness of this regimen for bone pain needs to be confirmed. Pamidronate cannot be infused subcutaneously.

Although some studies have compared clodronate and pamidronate in the setting of malignant hypercalcemia,[107,124] few have attempted direct comparison of their effect on bone pain. In a randomized double-blind study, the effects on hypercalcemia of single intravenous infusions of pamidronate and clodronate at doses of 90 mg and 1500 mg, respectively, were compared.[107] The control of hypercalcemia was associated with an improvement in the pain score in both treatment groups after 7 days, but was more marked in the pamidronate group. A recent study of the same doses found similar results.[125]

It now seems appropriate to consider the use of bisphosphonates earlier in the course of metastatic bone disease, to prevent skeletal morbidity.[94,95,99–101,117,126,127] Clodronate in oral doses of between 1600 mg and 2400 mg daily decreased the frequency of hypercalcemia, bone pain, and fractures in approximately 28% of patients with metastatic breast cancer and multiple myeloma.[98,117,126] Prevention of bone pain and skeletal complications was achieved in a large randomized placebo-controlled trial using 2.4 grams of clodronate orally daily for 2 years in patients with newly diagnosed myeloma.[94] The benefits of regular intravenous infusions of pamidronate on the prevention of skeletal events have also been reported.[100,114–116] These studies suggest that one-half to two-thirds of patients treated with pamidronate at doses that ranged from 30 mg to 90 mg and at intervals ranging from weekly to every 3 months had relief of bone pain.

Two recent large, prospective, controlled studies have confirmed the role of bisphosphonates in preventing skeletal events in patients with multiple myeloma and patients with breast cancer metastatic to bone.[96,102] In a double-blind study comparing multiple myeloma patients randomized to receive either 90 mg of pamidronate intravenously monthly for 9 cycles or placebo in addition to their regular chemotherapy,[96] patients who received pamidronate had lower bone pain and analgesic scores than patients receiving placebo. The proportion of patients experiencing any skeleton-related event was 22% for the pamidronate group, compared with 41% of those receiving placebo. In the second study, monthly infusions of pamidronate 90 mg were compared with placebo for the prevention of skeletal complications in breast cancer patients with lytic bone metastases.[102] The mean duration of participation in the study was 9.6 months and 48% of patients completed all 12 cycles of pamidronate or placebo. Overall morbidity from skeletal causes was reduced by approximately 30% by the end of 6 cycles in the pamidronate–treated group. The effects of pamidronate became more evident with successive treatments, and there were significant initial decreases in pain. It has been suggested that the use of bisphosphonates will not necessarily prevent spinal cord compression, since soft tissue epidural disease rather than bone collapse is often the underlying mechanism of spinal cord impingement. Moreover, repeated bisphosphonate administration does not seem to affect survival,[96,99,102,127,128] and two recent studies indicate that early use does not prevent bone metastases.[103,127] Whether the clinical benefits justify the high cost of treatment in asymptomatic patients with metastatic bone disease requires further study.[129–130]

In general, bisphosphonates are well tolerated when given intravenously. Symptomatic hypocalcemia rarely occurs.[131,132,133] A flu-like syndrome, which includes fever and myalgia, occurs in about 20% of cases of pamidronate therapy. It is transient, responds to acetaminophen, and occurs mainly after the first infusion. Nausea occurs in 5%–10% of patients treated with intravenous pamidronate.[133] Bisphosphonate administration is contraindicated in renal failure. If a decision is made to infuse a bisphosphonate in the presence of mild renal impairment, the infusion time should be increased and/or the dose reduced. Rehydration of dehydrated patients is essential.[134] The risk of renal impairment as a result of bisphosphonate infusion in patients with normal renal function appears minimal.[134]

The clinical usefulness of long-term oral dosing appears to be somewhat limited by the increased incidence of adverse gastrointestinal effects.[98,99,103,135] This is particularly true of amino-bisphosphonates such as pamidronate and alendronate. The digestive absorption of bisphosphonates varies, but is generally less than 5% of the administered dose with clodronate and as low as 0.3%–2% with the amino-bisphosphonates.[136] Significant interference by food intake is an added problem. Severe esophagitis has been described after oral administration of alendronate.[137]

Biochemical markers of bone resorption may offer an objective assessment of the effectiveness of bisphosphonates. Bone resorption results in the liberation of breakdown products of type I collagen into the circulation where they are then excreted, largely unchanged, in the urine. These markers, particularly the collagen peptide-bound cross-linked n-telopeptide (NTx) and c-telopeptide (Crosslaps), show promise as potential markers of response to bisphosphonate therapy.[106,124] In these studies, the changes in pain score seemed to follow the changes in resorption markers.[106,124] Plain radiographs and bone scintigraphy are not reliable indicators of response.[124]

"Newer generation" bisphosphonates such as ibandronate and alendronate are being studied in metastatic bone disease[138]. Some of the newer bisphosphonates may offer the option of effective oral therapy with fewer adverse effects. Transdermal formulations may also be developed.

Other inhibitors of bone resorption

Mithramycin is associated with significant nausea and bone marrow suppression[21,122] while the high toxicity of plicamycin precludes its long-term use. Calcitonin has been proposed as an adjuvant in malignant bone pain,[140–142] but the evidence of effectiveness in this role is mainly anecdotal and there are few published controlled studies.[141] The results of two randomized double-blind trials are contradictory.[140] Nausea, vomiting, and flushing are common side effects of calcitonin therapy, and its short duration of action and rapid development of tachyphylaxis are further limitations. Gallium nitrate is a newly developed agent which can also inhibit bone resorption in cancer patients; it has been proposed as an adjuvant analgesic for multifocal malignant bone pain.[143] However, clinical experience with it is limited and nephrotoxicity presents a problem.

Radiation Therapy

External radiotherapy

External beam irradiation is well established as a treatment of choice for localized bone pain associated with metastatic disease.[144,145] Prospective studies using validated patient assessments of pain have reported response rates of up to 90% and complete response rates of up to 45%.[146–151] The considerable variation in response rates is the result of varying methodology for measuring pain intensity, varied analgesic requirements, and the concurrent use of other treatment modalities. The analgesic mechanism of radiation is not clear, but may be secondary to tumor shrinkage and the inhibition of the release of chemical pain mediators from normal bone.[144,152] There may also be a direct effect on osteoclast activity. The degree of pain relief is independent of reduction in tumor size and cell kill. Wide individual variation is seen in reaction to radiation treatment, and parameters such as tumor histology, radiation dose, and type of irradiation do not appear to predict either response or duration of response.[153] There are limited data on length of response.

The optimal palliative dose and number of fractions remain controversial issues. Irradiation has traditionally been administered in multiple fractions over several days to weeks. Current evidence indicates that single fractions are as effective as multiple fractions when pain relief is the goal.[146,147,150,151] Response rates of 72%–90% have been reported. Moreover, single fractions are less demanding on the patient and resources. In a large prospective study, patients with a life expectancy of greater than 6 weeks were randomized to a single fraction of 8 Gy or 30 Gy over 2 weeks.[146] No difference could be seen between the 2 regimens, either for onset or duration of pain relief. Fifteen of the patients who received single fractions required repeat radiation to the painful site, whereas four of the patients who received multiple fractions required repeat radiation.

Small single doses of radiation for bone pain have also been reported.[150] Significantly better pain relief at 4 weeks with 8 Gy compared with 4 Gy was found. However, by 12 weeks, 8 Gy was only marginally superior. There was a significant increase in retreatment rate in the 4 Gy group. Pain relief with single doses, as with multiple fractions, generally occurs as soon as 48 hr after the start of radiotherapy, but may be seen up to 3 weeks after radiation.

Continued reservations concerning the use of single fractions for metastatic bone pain are based on doubts about efficacy and toxicity. However, these doubts are not well supported by the available data. There appears to be no difference in the incidence of side effects between single and multiple fraction regimens.[146] Only one prospective study[151] demonstrated differences in toxicity between single and multiple fractions. Concerns that a low total dose, as utilized in single-fraction regimens, will result in a higher relapse rate of pain is not well supported by data.[151] The recurrence rate of bone pain after single doses appears to be similar to that after multiple doses. Repeat radiation of an area previously radiated with a single fraction is feasible, particularly if there was a good response after the first treatment. One large prospective study[150] reported a 71% retreatment success rate after an initial single dose of 4 Gy, and 44% after a single dose of 8 Gy. Retreatment adverse effects appear to be minimal if the limits of radiation tolerance are not overstepped.[154]

Wide inter-individual variation in retreatment response has been noted. In a retrospective study, a total of 280 individual treatment sites were identified, of which 57 were retreated once and 8 were retreated twice.[155] The overall response rate to initial treatment was 84% for pain relief, and response at first retreatment was 87%. Seven of 8 patients retreated a second time also achieved some pain relief.

Other reasons for resisting the use of single fractions include the biases of departmental policy and training, attempts at promoting recalcification,[156,157] and reimbursement issues.[158] In general, single session palliative radiation therapy warrants wider adoption. However, fractionated regimens are the option of choice under certain circumstances, including lytic lesion liable to fracture (multi-fractions may promote recalcification) and spinal cord compression. The recommendation for multiple fractions in spinal cord compression is based on concern about acute edema during treatment with high doses, as well as the need to control soft tissue encroachment, which may be the underlying mechanism of compression.[32] Radiotherapy alone is effective in over 85% of cases of spinal cord compression if managed promptly.[159] There are, however, no valid randomized prospective studies comparing the effectiveness of surgical versus radiation decompression. Patients most suitable for management with radiation therapy are those with no structural compression or spinal instability, those with lesions of the cauda equina, those who are unfit for surgery, and those with multiple level compression. A wide variety of treatment schedules is used, but treatment often consists of a total of 20 Gy to 30 Gy distributed as 6–10 daily fractions over 1–2 weeks.[159]

Acute toxicity is dependent on the radiation dose and can either be confined to the irradiated area or present as a systemic effect, such as nausea or fatigue. Approximately 30% of patients experience nausea and vomiting.[144,145] Most studies suggest no difference in the frequency of this acute toxicity between single and multiple fractions. If the field involves extensive areas of bone marrow, myelosuppression may occur. Mucositis and dysphagia can result if the chest is irradiated. Severe reactions are not as common when palliative treatment uses smaller overall doses.[145]

Late damage to normal tissue can lead to progressive and irreversible changes. Structures such as the central nervous system, lung, kidney, the lens of the eye, and the microvasculature are especially vulnerable. Acute toxicity does not appear to predict late radiation damage. For terminally ill patients with a life expectancy of only weeks to months, the fear of late toxicity is not an issue in palliative radiation.

The prophylactic role of radiotherapy has not been well characterized. There may be a role for it in treating sites that appear to be at high risk for developing pathological fractures. Several retrospective studies have emphasized the importance of postoperative radiotherapy.[160,161] The rationale is the relief of local pain and the promotion of recalcification. In a patient with early vertebral collapse, it can be argued that it is not necessary to wait until the patient has pain or neurological symptoms and signs before giving radiotherapy.

Hemibody radiation

Hemibody radiation (HBI) offers an option in patients who require radiation to multiple sites. Excellent reported response rates are offset by a very high incidence of toxicity. Overall response rates of 73%–100% and complete response rates of 5%–57% have been reported in several studies.[162–168] Pain relief is often quite rapid, with the majority of patients responding within 48 hr. Proponents of this modality also suggest that local field irradiation can safely be given following HBI for those requiring retreatment.

HBI is conventionally given as a single fraction.[168] If both lower and upper body zones are to be radiated, sequential halves may be treated 4–6 weeks apart to allow hematological recovery. The potential for damage to the lungs limits the dose to the upper body to a single fraction of 6 Gy, while the maximum tolerated dose for the lower and mid hemibody is 8 Gy.[168]

The overall role of HIB is overshadowed by less toxic options such as the bisphosphonates. Because of the greater irradiated body volume, HBI-related toxicity is inevitably higher. This toxicity often includes nausea, vomiting, and diarrhea, particularly following lower hemibody treatment. Myelosuppression is not uncommon. Upper hemibody radiation may be associated with alopecia and pneumonitis. Although relatively infrequent ($\leq$ 16% of cases), pneumonitis is invariably fatal. HBI is not appropriate for patients with significantly reduced blood counts, those in generally poor condition, or those with a life expectancy of less than a few months.

Radioisotopes

Systemic administration of bone-seeking radioisotopes has been used to control pain associated with metastatic disease.[169–170] Several radioisotopes have been used for this purpose. Phosphorus (^{32}P) can be effective, but this drug shows nonspecific uptake in bone marrow and consequently causes significant bone marrow toxicity in 20% to 30% of cases.[171] Strontium chloride (^{89}Sr), a beta-particle-emitting calcium analogue, is preferentially taken up at sites of osteoblastic activity and is therefore best for tumors with increased osteoblastic activity such as prostate cancers.[169] Positive responses have also been noted in patients with primary breast and lung cancers.[169] It has been reported to relieve or reduce bone pain in 60%–90% of patients[172–176] and to yield complete pain relief in 10%–40%. Most studies have been small and non-comparative. In a placebo-controlled trial, the analgesic effect of ^{89}Sr was shown to be superior to placebo.[173]

A large randomized trial involving patients with painful metastatic prostatic cancer compared strontium with local irradiation and with hemibody radiation.[172] Pain relief a few months after treatment was similar in all groups. However, significantly fewer patients developed new painful sites after ^{89}Sr therapy, as compared with radiotherapy.

In another comparative study, ^{89}Sr was directly compared with external-beam radiation therapy.[175] Local field irradiation and ^{89}Sr were equally efficacious in reducing bone pain. At 12 weeks, 44.1% of the ^{89}Sr recipients and

36.4% of patients who received local field irradiation reported a dramatic reduction in pain. In another study, ^{89}Sr was evaluated as an adjuvant to local field irradiation.[176] There was no significant difference in survival or pain relief between the group that received ^{89}Sr and the group that did not, but the strontium recipients were less likely to develop new painful sites. Similar results were found in a comparison of ^{89}Sr and half body irradiation, and toxicity was lower in the ^{89}Sr–treated group.[177]

Repeated dosing with ^{89}Sr is not recommended at intervals of less than three months because of concerns for hematological toxicity. In most cases, pain relief begins in 10–20 days and lasts up to six months, and retreatment at a shortened interval is seldom needed. If the patient does not respond to the initial dose, it appears unlikely that a second administration will provide a favorable response.

The literature generally reports that adverse effects to systemic radioisotope administration tend to be mild to moderate.[170] One of the most common adverse effects reported is a transient increase in bone pain lasting 36–48 hours.[170] This "flare" response may be seen in 5% to 10% of patients one to two weeks after ^{89}Sr administration. It usually disappears within 48 hours and is often predictive of a positive clinical result. The majority of patients treated with ^{89}Sr have some reduction in platelet count. A reduction in the platelet count to <50 platelets/cu mm has been reported in 20%–30% of patients receiving ^{89}Sr, with the nadir occurring four to eight weeks after the injection.[170] Hemorrhage and excessive bruising have been observed only rarely. Reductions in the leukocyte count have also been reported.[120] Regular hematologic monitoring is therefore indicated for up to 12 weeks after therapy, and it is suggested that ^{89}Sr not be used in patients with initial platelet counts of <60000/cu mm or a leukocyte count of <2400 cells/cu mm.[170]

Generally, ^{89}Sr should be considered in patients with refractory multifocal pain caused by osteoblastic lesions. Eligible patients should have a life expectancy longer than three months, sufficient bone marrow reserve, and no further chemotherapy planned. The slow onset of effect makes this modality inappropriate as single therapy for patients with severe cancer pain. Clinical experience in the setting of palliative care and hospice does not seem to mirror the positive effects reported in the literature. Although it may be well tolerated in the short-term, data concerning late toxicity is very scant. Stratification of patients enrolled into these studies and the adequate quantification of toxicity and pain intensity are not well reported. In practice, it appears that ^{89}Sr may be less tolerated in patients with advanced cancer. Its role in these patients is overshadowed by other less toxic treatment modalities. Further drawbacks include high costs and the need for special precautions in handling, dispensing, and storage of the radioactive material and the urine of treated patients. Other isotopes, such as samarium ([153]Sm) and rhenium ([186]Re) are being investigated.[170,178] They appear to have a better side effect profile, a higher percentage of bone uptake, and a shorter half-life.

Hormonal Modalities

Cancers of the breast, prostate, and endometrium are, to varying degrees, responsive to hormonal manipulation.[179] Essentially, this therapy attempts to deprive tumor cells of the growth stimulus induced by hormones.

In prostate cancer, hormonal therapy can lead to sustained symptom relief in patients with widespread painful bone metastases.[7,180,181] It is estimated that this modality can relieve pain in more than 70%–80% of these patients for anywhere from 20 weeks to 2 years.[180] Hormonal manipulation can be affected by monotherapy or by combined therapy. Monotherapy attempts to either remove the testicular source of androgens by medical or surgical castration or to block the hormonal effects of androgens by administering an antiandrogen. In essence, combined therapy attempts to remove the testicular source of androgens (medical or surgical castration) and to block the effects of adrenal androgens with an antiandrogen.

Antiandrogens such as megesterol acetate and cyproterone acetate have steroidal structures while others such as flutamide are nonsteroidal. Flutamide acts peripherally rather than at the testicular or adrenal levels, and although it appears to cause an initial drop in prostatic dihydrotestosterone, the antiandrogen activity is later reversed by a compensatory increase in luteinizing hormone. Medical castration can be achieved by the administration of a luteinizing hormone–releasing hormone (LHRH) agonist such as leuprolide. There is an initial increase in testosterone production after initiating LHRH therapy. Because transient tumor growth can accompany this flare, it should not be given as monotherapy to patients with symptoms of cord compression. Castration levels of testosterone production are reached within 3–4 weeks. Surgical castration, on the other hand, has the advantage of a rapid onset of response–sometimes within hours or days. There is no convincing evidence that monotherapy, given early or late, alters the survival of patients with metastatic disease, and it is reasonable to delay monotherapy until the patient becomes symptomatic.

Combined therapy appears to offer no significant advantages over medical or surgical castration alone for patients with widespread bone or soft tissue involvement and poor performance status.[180] Responses to combined therapy in these patients are typically short. In patients without symptoms and with minimal bone metastases, combined therapy appears to give a longer duration of response (up to two years) and prolonged survival (up to six months) than monotherapy alone. However, the benefits of early initiation of androgen deprivation in asymptomatic patients with bone metastases compared with endocrine treatment delayed until complications or symptoms develop needs to be clarified. Unfortunately, most oncological trials do not focus on the assessment of symptoms as outcomes.

Recently, it has been suggested that a trial of flutamide withdrawal should be considered in patients with disease progression while on total androgen blockade (combined therapy) before more toxic therapies are initiated.[182] Second-line therapy after failure of androgen deprivation is rarely successful.[179] While hormonal therapy can provide substantial relief in prostate cancer, metastatic relapse is al-most inevitable. This can be explained by the presence of three different popula-tions of cells in normal and malignant prostatic epithelial cells: hormone–depend-ent, hormone–sensitive, and hormone–independent cells. Hormone–dependent cells die when androgen is withdrawn, and hormone–sensitive cells stop dividing until re-supplied with androgen. However, hormone–independent cells continue growing even after surgical castration and medical adrenalectomy.

The skeleton is the most common site of distant recurrence after primary treat-ment of breast cancer. Many patients with a first relapse confined to the skeleton are treated with endocrine therapy. Tamoxifen is the treatment of choice for post-menopausal women. Response to treatment is variable and ranges from 4% to 40%.[180] Such major differences in response rates might result from patient selec-tion and the fact that response assessment in the skeleton is difficult. Tamoxifen therapy may produce relief of metastatic bone pain in 50% of patients with estro-gen receptor–positive breast cancers, as compared with only 10% with estrogen re-ceptor–negative tumors.[179] If the receptor status is unknown, helpful predictors may be long disease-free intervals, late premenopausal or late postmenopausal status, bone and soft tissue metastases without visceral involvement, and slow pro-gression of metastatic lesions.[179] The optimal timing of initiation or discontinuation of this form of therapy is not well characterized. Hormonal therapy should be dis-continued where there is obvious rapid disease progression and deterioration of general status. Aminoglutethimide is an alternative where tamoxifen fails. Re-sponse rates to progestins, when used as a second-line therapy, also appears to vary considerably, ranging from 0% to 50% in phase 2 studies.

Chemotherapeutic Modalities

Chemotherapy has been used with limited success in the palliative treatment of pain associated with bone metastases.[183] High toxicity, coupled with poor effec-tiveness, has limited the general use of antineoplastic drugs in the management of malignant bone pain in patients with advanced cancer. The palliative benefit of chemotherapy is difficult to measure. Chemotherapy is usually reserved for endocrine-resistant disease in breast cancer patients with bone metastases. A review of several chemotherapy studies showed response rates ranging from 0% to 30%.[184] However, the low response rate in the skeleton compared with other sites of disease does not reflect the whole palliative effect, since patients occasion-ally experience pain relief without showing objective tumor response.[185]

Orthopedic Surgery

The major goals of orthopedic treatment are the control of pain and the mainte-nance of functional activity.[186] As with any treatment modality, the potential benefits of surgery need to be weighed against the potential risks and drawbacks; whether or not a patient should be referred for surgery depends on various factors, including the patient's overall fitness for surgery and the degree of pain and functional loss. In many cases, particularly those involving pathological fractures of the hips and lower extremities, surgery offers the only definitive therapy to control pain and provide mobility.[19] An expected survival of only weeks or months is not necessarily a contraindication to surgery. Surgical fixation of pathological fractures is best done with internal fixation using various devices such as intra- and extra-medullary pins, plates and screws, composite osteosynthesis, and hemi-joint replacements.[19] At the time of surgery, the tumor can be curetted and the defect filled with methyl methacrylate cement for strength.

Once a pathological fracture has occurred in the appendicular skeleton, surgical treatment should be considered. Up to 97% of patients with a pathological fracture have been reported to achieve good pain relief after internal fixation or prosthetic replacement.[187] Meticulous patient selection is paramount. A recent report suggested very poor success with rehabilitation in patients with Eastern Cooperative Oncology Group performance scores of 3 or more.[188]

Fractures of weight-bearing bones usually require surgical intervention. Pathological transcervical femoral fractures are usually treated with arthroplasty. If the acetabulum is involved, total hip replacement is indicated. Femoral shaft fractures are usually treated with an intramedullary nail, whereas fractures in the metaphysis may require plates and screws. Upper-extremity lesions are more amenable to bracing. Proximal humeral lesions can be supported with lightweight functional bracing. The majority of displaced humeral shaft and forearm pathological fractures, however, require intramedullary nailing.[189]

In the axial skeleton, conservative treatment of painful pathologic fractures usually suffices. Bones such as the vertebrae, clavicles, ribs, sternum, and pelvis have a good blood supply and heal more readily after fracture than do long bones. However, in a number of situations surgical management of spinal lesions may be necessary. These include the presence of neurological deficits that do not resolve rapidly with radiation therapy, bone destruction causing spinal instability, and vertebral body collapse resulting in retropulsion of bone fragments directly into the cord.[19,186] There are various surgical options. The treatment of choice appears to be anterior resection of the diseased vertebral body and reconstruction with bone grafting and fixation with instrumentation.[190] Where extreme instability is apparent, posterior instrumentation may be necessary. Radical resection of the vertebral body by a combined posterior and anterior and spinal reconstruction by internal fixation and grafting has been reported to be satisfactory in thoracic vertebral involvement.[191]

Postoperative irradiation is standard practice. However, the value of such treatment, especially in patients with a short life expectancy, has not been well documented. It appears to retard disease progression in the area. The optimal time for irradiation has not been clarified, but periods of two to six weeks after the fracture has occurred are commonly used.[192]

Prophylactic stabilization has been advocated in patients at high risk for pathological fracture.[19,193] A more conservative approach with radiotherapy was reported by one author to be as successful as surgery.[194] None of the patients with high risk osteolytic lesions developed pathological fractures after treatment with 30Gy given over 10 fractions.

In extreme and rare situations, palliative amputation of an extremity may be appropriate to provide pain control. This is particularly true of bulky, fungating, radio-resistant tumors exhibiting extensive soft tissue and bone involvement. Amputation or resection with reconstruction is occasionally the treatment of choice for primary bone tumors that have not metastasized.

An innovative approach to the treatment of fractures may involve the use of injectable bone mineral substitute. The fracture site is first anesthetized and a bone paste is injected into the checks of the fracture. The bone paste simply glues the fractured bone together and sets rapidly. This modality, however, has not been well reported and requires further evaluation.

Anesthetic and Neurosurgical Procedures

Local anesthetic blocks may provide analgesia where pain is localized to areas innervated by large, accessible nerves. Analgesia is achieved by blocking the primary afferent nerves.[195] The local anesthetic agent needs to be administered regularly. Data are limited to isolated case reports. Moreover, it is well recognized that chronic painful stimuli result in anatomical and biochemical changes within the central nervous system that cannot be reversed by peripheral nerve blockade. These changes, referred to as "plasticity" and "sensitization," are well documented and minimize the effectiveness of peripheral blocks.[196]

Intralesional methylprednisolone infiltration has been reported to be effective for painful metastatic lesions of the ribs.[197] In one study, this modality provided relief within 10 days in 70% of patients.[197] Pain recurred in about 10% of these patients. The procedure in this study involved an initial intercostal block with bupivacaine 0.5%, using up to 5 ml for each painful rib and a total maximum dose of 10 ml, followed by infiltration of the surrounding periosteum with 40 mg of methylprednisolone.[197] An alternative method of administering local anesthetic agents to painful rib lesions is by continuous infusion via pleural cavity catheters.[198,199] Potential complications include pneumothorax and overdose of the local anesthetic agents.

Continuous brachial plexus blocks, by various approaches, have been used to control upper limb pain.[200–202] Intermittent injections of a local anesthetic via a catheter in the supraclavicular area has been reported to control metastatic bone pain in the scapula.[195] Lumbar plexus blockade for analgesia of a pathological fracture of the femur is possible via an inguinal paravascular approach or a compartmental block.[195,203] Femoral nerve blocks have also been described.[204]

The use of the epidural or intrathecal routes for opioid administration has been advocated for patients with "intractable" pain and patients who are responsive to opioids but develop excessive side effects to oral or parenteral administration.[205–207] Advocates of this modality have reported that approximately 10% of patients with cancer pain may benefit from this form of opioid administration. Its mechanism is based on the concept of selective opioid binding to opioid receptors in the spinal cord.[208] However, some authors have reported the inability of this modality to control breakthrough and incident pain.[209,210] Additional analgesia may be obtained when low doses of a local anesthetic agent are added.[211] The addition of local anesthetics, however, may affect ambulation and bladder control. In selecting the appropriate analgesic for epidural or intrathecal administration, both the physical and chemical properties of the drug and its receptor and pharmacokinetic profiles need to be considered. Note that continuous epidural or intrathecal administration is associated with redistribution of drug to supraspinal sites via the cerebrospinal fluid and the systemic circulation.[212] Blood levels of epidural morphine may approach those achieved with parenteral dosing, losing the selective effect of spinal opioids.[213]

The widespread use of intraspinal therapy is limited by various factors, including very high cost, the need for specialized services, invasiveness, potential inconvenience, the potential for catheter blockage,[214] the risk of introducing infections into the spinal cord, and the lack of well demonstrated advantages over simpler methods such as systemic opioids. The availability of subcutaneous reservoirs to which the catheters are attached has decreased the incidence of infections and allowed patients to be fully ambulatory. Other difficulties arise with this route. Patients with back pain and vertebral body metastasis often have coexisting epidural metastases, which may complicate the use of spinal opioids.[36] Dose escalation may be required, and as patients require higher doses, the selective spinal effects of the drug can be lost.[213] This is particularly true when patients have received large doses of systemic opioids.[215] The conversion from systemic to epidural and spinal opioid administration still presents a dilemma.[216] Simple and effective strategies, such as opioid rotation, are available to manage the neuroexcitatory adverse effects of systemic opioids when they do arise, negating the need for spinal administration to minimize toxicity.[40] Ongoing studies, including comparative studies using appropriate clinical analgesic designs with clear definitions of intractable pain, are required to clarify the exact role of these techniques in cancer pain.

When all other treatment modalities have failed, unilateral destruction of the lateral spinothalamic tract in the anterolateral column of the cervical spinal cord has been advocated for pain relief.[217,218] This neurosurgical modality, referred to as a cordotomy, may be considered for unilateral incident pain below the waist and is generally done percutaneously under localized anesthesia at the level of the upper cervical spine. Analgesia has been reported to be prompt and significant in up to 90% of well-selected patients.[219] The potential for neurological complications, including hemiparesis, urinary retention, and the unmasking of contralateral pain, limit the applicability of this modality.[219] High complication rates limit the use of bilateral cordotomies. Apart from meticulous patient selection, the effectiveness of a cordotomy depends on physician expertise and patient endurance.

In the case of refractory chest or limb pain, segmental or multisegmental destruction of the dorsal sensory roots can be performed. Occasionally, neurolysis of a peripheral nerve is possible. Rhizotomy can be achieved by surgical section, chemical neurolysis, or radiofrequency. Chemical rhizotomy is produced by the instillation of a neurolytic solution into either the epidural or intrathecal space.[217] Satisfactory analgesia is reported in about 50% of patients, and the average duration of relief is 3–4 months. However, there is a high incidence of side effects, including paresis (5%–20%), sphincter dysfunction (5%–60%), impairment of touch and proprioception, and dysesthesias. In some cases, a severe neuropathic pain develops from irritation of the nerve roots. These adverse effects limit the use of this modality. Pituitary ablation has been suggested as a last resort to control refractory pain from disseminated bone metastases, but requires special expertise and is invasive.

Conclusion

Malignant bone pain is the result of a complex cascade of events, including osteolysis. Opioid analgesics remain the mainstay of pharmacological therapy for both localized and multifocal bone pain. Adjuvant analgesics must occasionally be added. The most commonly used are the corticosteroids and the NSAIDs. The specific role of NSAIDs in bone pain is not well documented and toxicity remains problematic. These drugs appear to be quite helpful in some cases. A newer generation of NSAIDs, more specific to the COX-2 enzyme, may circumvent these toxicities. External irradiation remains a key treatment modality for malignant bone pain, and the use of single fraction therapy for palliation should be adopted more widely. In the setting of multifocal bone pain, bisphosphonates as a group are useful, and their role in preventing skeletal events associated with metastatic bone disease needs to be considered more seriously. Future comparative studies should try to better define the role of other modalities, such as systemic radionuclide administration, hemibody irradiation, and anesthetic and neurosurgical modalities.

References

1. Vainio A, Auvinen A, Ahmedzai S, et al. Prevalence of symptoms among patients with advanced cancer: an International Collaborative Study. *J Pain Symptom Manage* 1996; 12:3–10.

2. *Cancer Pain Relief*, 2nd Ed. Geneva, Switzerland: World Health Organization, 1996.

3. Lote K, Walloe A, Bjersand A. Bone metastases: prognosis, diagnosis and treatment. *Acta Radiol Oncol* 1986; 25:227–232.

4. Galasko CSB. Skeletal metastases. *Clin Orthop* 1986; 210:18–30.

5. Koenders PG, Beex LV, Kloppenborg PWC, Smals AGH, Benraad THJ. Human breast cancer: survival from metastases. *Breast Cancer Res Treat* 1992; 21:173–180.

6. Nielson OS, Munro AJ, Tannock IF. Bone metastases: pathophysiology and management policy. *J Clin Oncol* 1991; 9:509–524.

7. Perez CA, Fair WR, Ihde DC. Carcinoma of the prostate. In: DeVita VT Jr, Heliman H, Rosenberg SA, eds. *Cancer: Principles and Practice of Oncology,* 3rd ed. Philadelphia: JB Lippincott Co., 1989:1023–1058.

8. Mundy GR. Mechanisms of osteolytic bone destruction. *Bone* 1991; 12(suppl 1):S1–S6.

9. Garrett IR. Bone destruction in cancer. *Semin Oncol* 1993; 20(suppl 2):4–9.

10. Front D, Schneck SO, Frankel A, Robinson E. Bone metastases and bone pain in breast cancer. *JAMA* 1979; 2242:1747–1748.

11. Osler MW, Vizel M, Turgeon LR. Pain of terminal cancer patients. *Arch Intern Med* 1978; 138:1801–1802.

12. Bennett A. The role of biochemical mediators in peripheral nociception and bone pain. *Cancer Surv* 1988; 7:55–67.

13. Hungerford DS. Bone marrow pressure and intramedullary venography. In: Owen R, Goodfellow J, Bullough P, eds. *Scientific Foundations of Orthopaedics and Traumatology*. London: Heinemann, 1980:357–361.

14. Aaron AD. The management of cancer metastatic to bone. *JAMA* 1994; 272:1206–1209.

15. Garfunkel L. Statistics and trends. In: Holleb AI, Fink DJ, Murphy GP, eds. *Textbook of Clinical Oncology*. Atlanta: American Cancer Society, 1991:1–6.

16. Portenoy RK, Hager N. Breakthrough pain: definition, prevalence and characteristics. *Pain* 1990; 41:273–283.

17. Bruera E, Schoeller T, Werk R, MacEachern T, Marcelino S, Suarez-Almazor M, Hanson J. A prospective multicenter assessment of the Edmonton staging system for cancer pain. *J Pain Symptom Manage* 1995; 5:348–355.

18. Helweg-Larsen S, Sorensen PS. Symptoms and signs in metastatic spinal cord compression: a study of progression from first symptom until diagnosis in 153 patients. *Eur J Cancer* 1994; 30:396–398.

19. Harrington KD. Orthopaedic management of metastatic bone disease. St. Louis, Mo. CV Mosby, 1988:7–14.

20. Fidler MW. Incidence of fracture through metastases in long bones. *Acta Orthop Scand* 1981; 52:623–627.

21. Ralston SH. Management of cancer-associated hypercalcemia. *Eur J Palliat Care* 1994; 1:170–174.

22. Grant R, Papadopoulos SM, Sandler HM, Greenberg HS. Metastatic epidural spinal cord compression: Current concepts and treatment. *J Neuro–Oncol* 1994; 19:79–92.

23. Rodichok LD, Ruekdeschel JC, Harper GR, Cooper G, Prevosti L, Fernando L, Baxter DH. Early detection and treatment of spinal epidural metastases: the role of myelography. *Ann Neurol* 1986; 20:696–702.

24. Frassica FJ, Gitelis S, Sim FH. Metastatic bone disease: general principles, pathophysiology, evaluation and biopsy. *Instr Course Lect* 1992; 41:293–300.
25. Peter JE. Skeletal imaging in metastatic disease. *Curr Opin Radiol* 1991; 3:791–796.
26. Wilkens RF. The selection of a nonsteroidal antiinflammatory drug. Is there a difference? *J Rheumatol* 1992; 19:9–12.
27. Mirels H. Metastatic disease in long bones. *Clin Orthop* 1989; 249:256–264.
28. Brown ML. Bone scintigraphy in benign and malignant tumors. *Radiol Clin North Am* 1993; 31:731–738.
29. Perez DJ, Milan J, Ford HT, et al. Detection of breast carcinoma metastases in bone. Relative merits of x-rays and skeletal scintigraphy. *Lancet* 1983; 2:613–616.
30. Gold RI, Seeger LL, Bassett LW, Steckel RJ. An integrated approach to the evaluation of metastatic bone disease. *Radiol Clin North Am* 1990; 28:471–483.
31. Portenoy RK, Lipton RB, Foley KM. Back pain in the cancer patient. An algorithm for evaluation and management. *Neurology* 1987; 37:134–138.
32. Pigott KH, Baddeley H, Maher EJ. Pattern of disease in spinal cord compression on MRI scan and implications for treatment. *Clin Oncol* 1994; 6:7–10.
33. Kattapuram SV, Khurana JS, Scott JA, Khourygy E. Negative scintigraphy with positive magnetic resonance imaging in bone metastases. *Skeletal Radiol* 1990; 19:113–116.
34. Jacobson H, Goransson H. Radiological detection of bone and bone marrow metastases. *Med Oncol Tumor Pharmacol Ther* 1991; 4:253–260.
35. Yamagucchi T, Tamai K, Yamato M, et al. Intertrabecular pattern of tumors metastatic to bone. *Cancer* 1996; 78:1288–1394.
36. Campa JA, Payne R. The management of intractable bone pain: a clinician's perspective. *Semin Nucl Med* 1992; 22:3–10.
37. Hanks GW. Pharmacological treatment of bone pain. *Cancer Surv* 1988; 7:87–101.
38. *Cancer pain: a monograph on the management of cancer pain*. Health and Welfare Canada: Minister of Supply and Services Canada, Ottawa. H42-2/5 1984E.
39. Portenoy RK. Management of common opioid side effects during long term therapy of cancer pain. *Ann Acad Med Singapore* 1994; 23:160–170.
40. Pereira J, Bruera E. Emerging neuropsychiatric toxicities of opioids. *J Pharm Care Pain Sympt Control* 1997; 5(4):3–29.
41. Pace V. Use of nonsteroidal anti-inflammatory drugs in cancer. *Palliat Med* 1995; 9:273–286.
42. Stambaugh JE. Role of non steroidal anti-inflammatory drugs in the management of cancer pain. In: Patt R, ed. *Cancer Pain*. Philadelphia: JB Lippincott Co., 1993:105–117.
43. Ventafridda V, Jamburini M, Caraceni A, et al. A validation study the WHO method for cancer pain relief. *Cancer* 1987; 59:850–856.
44. Ferrer-Brechner T, Ganz P. Combination therapy with ibuprofen and methadone for chronic cancer pain. *Am J Med* 1984; 77:78–83.
45. Sunshine A, Olson NZ. Analgesic efficacy of ketoprofen in postpartum, general surgery and chronic cancer pain. *J Clin Pharmacol* 1988; 28:S47–S54.
46. Martino G, Emanueli A, Mandelli V, Vertafridda V. A controlled study of the analgesic effect of two non-steroidal anti-inflammatory drugs in cancer pain. *Arzneim Forsche* 1978; 28:1657–1659.
47. Stambaugh JE, Drew J. A double-blind parallel evaluation of the efficacy and safety of a single dose of ketoprofen in cancer pain. *J Clin Pharmacol* 1988; 28:S34–S39.

48. Stambaugh JE, Tejada F, Trundowski RJ. Double-blind comparison of zomepirac and oxycodone with APC in cancer pain. *J Clin Pharmacol* 1980; 20:261–270.
49. Stambaugh JE, Sarajian C. Analgesic efficacy of Zomepirac sodium in patients with pain due to cancer. *J Clin Pharmacol* 1981; 21:501–507.
50. Ventafridda V. Diflusinal in the treatment of cancer pain. In: Huskisson EC, Calwell ADS, eds. *Diflusinal: New Perspectives in Analgesia.* London: Royal Society of Medicine, 1979:177–179.
51. Staquet MJ. A double blind study with placebo control of intramuscular ketorolac trumethamine in the treatment of cancer pain. *J Clin Pharmacol* 1989; 29:1031–1036.
52. Minotti V, Patoia L, Roila F, et al. Double-blind evaluation of analgesic efficacy of orally administered dicloferac, nefopam and acetylsalicylic acid (ASA) plus codeine in chronic cancer pain. *Pain* 1989; 36:177–183.
53. Stambaugh JE, Drew JA. The combination of ibuprofen and oxycodone/acetamino-phen in the treatment of chronic cancer pain. *Clin Pharmacol Ther* 1988; 44:665–669.
54. Tonachella R, Gallo Curcio C, Grossi E. Diclofenac sodium in cancer pain: a double blind within patients comparison with pentazocine. *Curr Ther Res* 1985; 37:1130–1133.
55. Carlson RW, Borrison RA, Sher HB, et al. A multi-institutional evaluation of the analgesic efficacy and safety of ketorolac tromethamine, acetaminophen plus co-deine, and placebo in cancer pain. *Pharmacotherapy* 1990; 10:211–216.
56. Weingart WA, Sorkness CA, Eahart RH. Analgesia with oral narcotics and added ibuprofen in cancer patients. *Clin Pharm* 1985; 4:53–58.
57. Ventafridda V, De Conno F, Panerai AE, Maresca V, Monzagc, Ripamonti C. Non-steroidal anti-inflammatory drugs as the first step in cancer pain therapy: double-blind, within-patient study comparing nine drugs. *J Int Med Res* 1990; 18:21–29.
58. Saxena A, Andley M, Granasekaran N. Comparison of piroxicam and acetyl salicylic acid for pain in head and neck cancers: a double-blind study. *Palliat Med* 1994; 8:223–229.
59. Ventafridda V, Toscani F, Tamburini M, et al. Sodium naproxen versus sodium diclofenac in cancer pain control. *Arzneim Forsche* 1990; 40:1132–1134.
60. Toscani F, Barosi K, Scazzina M, Camerini S, Gallucci M. Sodium naproxen: continu-ous subcutaneous infusion in neoplastic pain control. *Palliat Med* 1989; 3:207–211.
61. Hall E. Subcutaneous diclofenac: an effective alternative? [letter]. *Palliat Med* 1993; 7:339–340.
62. Blackwell N, Bangham L, Hughes M, Melzack D, Trotman I. Subcutaneous ketoro-lac—a new development in pain control. *Palliat Med* 1993; 7:63–65.
63. Myers KG, Trotman IF. Use of ketorolac by subcutaneous infusion for the control of cancer-related pain. *Postgrad Med J* 1994; 70:359–362.
64. Eisenberg E, Berkey CS, Carr DB, Mosteller F, Chalmes T. Efficacy and safety of nonsteroidal anti-inflammatory drugs for cancer pain: a meta-analysis. *J Clin Oncol* 1994; 12:2756–2765.
65. Max MB, Laska EM. Single-dose analgesic comparisons. In: Max M, Portenoy R, Laska E, eds. *Advances in Pain Research and Therapy*; Vol 18. New York: Raven Press Ltd, 1991:55–95.
66. Levick S. Jacobs C, Loukas DF, et al. Naproxen sodium in treatment of bone pain due to metastatic cancer. *Pain* 1988;35:353–358.

67. Sachetti G, Camera P, Rossi AP. Injectable ketoprofen vs acetyl salicylic acid for the relief of severe cancer pain: A double-blind trial. *Drug Intell Clin Pharm* 1984; 18:403–406.

68. Lomen PL, Samal BA, Lamborn KR. Flubiprofen for the treatment of bone pain in patients with metastatic breast cancer. *Am J Med* 1986; 80:83–87.

69. Ellis GA, Blake DR. Why are non-steroidal anti-inflammatory drugs so variable in their efficacy? A description of ion trapping. *BMJ* 1993; 10:241–243.

70. Ferreira SH. Prostaglandins, aspirin-like drugs and analgesia. *Nature [New Biol]* 1972; 240:200–203.

71. McCormack K. Non-steroidal anti-inflammatory drugs and spinal nociceptive processing. *Pain* 1994; 59:9–43.

72. Bjorkman R, Ullman A, Hedner J. Morphine-sparing effect of diclofenac in cancer pain. *Eur J Clin Pharmacol* 1993; 44:1–5.

73. Duncan A, Hardy JR, Davis CL. Subcutaneous ketorolac [letter]. *Palliat Med* 1995; 9:77–78.

74. Hollander D. Gastrointestinal complications of non-steroidal anti-inflammatory drugs: Prophylactic and therapeutic Strategies. *Am J Med* 1994; 96:274–280.

75. Simon L. Non-steroidal anti-inflammatory drug toxicity. *Curr Opin Rheumatol* 1993; 5:265–275.

76. Nuki G. Pain control and the use of non-steroidal analgesic anti-inflammatory drugs. *Br Med Bull* 1990; 46:262–278.

77. Whelton A, Hamilton CW. Nonsteroidal anti-inflammatory drugs: effects on kidney function. *J Clin Pharmacol* 1991;31:588–598.

78. Koch M, Dezi A, Ferrario F, Capurso L. Prevention of nonsteroidal anti-inflammatory drug-induced gastrointestinal mucosal injury: a meta-analysis of randomized controlled clinical trials. *Arch Intern Med* 1996; 156:2321–2332.

79. Friedel HA, Langtry HD, Buckley MM. Nabumetone: a reappraisal of its pharmacology and therapeutic use in rheumatic diseases. *Drugs* 1993; 45:131–156.

80. Xie W, Robertson DL, Simmons D. Mitogen-inducible prostaglandin G/H Synthase: a new target for nonsteroidal antiinflammatory drugs. *Drug Dev Res* 1992; 25:249–253.

81. Glaser K, Sung ML, O'Neill K, et al. Etodolac selectively inhibits human prostaglandin G/H Synthase 2 (PGHS-2) versus human PGHS-1. *Eur J Pharm* 1995; 281:107–111.

82. Watanabe S, Bruera E. Corticosteroids as adjuvant analgesics. *J Pain Symptom Manage* 1994; 9:442–445.

83. Twycross R. The risks and benefits of corticosteroids in advanced cancer. *Drug Saf* 1994; 11:163–178.

84. Bruera E, Roca E, Cedaro L, Carraro S, Chacon R. Action of oral methylprednisolone in terminal cancer patients: a prospective randomized double-blind study. *Cancer Treat Rep* 1985; 69:751–754.

85. Haynes JRC. Adrenocortical steroids. In: Goodman R, et al., eds. *The Pharmacological Basis of Therapeutics*. New York: Pergamon Press, 1990:1436–1458.

86. Levy M. Pharmacological treatment of cancer pain. *N Engl J Med* 1996; 335:1124–1132.

87. Vecht CJ, Haaxma-Reiche H, van Putten WLJ, et al. Initial bolus of conventional versus high-dose dexamethasone in metastatic spinal cord compression. *Neurology* 1989; 39:1255–1257.

88. Grant R, Papadopoulos SM, Sandler HM, Greenberg HS. Metastatic epidural spinal cord compression: current concepts and treatment. *J Neurooncol* 1994; 19:79–92.

89. Stiefel FC, Breitbart WS, Holland JC. Corticosteroids in cancer: neuropsychiatric complications. *Cancer Invest* 1989; 7:479–491.

90. Conn HO, Poynard T. Corticosteroids and peptic ulcer: meta-analysis of adverse events during steroid therapy. *J Intern Med* 1994; 236:619–632.

91. Piper JM, Ray WA, Daugherty JR, Griffin MR. Corticosteroid use and peptic ulcer disease: role of nonsteroidal anti-inflammatory drugs. *Ann Intern Med* 1991; 114:735–740.

92. Coleman R, Purohit K, Vinholes J. New roles for bisphosphonates in cancer therapy. *Prog Palliat Care* 1996; 4:39–43.

93. Body JJ. Pathophysiology of osteolysis: the putative mode of action of bisphosphonates. *Eur J Palliat Care* 1994; 1:116–120.

94. Lahtinen R, Laakso M, Palva I, et al. Randomized, placebo-controlled multicentre trial of clodronate in multiple myeloma. *Lancet* 1992; 340:1049–1052.

95. McClosky EV, MacLennan ICM, Drayson M, Chapman C, Dunn J, Kanis JA. Effect of clodronate on progression of skeletal disease in multiple myelomatosis. *Eur J Cancer* 1995; 31A(suppl 5):162.

96. Berenson JR, Lichterstein A, Porter L, et al. Efficacy of pamidronate in reducing skeletal events in patients with advanced multiple myeloma. *N Engl J Med* 1996; 334:488–493.

97. Cascinu S, Casadei V, Del Forro E, Alexandroni P, Catalano G. Pamidronate in patients with painful bone metastases who failed initial treatment with hormones and/or chemotherapy. *Support Care Cancer* 1996; 4:31–33.

98. Paterson AHG, Powles TJ, Kanis JA, et al. Double-blind controlled trial of oral clodronate in patients with bone metastases from breast cancer. *J Clin Oncol* 1993; 11:59–65.

99. van Holten-Verzantvoort ATM, Kroon HM, Bijvoet OLM, et al. Palliative pamidronate treatment in patients with bone metastases from breast cancer. *J Clin Oncol* 1993; 11:491–498.

100. Conte PF, Latreille J, Mauriac F, et al. Delay in progression of bone metastases in breast cancer patients treated with intravenous pamidronate: results from a multinational randomized control trial. *J Clin Oncol* 1996; 14:2552–2559.

101. van Holten-Verzantvoort ATM, Zwinderman AH, Aaronson NK, et al. The effect of supportive pamidronate treatment on aspects of quality of life of patients with advanced breast cancer. *Eur J Cancer* 1991; 27:544–549.

102. Hortobagyi GN, Thierault RL, Porter L, et al. Efficacy of pamidronate in reducing skeletal complications in patients with breast cancer and lytic bone metastases. *N Engl J Med* 1996; 335:1785–1791.

103. van Holten-Verzantvoort ATM, Hermans J, Beex LVAM, et al. Does supportive Pamidronate treatment prevent or delay the first manifestations of bone metastases in breast cancer patients? *Eur J Cancer* 1996; 32A(3):450–454.

104. van Holten-Verzantvoort ATM, Bijvoet OLM, Cleton FJ, et al. Reduced morbidity from skeletal metastases in breast cancer patients during long term bisphosphonate (APD) treatment. *Lancet* 1987; 2:983–985.

105. Ernst DS, MacDonald N, Paterson AHG, Jenson J, Brasher P, Bruera E. A double blind, crossover trial of intravenous clodronate in metastatic bone pain. *J Pain Symptom Manage* 1992; 7:4–11.

106. Vinholes J, Guo C-Y, Purohit OP, et al. Metabolic effects of pamidronate in patients with metastatic bone disease. *Br J Cancer* 1996; 73:1089–1095.
107. Purohit OP, Radstone CR, Anthony C, et al. A randomized double-blind comparison of intravenous pamidronate and clodronate in the hypercalcemia of malignancy. *Br J Cancer* 1995; 72:1289–1293.
108. Lipton A, Glover D, Harvey H, Grabelsky S, et al. Pamidronate in the treatment of bone metastases: results of 2 dose-ranging trials in patients with breast or prostate cancer. *Ann Oncol* 1994; 5(suppl 7):531–535.
109. Merlini G, Parrinello GA. Long-term effect of parenteral dichloromethylene bisphosphonate on bone disease of myeloma patients treated with chemotherapy. *Hematol Oncol* 1990; 8:23–30.
109. Clarke NW, Holbrook J, McClure J, et al. Osteoclast inhibition by pamidronate in metastatic prostate cancer: a preliminary study. *Br J Cancer* 1991; 63:420–423.
110. Adami S, Salvagno G, Guerrera G. Dichloromethylene diphosphonate in patients with prostatic carcinoma metastatic to the skeleton. *J Urol* 1985; 134:1152–1154.
111. Belch AR, Bergsagel DE, Wilson K, et al. Effect of daily Etidronate on the osteolysis of multiple myeloma. *J Clin Oncol* 1991; 9:1397–1402.
112. Purohit OP, Anthony C, Radstone CR, Owen J, Coleman RE. High-dose intravenous Pamidronate for metastatic bone pain. *Br J Cancer* 1994; 70:554–558.
113. Thurlimann B, Morant R, Jungi WF, Radziwill A. Pamidronate for pain control in patients with malignant osteolytic bone disease: a prospective dose-effect study. *Support Care Cancer* 1994; 2:61–65.
114. Coleman RE, Woll PJ, Miles M, et al. Treatment of bone metastases from breast cancer with 3-amino-1-hydroxypropylidene)-1, 1-bisphosphonate (APD). *Br J Cancer* 1988; 58:621–625.
115. Thiebaud D, Leyvraz S, von Fliedner V, et al. Treatment of bone metastases from breast cancer and myeloma with pamidronate. *Eur J Cancer* 1991; 27:37–41.
116. Glover D, Lipton A, Keller A, et al. Intravenous Pamidronate disodium treatment for bone metastases in patients with breast cancer: a dose seeking study. *Cancer* 1994; 74:2949–2955.
117. Elomaa I, Blomquist C, Grohn P, et al. Long-term controlled trial with diphosphonate in patients with osteolytic bone metastases. *Lancet* 1983; 1:146–149.
118. Adami S, Miar M. Clodronate therapy of metastatic bone disease in patients with prostatic carcinoma. *Cancer Res* 1989; 116:67–72.
119. Vorreuther R. Bisphosphonates as an adjunct to palliative therapy of bone metastases from prostate carcinoma. A pilot study on clodronate. *Br J Urology* 1993; 72:792–795.
120. Elomaa I, Kylmala T, Tammela T, et al. Effect of oral clodronate on bone pain: a controlled study in patients with metastatic prostate cancer. *Int Urol Nephrol* 1992; 24:159–166.
121. Robertson AG, Reed NS, Ralston SH. Effect of oral clodronate on metastatic bone pain: a double-blind, placebo controlled study. *J Clin Oncol* 1995; 13:2427–2430.
122. Portenoy RK. Adjuvant analgesic agents. In: Cherny N, Foley K, eds. *Hematol Oncol Clin North Am: Pain and Palliative Care* 1996; 10:103–119.
123. Walker P, Watanabe S, Lawlor P, Hanson J, Pereira J, Bruera E. Subcutaneous clodronate: A study evaluating efficacy in hypercalcemia of malignancy and local toxicity. *Ann Oncol* 1997; 8:915–916.

124. Ralston SH, Gallacher SJ, Patel U, et al. Comparison of three intravenous bisphos-phonates in cancer-associated hypercalcemia. *Lancet* 1989; 2:1180–1182.

125. Vinholes J, Guo C-Y, Purohit OP, et al. Evaluation of new bone resorption markers in a randomized comparison of pamidronate or clodronate for hypercalcemia of malignancy. *J Clin Oncol* 1997; 15:131–138.

126. Clemens MR, Fessele K, Heim ME. Multiple myeloma: effect of daily dichloro-methyle bisphosphonate on skeletal complications. *Ann Hematol* 1993; 66 141–146.

127. Kanis JA, Powles T, Paterson AHG, et al. Clodronate decreases the frequency of skeletal metastases in women with breast cancer. *Bone* 1996; 19:663–667.

128. Man Z, Otero AB, Rendo P, et al. Use of pamidronate for multiple myeloma osteolytic lesions. *Lancet* 1990; 335:663.

129. Richards MA, Braysher S, Gregory WM, et al. Advanced breast cancer: use of resources and cost implications. *Br J Cancer* 1993; 67:856–860.

130. Biermann WA, Cantor RI, Fellin FM, et al. An evaluation of the potential cost reductions resulting from the use of clodronate in the treatment of metastatic carcinoma of the breast bone. *Bone* 1991; 12 suppl 1, S37–S42.

131. McIntyre E, Bruera E. Symptomatic hypocalcemia after intravenous pamidronate. *J Palliat Care* 1996; 12:46–47.

132. Jodrell DJ, Iveson TJ, Smith IE. Symptomatic hypocalcemia after treatment with high-dose aminohydroxypropylidere diphosphonate. *Lancet* 1987; I: 622.

133. Tyrrell CJ, Bruning PF, May-Levi F, et al. Role of pamidronate in the management of bone metastases from breast cancer: Results of a non-comparative multicenter phase II trial. *Ann Oncol* 1994; 5(suppl 7):S37–S40.

134. Tyrrell CJ, Collinson M, Madsen EL, et al. Intravenous pamidronate: infusion rate and safety. *Ann Oncol* 1994; 5(Suppl 7):27–29.

135. Coleman RE, Rubers RD, Rose C, et al. A randomized phase II evaluation of oral pamidronate for advanced bone metastases from breast cancer. *Breast* 1995; 4:235.

136. Daley-Yates PT, Dodwell DJ, Pongchaidecha M, et al. The clearance and bioavail-ability of pamidronate in patients with breast cancer and bone metastases. *Calcif Tissue Int* 1991; 49:433–435.

137. DeGroen PC, Lubbe DF, Hirsch L, et al. Esophagitis associated with the use of alendronate. *N Engl J Med* 1996; 335:1016–1021.

138. Burkhardt P. Ibandronate in oncology. *Cancer* 1997; 80(suppl 8):1696–1698.

140. Roth A, Kolaric K. Analgesic activity of calcitonin in patients withe painful osteolytic metastases of breast cancer: Results of a controlled randomized study. *Oncology* 1986; 43:283–286.

141. Hindley AC, Hill AB, Leyland MJ, et al. A double-blind controlled trial of salmon calcitonin in pain due to malignancy. *Cancer Chemother Pharmacol* 1982; 9:71–74.

142. Szanto J, Ady N, Jozef S. Pain killing with calcitonin nasal spray in patients with malignant tumors. *Oncology* 1992; 49:180–182.

143. Warrell RP, Lovett D, Dilmarian FA, et al. Low-dose gallium nitrate for prevention of osteolysis in myeloma: results of a pilot randomized study. *J Clin Oncol* 1993; 11:2443–2446.

144. Hoskin PJ. Radiotherapy for bone pain. *Pain* 1995; 63:137–139.

145. Ashby M. Radiotherapy in the palliation of cancer. In: Patt RB, ed. *Cancer Pain.* Philadelphia: JB Lippincott Co. 1993:235–249.

146. Price P, Hoskin PJ, Easton D, et al. Prospective randomized trial of single and multifraction radiotherapy schedules in the treatment of painful bony metastases. *Radiother Oncol* 1986; 6:247–255.

147. Price P, Hoskin PJ, Easton D, et al. Low dose single fraction radiotherapy in the treatment of metastatic bone pain: a pilot study. *Radiother Oncol* 1988; 12:297–300.

148. Okawa T, Kita M, Goto M, et al. Randomized prospective clinical study of small, larger and twice-a-day fraction radiotherapy for painful bone metastases. *Radiother Oncol* 1988; 13:99–104.

149. Madsen LE. Painful bone metastases. Efficacy of radiotherapy assessed by the patients: A randomized trial comparing 4 gy × 6 versus 10 gy × 2. *Int J Radiat Oncol Biol Phys* 1983; 9:1775–1779.

150. Hoskin PJ, Price P, Easton D, et al. A prospective randomized trial of 4 gy or 8 gy single doses in the treatment of metastatic bone pain. *Radiother Oncol* 1992; 23:74–78.

151. Cole DJ. A randomized trial of a single treatment versus conventional fractionation in the palliative radiotherapy of painful bone metastases. *Clin Oncol* 1989; 1:59–62.

152. Poulson HS, Nielson OS, Klee M, et al. Palliative irradiation of bone metastases. *Cancer Treat Rev* 1989; 16:41–48.

153. Arcangeli G, Micheli A, Giannarelli D, et al. The responsiveness of bone metastases to radiotherapy. The effect of site, histology and radiation done on pain relief. *Radiother Oncol* 1989; 14:95–101.

154. Maher E. The use of palliative radiotherapy in the management of breast cancer. *Eur J Cancer* 1992; 28:206–210.

155. Mithal N, Needham PR, Hoskin PJ. Retreatment with radiotherapy for painful bone metastases. *Int J Radiation Oncol Biol Phys* 1994; 29:1011–1014.

156. Crellin AM, Marks A, Maher EJ. Why don't British radiotherapists give single fractions of radiotherapy for bone metastases? *Clin Oncol* 1989; 1:63–66.

157. Priestman TJ. Palliative radiotherapy in the UK. In: Mackillop W, Kirkbride P, eds. *Controversies in Palliative Radiotherapy. Can J Oncol* 1996; 6(suppl 1):69–73.

158. Coia LR. Palliative radiation therapy in the United States. In: MacKillop W, Kirkbride P, eds. *Controversies in Palliative Radiotherapy. Can J Oncol* 1996; 6(suppl 1):62–68.

159. Janjan NA. Radiotherapeutic management of spinal metastases. *J Pain Symptom Manage* 1996; 11:47–56.

160. Blake DD. Radiation treatment of metastatic bone disease. *Clin Orthop* 1970; 73:89–100.

161. Galasko CSB. The management of skeletal metastases. *J R Coll Surg Edinb* 1980; 25:143–161.

162. Hoskin PJ, Ford HT, Harmer CL. Hemibody irradiation (HBI) for metastatic bone pain in two histologically distinct groups of patients. *Clin Oncol* 1989; 1:67–69.

163. Rowland CG, Bullimore JA, Smith PJB, Roberts JBM. Half-body irradiation in the treatment of metastatic prostatic carcinoma. *Br J Urol* 1981; 53:628–629.

164. Salazar OM, Rubin P, Keller B, Scarantino C. Systemic (half-body) radiation therapy: response and toxicity. *Int J Radiat Oncol Biol Phys* 1978; 4:937–950.

165. Wilkins MF, Keer CW. Hemibody radiotherapy in the management of metastatic carcinoma. *Clin Radiol* 1987; 38:267–268.

166. Kuban DA, Delbridge T, El-Mahdi AM, Schellhammer PF. Half-body irradiation for the treatment of widely metastatic adenocarcinoma of the prostate. *J Urol* 1989; 141:572–574.

167. Zelefsky MJ, Scher HI, Forman JD, et al. Palliative hemiskeletal irradiation for widespread metastatic prostate cancer: a comparison of single dose and fractionated regimes. *Int J Radiat Oncol Biol Phys* 1989; 17:1281–1285.

168. Salazar OM, Rubin P, Hendrickson FR, et al. Single-dose half-body irradiation for palliation of multiple bone metastases from solid tumors. *Cancer* 1986; 58:24–36.

169. Robinson RG, Preston DF, Margi Schiefelbain BHS, Baxter K. Strontium-89 therapy for the palliation of pain due to osseous metastases. *JAMA* 1995; 274:420–424.

170. Nightengale B, Brune M, Blizzard S, et al. Strontium chloride Sr^{89} for treating pain from metastatic bone disease. *Am J Health - Syst Pharm* 1995; 52:2189–2195.

171. Silverstein EB. The treatment of painful osseous metastases with phosphorus-32-labeled phosphates. *Semin Oncol* 1993; 20(suppl 3):10–21.

172. Quilty PM, Kirk D, Bolger JJ, et al. A comparison of the palliative effects of strontium-89 and external beam radiotherapy in metastatic prostate cancer. *Radiother Oncol* 1994; 31:33–40.

173. Lewington VJ, McEwan AJB, Ackery DM, et al. A prospective, randomized double-blind crossover study to examine the efficacy of strontium-89 in pain palliation in patients with advanced prostate cancer metastatic to bone. *Eur J Cancer* 1991; 27:954–958.

174. Laing AH, Ackery DM, Bayly RJ, et al. Strontium-89 chloride for pain palliation in prostate skeletal malignancy. *Br J Radiol* 1991; 64:816–822.

175. The correct reference is: Bolger JJ, Dearnaley DP, Kirk D, et al. Strontium 89 (Metastron) versus external beam radiotherapy in patients with painful bone metastases secondary to prostatic cancer: a preliminary report of a multicenter trial. *Semin Oncol* 1993; 20(Suppl 2):32–33.

176. Porter AT, McEvan AJB, Powe JE, et al. Results of a randomized phase III trial to evaluate the efficacy of strontium-89 adjuvant to local field external beam irradiation in the management of endocrine resistant metastatic prostate cancer. *Int J Radiat Oncol Biol Phys* 1993; 25:805–813.

177. Dearnaley DP, Bayly RJ, A'Hern RP, et al. Palliation of bone metastases in prostate cancer. Hemibody irradiation or strontium-89. *Clin Oncol* 1992; 4:101–107.

178. Maxon HR, Thomas SR, Hertzbeg VS, et al. Rhenium-186 hydroxyerhylidase 6. Disphosphonate for the treatment of painful osseous metastases. *Semin Nucl Med*, 1992; XXII:33–40.

179. Wood BC. Hormone treatments in the common "hormone dependent" carcinomas. *Palliat Med* 1993; 7:257–272.

180. Dearnaley DP. Cancer of the prostate. *BMJ* 1994; 308:780–784.

181. Gallagher CJ. The role of gondotrophin-releasing hormone analogues in the management of prostate cancer (Editorial). *Clin Oncol* 1992; 4:137–138.

182. Scher HI, Kelly WK. Flutamide withdrawal syndrome: its impact on clinical trials in hormone-refractory prostate cancer. *J Clin Oncol* 1993; 11:1566–1572.

183. Kearsley JH. Some basic guidelines in the use of chemotherapy for patients with incurable malignancy. *Palliat Med* 1994; 8:11–17.

184. Whitehouse JMA. Site-dependent response to chemotherapy for carcinoma of the breast. *J R Soc Med* 1985; 78(suppl 9):18–22.

185. Hoy AM. Radiotherapy, chemotherapy and hormone therapy: treatment for pain. In: Well PD, Melzack R, eds. *Textbook of Pain*. Edinburgh: Churchill Livingstone, 1989:966–978.

186. Rosier RN. Orthopedic management of cancer pain. In: Patt RB, ed. *Cancer Pain*. Philadelphia: JB Lipincott Co., 1993:461–468.

187. Habermann ET. The pathology and treatment of metastatic disease of the femur. *Clin Orthop* 1982; 169:70–82.

188. McNamara P, Sharma K. Fractures in the palliative setting: a study of management and outcome. *Palliat Med* 1996; 10(1):59.

189. Pritchard DJ. Pathological fractures of the humerus. *Orthopedics* 1992; 15:557–562.

190. Siegel T. Vertebral body resection of epidural compression by malignant tumor. Results of forty-seven consecutive operative procedures. *J Bone Joint Surg* 1985; 67A:375–382.

191. Fidler MW. Radical resection of vertebral body tumours. *J Bone Joint Surg* 1994; 76B:765–772.

192. Galasko CSB. Orthopedic principles and management. In: Doyle D, Hanks GW, MacDonald N, eds. *Oxford Textbook of Palliative Medicine*. Oxford: Oxford Medical Publications, 1993; 274–282.

193. Keene JS, Sellinger DS, McBeath AA, Engber WD. Metastatic breast cancer in the femur: a search for the lesion at risk for fracture. *Clin Orthop* 1986; 203:282–288.

194. Cheng DS, Seitz CB, Eyre HJ. Nonoperative management of femoral, humeral and acetabular metastases in patients with breast carcinoma. *Cancer* 1980; 45:1533–1537.

195. Mercadante S. Analgesic blocks in palliative care. *Eur J Palliat Care* 1995; 2:103–106.

196. Hanks GW, Justins DM. Cancer pain: management. *Lancet* 1992; 339:1031–1036.

197. Rowell NP. Intralesional methylprednisolone for rib metastases: an alternative to radiotherapy? *Palliat Med* 1988; 2:153–155.

197. Myers DP, Lema MJ, de Leon-Casasola OA, et al. Intrapleural analgesia for the treatment of severe cancer pain in terminally ill patients. *J Pain Symptom Manage* 1993; 8:505–510.

199. Aguilar JL, Montes A, Samper D, et al. Interpleural analgesia through a DuPen catheter in lung cancer pain. *Cancer* 1992; 7:2621–2623.

200. Pham-Dang C, Meunier JF, Poirier P, et al. A new axillary approach for continuous brachial plexus block. A clinical and anatomic study. *Anesth Analg* 1995; 81:686–693.

201. Cooper MG, Keneally JP, Kinchington D. Continuous brachial plexus neural blockade in a child with intractable cancer pain. *J Pain Symptom Manage* 1994; 9:277–281.

202. Sato S, Yamashita S, Iwai M, et al. Continuous interscalene block for cancer pain. *Reg Anesth* 1994; 19:73–75.

203. Woodham MJ, Hanna M. Psoas compartment block in malignant pain. *Pain Clin* 1988; 2:219–224.

204. Khor KE, Ditton JN. Femoral nerve blockade in the multidisciplinary management of intractable localized pain due to metastatic tumor: a case report. *J Pain Symptom Manage* 1996; 11:57–60.

205. Devulder J, Ghys L, Dhondt W, et al. Spinal analgesia in terminal care: risk versus benefit. *J Pain Symptom Manage* 1994; 9:75–81.
206. Boys L, Peat SJ, Hanna MH, et al. Audit of neural blockade for palliative care patients in an acute unit. *Palliat Med* 1993; 7:205–211.
207. Samuelsson H, Malmberg F, Eriksson M, et al. Outcomes of epidural morphine treatment in cancer pain: nine years of clinical experience. *J Pain Symptom Manage* 1995; 10:105–112.
208. Yaksh TL. Spinal opiate analgesics: characteristics and principles of action. *Pain* 1981; 11:293–346.
209. Arner S, Amer B. Differential effects of epidural morphine in the treatment of cancer-related pain. *Acta Anaesthesiol Scand* 1985; 29:32–36.
210. Samuelsson H, Hedner T. Pain characterization in cancer patients and the analgesic response to epidural morphine. *Pain* 1991; 46:3–8.
211. Du Pen SL, Kharasch ED, Williams A, et al. Chronic bupivacaine–opioid infusion in intractable cancer pain. *Pain* 1992; 49:293–300.
212. Moulin DE, Inturrisi CE, Foley KM. Epidural and intrathecal opioids: cerebrospinal fluid and plasma pharmacokinetics in cancer pain patients. In: Foley KM, Inturrisi CE, ed. *Advances in Pain Research and Therapy*, Vol 8: *Opioid Analgesics in the Management of Clinical Pain*. New York: Raven Press, 1986:369–384.
213. Foley KM. Pharmacologic approaches to cancer pain management. In: Fields HL, Dulner R, Cervero F, eds. *Advances in Pain Research and Therapy, Vol 9*. New York: Raven Press, 1984:629–653.
214. Tanelian DL, Cousins MJ. Failure of epidural opioid to control cancer pain in a patient previously treated with massive doses of intravenous opioid. *Pain* 1989; 36:359–362.
215. Aldrete JA. Epidural fibrosis after permanent catheter insertion and infusion. *J Pain Symptom Manage* 1995; 10:624–631.
216. Du Pen SL, Williams AR. The dilemma of conversion from systemic to epidural morphine: a proposed conversion tool for treatment of cancer pain. *Pain* 1994; 56:112–118.
217. Cherny N, Arbit E, Jain S. Invasive techniques in the management of cancer pain. In Cherny N, Foley KM, eds. *Hematology Oncology Clinics in North America: Pain and Palliative Care*. Philadelphia: WB Saunders, 1996:10:121–137.
218. Tasker R. Neurosurgical and neuroaugmentative intervention. In Patt RB, ed. *Cancer Pain*. Philadelphia: JB Lippincott Co., 1993:471–500.
219. Sanders M, Zuurmond W. Safety of unilateral and bilateral percutaneous cervical cordotomy in 80 terminally ill cancer patients. *J Clin Oncol* 1995; 13:1509–1512.

5

Role of Bisphosphonates and Other Bone Resorption Inhibitors in Metastatic Bone Pain

D. SCOTT ERNST

Bone metastases are a frequent occurrence in patients with advanced cancer, usually developing from primary malignancies of the breast, prostate, and lung.[1–3] Indeed, autopsy studies suggest that bone metastases occur in up to 85% of patients who die from these primaries.[4] Other primary tumors, such as kidney, bladder, and neoplasms of the gastrointestinal tract, also metastasize to bone and account for up to 20% of those patients with bone lesions.[3] Of the hematological malignancies, multiple myeloma typically has extensive bone involvement, which contributes significantly to the morbidity of the disease.[2]

Survival after the development of bone disease is quite variable. In patients with breast and prostate cancer, the median survival with metastatic bone disease is approximately two years.[2,5,6,7] The development of bone involvement in renal, lung, and gastrointestinal tract malignancies is ominous, and life expectancy is generally less than six months.[1] Irrespective of survival, complications due to the bone disease often contribute greatly to the morbidity of the malignancy and can severely impair the quality of life for these patients.[8–10]

Pathogenic Mechanisms

Bone pain is the most common sequela of metastatic bone disease.[11] Nonetheless, other problems, such as pathological fractures, spinal cord compression, nerve root entrapment, hypercalcemia, and general debility, can also develop and contribute significantly to the morbidity of the malignant disease.[3] Pain may be a predominant feature of any one or all of these complications and, therefore, the optimal management of the various pain syndromes associated with metastatic bone disease often becomes a central component in patients' overall oncological and symptom control.[9]

Most bone metastases are not painful and the discomfort experienced by the patient may be independent of the anatomical location, extent, or appearance of the metastatic bone lesions. Extensive axial or appendicular skeletal lesions may cause only mild pain which can be easily controlled, or may cause unrelenting symptoms refractory to a variety of management strategies.[12] Lytic or blastic bone disease can be equally debilitating.[2,13–15]

Pain from bone metastases can occur through a variety of mechanisms. Local osteolysis can result in bone pain and is likely mediated through interaction between the tumor and the bone mineral and cellular infrastructure.[10] Bone destruction is mediated principally by osteoclasts, which are stimulated either directly through mediators produced by the tumor, such as the osteoclast activating factor produced by some lymphomas and multiple myeloma, or indirectly by products which stimulate intermediary cells leading to osteoclast activation.[15–17] Local bone destruction results in release of chemical mediators, such as histamine, bradykinins, and substance P, which may stimulate nociceptive nerve endings in the endosteum.[18] Prostaglandins may also play a pathogenic role by sensitizing free nerve endings to the various vasoactive amines and kinins released.[19] The precise interaction between tumor and bone microenvironment is unknown.

Distortion of the periosteum and stimulation of mechanoreceptors, either by enlarging tumor mass or surrounding edema, may result in pain.[20] Direct tumor extension into surrounding tissues may cause pain through nerve or root entrapment syndromes or spinal cord compression.[1,21,22] Localized pain can occur with the development of micro- or macropathological fractures and regional muscle spasms.[9]

It is useful for the clinician to differentiate among the potential mechanisms, as there are different approaches to management. Of particular importance is ruling out the possibility of nerve root or spinal cord compression. Early intervention may avert the development of progressive neurological dysfunction and concomitant neuropathic pain.[23–25]

Clinical Characteristics

Bone pain is often described by patients as a dull ache localized to a specific osseous site, which may be aggravated with movement, weight bearing, or both. Some patients report more intense discomfort at night. Local bony tenderness may be present.[25,26] Incident pain is characteristic of bone pain, and can best be defined as pain that intensifies or appears for a short time after movement. The degree of pain accentuation is out of keeping with the nature of the associated movement.[27] The presence of incident pain predicts a poor outcome for eventual symptom control.[28,29] Breakthrough doses of opioids are often insufficient to alleviate these transient but severe pain episodes.

Treatment Strategies

Similar to the management of other cancer pain syndromes, a stepwise approach to controlling bone pain is recommended.[9] Non-opioid analgesics, such as acetaminophen or nonsteroidal anti-inflammatory drugs (NSAIDs), may initially be useful. Acetaminophen acts primarily in the central nervous system (CNS) and NSAIDs appear to act both centrally and peripherally. The so-called "weak opioids," such as codeine, may provide adequate and consistent relief from bone pain. The "strong opioids" are usually required; however, they should be carefully titrated to balance optimal analgesia with tolerated and manageable side effects. Bone pain is frequently responsive to opioids, particularly when given with adjunctive agents, such as NSAIDs and corticosteroids.[30–33]

In addition to systematic application of analgesic strategies, systemic treatment of the underlying malignancy with chemotherapy or hormonal therapy is potentially beneficial in the palliation of bone pain. Antineoplastic therapy for carcinomas of the breast, prostate, thyroid, and multiple myeloma can provide particularly dramatic relief from bone pain if the tumor proves to be sensitive.[3,34,35] Radiotherapy and surgery can be effective for bone pain, irrespecitive of the nature of the primary tumor. Local radiotherapy has long been used to reduce bone pain in localized sites. Although the optimal dose and fractionation have yet to be clearly established, radiotherapy has been reported to benefit up to 80% of patients.[3,36,37] However, the degree and duration of pain relief varies greatly, and may depend on both the tumor site and dosing schedule.[38] Radiotherapy has prompt analgesic effects for most patients, even if the primary tumor is apparently radioresistant. When radiation is given as a single fraction the short-term toxicity tends to be low.[39] Multiple lower dose fractions are similarly effective in providing pain relief with reduced long-term potential for normal tissue injury.[40,41]

Surgery is sometimes required in the management of bone pain. Large lytic lesions that involve cortical bone can cause increasing pain prior to the development of a pathological fracture.[42] In Mirels's scoring system for pathological fractures, pain, radiological appearance, and anatomical location are used to predict an impending fracture of long bones.[43] Prophylactic internal fixation may help to prevent fracture and reduce bone pain.[44]

Spinal instability can result in severe back pain. Vertebral collapse may be variably present and no discrete fractures may be apparent. A variety of surgical procedures can be used to stabilize the spine and subsequently relieve the intensity of symptoms.[45,46] As previously mentioned, surgical decompression of spinal cord or nerve root compression can lead to significant pain relief and restore or improve neurological function.[23–25] Physical therapy, such as local heat, transcutaneous electronic nerve stimulation, and immobilization devices such as collars or splints, can also be useful for patients with mild to moderate bone pain.[47,48]

In spite of systematic deployment of these therapeutic maneuvers, there remains a subpopulation in whom bone pain is refractory and whose quality of life is impaired by the distress and debility associated with uncontrolled chronic pain.[28] In particular, patients with significant incident pain may become limited in their activities. Furthermore, some patients are very sensitive to the adverse effects of opioids, and difficulties emerge in optimizing their analgesic treatment because of dose-limiting toxicity.[21,26] Consequently, supplementary agents or measures are required to improve pain control, mobility, and quality of life for patients with apparently refractory bone pain.

Bone Resorption Inhibitors

In normal bone, remodeling occurs continuously through carefully regulated processes. Bone resorption is mediated primarily through osteoclasts, and new bone formation is promoted by osteoblasts.[49,50] With malignant infiltration of tumor cells into bone, both focal and generalized increase in bone resorption can occur. Focal resorption processes can be altered, either through local mediators produced by tumour cells or through direct bone destruction by tumor. Generalized resorption can be stimulated by hormonal factors secreted by the tumor cells.[10] In lung carcinomas and multiple myeloma, osteolytic processes predominate; in prostate and some breast cancers, osteoblastic lesions are more apparent.[2,51,52] However, in both osteolytic and osteoblastic bone disease, local bone resorption appears to be increased. Markers of enhanced bone resorption, such as urinary calcium and urinary hydroxyproline: urinary creatinine ratios, and pyridoline cross-links, are enhanced in the presence of metastatic bone disease.[53–55]

Agents that specifically inhibit or reduce bone resorption have potential therapeutic use. Bone resorption inhibitors (BRI) may decrease the extent of bone destruction and, thereby, reduce associated clinical problems, such as pathological fractures, hypercalcemia, and pain.[18] BRI can reduce the effect on normal bone from systemic promoters of bone resorption such as parathyroid hormone-related peptide (PTH-rP), and may reduce the incidence of new metastatic bone lesions by rendering the bone matrix less amenable to tumor adhesion and local growth. In order to be effective and clinically relevant, however, BRI must have a favorable acute and chronic toxicity profile and, specifically, must not significantly interfere with new bone formation.[56]

Three main classes of BRI are available for clinical use: calcitonin, gallium nitrate, and the bisphosphonates. All of these agents have been used in the management of hypercalcemia of malignancy.[57,58] Whether the hypercalcemia has resulted from tumor-associated humeral mechanisms, such as ectopic PTH-rP production, or from direct tumor osteolysis, BRI can be effective in reducing loss of calcium and other minerals from bone and facilitating the re-establishment of normal calcium homeostasis. BRI have proven to be so effective in managing hypercalcemia of malignancy that the bisphosphonates, in particular, have become the agents of choice in this context.[59] Because these agents have no effect on renal calcium reabsorption, attention is still required to restoring intravascular fluid volume, optimizing renal perfusion, and treating the underlying malignant process where possible.[60]

In uncontrolled studies that evaluated BRI in the management of hypercalcemia, bone pain decreased in some patients as normocalcemia was achieved. In 1983, Siris et al. reported a placebo-controlled, cross-over study of 10 women with metastatic breast cancer and hypercalcemia or hypercalciuria.[61] In the eight patients who were described as having moderate to severe bone pain, after receiving the oral bisphosphonate all had "definite" pain relief in conjunction with normalization of their serum calcium.

In a placebo-controlled trial of patients with prostate cancer and painful bone metastases, Elomaa et al. found that patients who received the bisphosphonate, clodronate, had significantly lower analgesic requirements over the first three months of treatment.[62] Thirty percent of the clodronate group were pain-free at one month, compared with 15% of the placebo group. Similarly, in a controlled trial of 131 patients with osteolytic bone metastases from breast cancer, Van Holten-Verzantvoort et al. reported that women who received the bisphosphonate, pamidronate, had less frequent episodes of severe bone pain than those who received the placebo.[63]

The utility of BRI in the management of patients with metastatic bone pain has been the subject of ongoing evaluation. Evidence of analgesic efficacy, and practical implications, are reviewed below.

Calcitonin

Calcitonin plays a physiological role in maintaining skeletal integrity by inhibiting osteoclast function.[64] Although found in many tissues, calcitonin is primarily released into the circulation from C cells (parafollicular cells) within the thyroid, in response to increases in serum ionized calcium.[65,66] The precise control of calcitonin is not well understood, and the relationship between serum calcium and calcitonin secretion is inconsistent. Small, sudden changes in serum calcium do not alter calcitonin levels, leading investigators to conclude that calcitonin does not appear to have a role in the fine control of serum calcium.[67] In addition to inhibiting osteoclast function, calcitonin decreases renal tubular reabsorption of calcium and phosphate, and increases excretion of sodium, potassium, and magnesium.[68]

Calcitonin may also play a role in pain transmission and modulation in the CNS. Pecile et al. first demonstrated a central analgesic effect with intraventricular infusions of calcitonin in a rabbit model.[69] This central effect appeared to be independent of central opiate receptors, although increased levels of beta-endorphin in serum have been observed following calcitonin infusions.[70,71] Other studies involving animal models have suggested that calcitonin inhibits cyclo-oxygenase and, hence, reduces prostaglandin synthesis.[72]

Synthetic salmon calcitonin (sCT) is available for pharmacological use. sCT differs from the human peptide in 16 of the 32 amino acids. It also has greater hypocalcemic potency, enhanced affinity for target tissues, and slower degradation and clearance. sCT can be administered parenterally or intranasally. Local irritation commonly occurs at injection sites. Flushing, nausea, and vomiting can also develop, but all side effects usually diminish over time.[64]

The primary oncological indication of sCT has been in the management of hypercalcemia. sCT is particularly helpful in the acute reduction of serum calcium; reports indicate that sCT can reduce the calcium levels by 0.5–1.5 mg/dl in 75% of cases, irrespective of the underlying mechanism.[73–75] It is well tolerated even in settings of renal failure and congestive heart failure; however, its utility is limited by the magnitude and duration of the hypocalcemic effect. Osteoclasts appear to escape the inhibitory effects of sCT with continued exposure. This phenomenon may be due to downregulation of the calcitonin receptor number or binding, or to the emergence of a population of osteoclasts that are insensitive to calcitonin.[75–77]

The potential for pain mediation by CNS effects or by altered prostaglandin production has led to several studies of the role of calcitonin in modulating metastatic bone pain. Uncontrolled studies of doses of 100–400 IU suggested that calcitonin was efficacious in intractable pain.[78,79] In an open label study of 34 patients with metastatic bone disease from lung cancer, Schiraldi et al. assessed pain response using intravenous sCT 400 IU/day for three days or intravenous sCT 200 IU/day for six days.[80] Hydrocortisone 100 mg intravenous was given to both groups prior to each infusion. In both groups, a significant reduction in visual analogue scores (VAS) was apparent after five days and was sustained to 15 days.

In the first published controlled study, Hindley et al. evaluated 25 patients with various malignancies and pain.[81] Sixteen (64%) patients had pain attributable to bone metastases, and 8 of the 13 patients receiving sCT 200 IU subcutaneously every 6 hr for 48 hr showed an improvement in pain at week 1, compared with only 2 of 12 in the placebo group. This difference was not statistically significant. All 4 patients who had sustained pain relief for 2 weeks had bone metastases. Eight of 13 patients who received sCT had severe nausea during the first 24 hr.

More recently, Roth reported a double-blind, placebo-controlled study of 40 women with painful osteolytic metastases from breast cancer.[82] The sCT group received 100 IU subcutaneously daily for 28 days. The daily analgesic requirement in the sCT group decreased by a mean of 44% and increased by 8% in the placebo group. In a blinded assessment of efficacy, the investigators described sCT as moderately useful in 11 of 20 patients, and placebo as moderately useful in 3 of 20 patients. No difference in functional capability was observed in either group during the treatment period.

In another controlled study by Blomqvist et al., 50 patients with painful bone metastases from breast cancer were randomized to receive intravenous sCT 100 mg daily or saline placebo for three of four weeks during a 3-month period.[83] No improvement in general performance scores or bone pain was detected. Also, sCT had no effect on disease progression, as evaluated through bone scintigrams and radiographs. In fact, biochemical markers of bone resorption were unchanged by sCT and would suggest that sCT was ineffective, possibly because of a relatively low level of bone turnover at baseline in these patients or because of calcitonin receptor downregulation.

The analgesic efficacy of sCT has yet to be defined for bone pain, and definition of a dose-response relationship requires further exploration. It would appear that the effect, if present, is modest and is dependent upon the pretreatment rate of bone turnover.

Gallium nitrate

Gallium nitrate was initially investigated as an antineoplastic agent and was subsequently found to have marked hypocalcemic effects, primarily by inhibiting bone resorption.[84,85] Gallium is avidly incorporated into the bone mineral matrix and preferentially localizes to regions of increased bone turnover.[86] Gallium reduces the solubility of existing hydroxyapatite and renders mineralized bone more resistant to osteoclastic resorption.[87,88] It does not appear to have any direct cytotoxic activity, and no changes in bone cellular morphology are apparent following gallium administration.[84]

Gallium nitrate is only available as a parenteral solution; following bolus infusion, 65% is excreted unchanged in the urine after 24 hours.[89] Clinical use has been largely confined to the management of hypercalcemia of malignancy. In this context, a dose-response relationship is apparent.[90] The optimal dose appears to be 200 mg/m² daily continuous intravenous for 5 days; the maximal hypocalcemic effect is observed within 24–48 hr of initiating therapy.[85,90,91] Nephrotoxicity is the primary dose limitation; this adverse effect occurs in up to 13% of cases and is usually reversible.[84]

Scher et al. reported some improvement in bone pain in a phase 2 study of 23 normocalcemic patients with hormone refractory metastatic carcinoma of the prostate.[92] Gallium 200 mg/m² was given by continuous infusion over 7 days every 28 days, and the dose was escalated in accordance with stable renal function. Seven of 23 patients (30%) had diminution in pain, but the methods of pain assessment, and the extent and duration of pain relief, were not provided. Two patients with bidimensionally measurable disease achieved partial responses. Symptomatic episodes of hypocalcemia occurred in 2 patients, and renal toxicity occurred in 3 patients.

Although gallium has antiresorptive capabilities, no controlled studies with bone pain as a primary endpoint have been completed. Factors limiting its potential in treating metastatic bone disease include the need for continuous intravenous administration and renal toxicity.

Bisphosphonates

Bisphosphonates have a double phosphonate group (P-C-P) and are chemically similar to organic pyrophosphate.[57] The phosphonate groups confer binding affinity for calcium phosphate within the mineralized bone matrix.[93] Bisphosphonates are readily cleared from blood and are incorporated predominantly in bone tissue. Peak concentrations in bone appear several hours after intravenous administration.[57,94] Bioavailability following oral administration is low (1%–2%) and is reduced further with food, particularly dairy products.[95–97] The bisphosphonates are primarily eliminated unchanged in the urine, and doses must be reduced in patients with markedly impaired renal function.[98] Two to three days following an intravenous dose, 20%–50% of the bisphosphonate remains in the bones, from which it is slowly released over subsequent weeks and months.[96] Rapid intravenous infusions of a bisphosphonate have precipitated acute renal failure in some patients by causing acute tubular necrosis.[99] This problem can be averted by administering these agents over several hours.[100] The newer and more potent bisphosphonates can be given more rapidly without the same apparent risk.[101] Transient proteinuria can occur, and is not generally associated with renal dysfunction.[102] Fever can occur following administration of the amino bisphosphonates, such as pamidronate and alendronate.[103,104]

When bone resorption occurs, the bisphosphonates are released from the bone matrix into the surrounding solution at high concentrations and are taken up by the osteoclasts either as free drug or bound to hydroxyapatite crystals.[57,94] These agents appear to have a direct inhibitory effect on osteoclast function. Both alterations in osteoclast morphology and numbers have been described in vivo, but the precise cellular mechanism of action remains unknown.[105–107]

An increasing number of bisphosphonate analogues have been developed and are available for clinical use (Fig. 5.1). The various agents differ structurally in the nature of the central carbon side-chain and also contrast markedly in their relative potency in vivo (Table 5.1). The pharmacological basis for differences in potency among the bisphosphonates is not known, but may be related to the biodistribution and differential effects on osteoclastic development or function.[57,108,109] The first bisphosphonate available for clinical use, etidronate (methylbisphosphonate), has the lowest antiresorptive potency, but also appears to inhibit normal mineralization of bone.[110] In some studies of long-term use, this drug has produced osteomalacia.[111] In oncology, etidronate has largely been replaced by newer and more efficacious bisphosphonates that do not impair new bone formation.[57,58,112] In North America, etidronate, clodronate, pamidronate, and alendronate are currently approved for clinical use.

Although the utility of bisphosphonates in the treatment of hypercalcemia of malignancy is now well established, the role in normocalcemic patients with bone

ETIDRONATE

$$\begin{array}{ccc} OH & CH_3 & OH \\ | & | & | \\ O=P-&C-&P=O \\ | & | & | \\ OH & OH & OH \end{array}$$

CLODRONATE

$$\begin{array}{ccc} OH & Cl & OH \\ | & | & | \\ O=P-&C-&P=O \\ | & | & | \\ OH & Cl & OH \end{array}$$

PAMIDRONATE

$$\begin{array}{c} NH_2 \\ | \\ (CH_2)_2 \end{array}$$
$$\begin{array}{ccc} OH & & OH \\ \backslash & | & / \\ O=P-&C-&P=O \\ | & | & | \\ OH & OH & OH \end{array}$$

ALENDRONATE

$$\begin{array}{c} NH_2 \\ | \\ (CH_2)_3 \end{array}$$
$$\begin{array}{ccc} OH & & OH \\ \backslash & | & / \\ O=P-&C-&P=O \\ | & | & | \\ OH & OH & OH \end{array}$$

RISEDRONATE

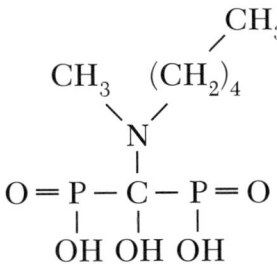

IBANDRONATE

Figure 5.1. Structural formulae of bisphosphonates.

pain is less well defined. Most of the studies that have measured pain evaluate clodronate or pamidronate. Few have been controlled and even fewer have used validated endpoints of symptom control or quality of life. Many doses, schedules, and modes of administration have been reported, with varying degrees of analgesic efficacy (Table 5.2).

In the first controlled trial in which pain was a primary endpoint, Delmas et al. randomized 13 patients with multiple myeloma to receive either oral clodronate 1600 mg/day or placebo.[113] Within the first six months, the mean pain index in the clodronate patients decreased from 4.43 to 0.86 (maximum score: 9);

Table 5.1 Relative potency of bisphosphonates

	Relative antiresorptive potency
Etidronate	1
Clodronate	10
Pamidronate	100
Alendronate	1,000
Risedronate	5,000
Ibandronate	10,000

the mean pain index in the placebo group increased from 3.17 to 5.83. This pain index incorporated not only the degree of pain but also the association with movement (incident pain). In an unblinded, comparative trial of oral versus intravenous clodronate in patients with metastatic prostate cancer, Adami and Milan demonstrated a minimal and transient reduction in self-reported visual analogue scores (VAS) in patients who received oral clodronate 1200 mg/day for two weeks.[114] A sustained (<6 weeks) improvement was seen in patients who received intravenous clodronate 300 mg/day for two weeks.

In 1992, Ernst et al. reported a placebo-controlled, double-blind crossover trial of 24 patients with metastatic bone disease from a variety of primary tumor sites.[115] All patients had refractory bone pain. Blinded patient selection of the more effective agent was the primary endpoint for the trial in which intravenous clodronate 600 mg or placebo was given. Daily VAS scores were collected on a variety of symptom measures, including pain, and analgesic diaries were recorded for each patient. Twelve (57%) of 21 evaluable patients selected the clodronate infusion as beneficial; 4 (19%) chose placebo; and 5 (24%) had no preference. A significant decrease in pain scores and increase in activity levels were also noted. In another study of similar design, 59 patients were randomized to receive either clodronate 600 mg or 1500 mg, or placebo.[116] Of the 46 evaluable patients, 26 (57%) chose clodronate; 12 (26%) chose placebo; and 8 (17%) could not distinguish a difference. No dose effect could be discerned in the trial, although a carry-over effect was apparent with the cross-over at 2 weeks.

The analgesic activity of pamidronate in metastatic bone pain has also been evaluated in controlled clinical trials. Using a parallel design, Glover et al. randomized 61 patients with metastatic breast cancer of 4 different dose schedules of intravenous pamidronate: 30 mg every 2 weeks, 60 mg every 4 weeks, 60 mg every 2 weeks, and 90 mg every 4 weeks.[117] At 3 months, there was a significant reduction in pain scores at all dose levels except the 30 mg every 2 weeks. Although analgesic scores were secondary endpoints of efficacy, no other treatment effect was apparent. Similarly, a dose-response relationship was evaluated by Thurlimann et al. in a dose escalation study of 80 patients with osteolytic bone metastases and pain.[118] Patients who received pamidronate doses

Table 5.2 Randomized, placebo-controlled trials of bisphosphonates for metastatic bone pain

Reference	Disease	No. of patients	Design	Daily dose	Duration of Rx	Outcome
Clordonate Siris (1983)[61]	Breast	34	Parallel	1.6 gm PO	12 mo	↓ New bone mets ↓ Analgesic use
Elomaa (1983)[62]	Breast	10	Cross-over	3.2 gm PO	2 mo	↓ Self reports of pain intensity
Siris (1980)[137]	M myeloma°	10	Cross-over	3.2 gm PO	2 mo	↓ Pain intensity on self reports
Ernst (1992)[115]	Various 1° sites	24	Cross-over	600 mg IV	1 day	↓ VAS pain scores ↑ VAS activity scores Preference: NS difference
Lahtinen (1992)[134]	M myeloma	350	Parallel	2.4 gm PO	24 mo	↓ Pain score ↓ Progression of bone lesions
Elomaa (1992)[135]	Prostate	75	Parallel	3.2 gm PO 1.6 gm PO	1 mo 5 mo	↑ Self report of pain-free ↓ Analgesics
Peterson (1993)[131]	Breast	173	Parallel	1.6 gm PO	36 mo	↓ Vertebral fractures
Robertson (1995)[121]	Various 1° sites	55	Parallel	1.6 gm PO	Indefinite	↓ VAS pain scores Analgesics: NS difference
Ernst (1997)[116]	Various 1° sites	44	Cross-over	600 mg or 1500 mg IV	1 day	Clodronate preference ↓ Analgesics
Pamidronate Van Holten - Verzantvoort (1993)[138]	Breast	161	Parallel	300 mg PO	Indefinite	↓ RT for severe pain ↓ Symptomatic pending fractures
Coleman (1996)[122]	Various 1° sites	52	Parallel	120 mg IV	1 day	↓ Pain score (intensity, analgesics, performance status)
Berenson (1996)[133]	M myeloma	377	Parallel	90 mg IV	Q4 wk × 9	↓ Pain score

°M myeloma - multiple myeloma; NS difference - no statistically significant difference; RT - radiotherapy; VAS - visual analogue score.

less than 10 mg/week or single doses of 30 mg had no apparent benefit. Patients who received doses of 25–45 mg/week had improvement in their pain control.

Purohit et al. reported that after a single dose of pamidronate 120 mg intravenously, 20 of 34 (59%) patients with metastatic bone disease showed a <20% improvement in patient-completed pain scores reflecting pain, analgesic use, and performance status.[119] The mean duration of response was 12 weeks (range: 4–24 + weeks). The investigators also assessed changes in the Rotterdam Symptom Checklist instrument and the Oswestry Mobility questionnaire, and found that those patients who had responded to the pamidronate also demonstrated significant improvement in the domains of physical activity, psychological profile, social functioning, and activities of daily living.

In van Holten-Verzantvoort's controlled study of oral pamidronate in 144 patients with advanced breast cancer, the quality of life instrument specifically designed for the trial evaluated the impact of treatment on four separate scales: mobility impairment, gastrointestinal toxicity, bone pain, and fatigue.[120] The investigators found that the mean mobility impairment score was significantly higher in the control group, and a rapid and then sustained improvement in mobility scores occurred in the pamidronate group. Interestingly, there was no difference in fatigue and gastrointestinal scores between groups, despite the observation that 23% of pamidronate patients were discontinued from the study because of gastrointestinal toxicity.

In 1995, Robertson et al. published findings of a double-blind, placebo-controlled trial of oral clodronate 1600 mg/day in 55 patients with metastatic bone disease.[121] Patients were stratified by primary tumor site (breast, lung, or other). The pain response was determined by 10 cm linear VAS completed at each monthly visit. Although significant improvements in pain were observed at one month, 37% of clodronate and 46% of placebo patients had to withdraw prematurely, most commonly because of difficulties in swallowing the capsules.

Most recently, Coleman reported preliminary findings in a phase 3 study of pamidronate 120 mg intravenously versus placebo in 52 patients with painful and progressive bone metastases from a variety of primary sites, predominantly breast and prostate.[122] A response defined as a >20% reduction in pain score measured on two consecutive occasions was achieved by five of the 21 patients (24%) receiving pamidronate and by only one of the 25 patients (4%) receiving placebo. N-terminal and C-terminal peptide–bound collagen cross-links were measured in all patients. Patients with levels of cross-links and presumably higher bone resorptive activity were more likely to have a symptomatic response to the pamidronate. These findings suggest that it may become possible to select those patients more likely to achieve an improvement in pain with bisphosphonate therapy.

Clinical studies evaluating other bisphosphonates, including alendronate, neridronate, and ibandronate, have primarily focused on their utility in hypercalcemia.[123–127] The duration of the hypocalcemic response appears to be consistently related to the parenteral dose of the specific bisphosphonate; a maximal effective dose was also apparent. In these studies, pain control was not an endpoint and, therefore, it is difficult to extrapolate a similar dose-response relationship for pain control. Nevertheless, multiple doses could be safely given by slow bolus infusions, and their role in treating refractory bone pain requires further exploration.

Radiolabeled bisphosphonates such as 186-rhenium hydroxyethylidene diphosphonate have been developed, and have undergone early clinical evaluation specifically for pain control.[128] In a phase 2 trial of 186-rhenium in 27 patients with hormone refractory metastatic carcinoma of the prostate, Curley et al. found that 67% of patients had a significant decrease in pain VAS.[129] The maximum benefit appeared to occur by day 7, and was maintained for three weeks. Similarly, in an open label study, Maxon et al. reported a decrease in pain in 24 of 43 patients (56%) with metastatic bone disease from a variety of primaries.[130] Myelosuppression was only problematic in those patients who received concomitant external beam radiotherapy or chemotherapy.

Bone Pain Prevention

A potential novel use of bisphosphonates is the prevention of bone metastases or complications of bone disease, such as bone pain. Several controlled studies in populations with multiple myeloma, breast cancer, or prostate cancer suggest that regular bisphosphonate administration can lead to a reduction in the frequency of clinical problems associated with metastatic bone disease. In 1993, Paterson et al. reported on a placebo-controlled trial of oral clodronate 1600 mg/day in women with known bone metastases from breast cancer.[131] They found a reduction in the incidence of vertebral fractures and the rate of vertebral deformity in the clodronate group. The overall rate of adverse skeletal events, including the need for local radiotherapy, was decreased in the patients who received clodronate. A similar reduction in morbidity from skeletal disease was observed in placebo-controlled studies with pamidronate in breast cancer, with clodronate and pamidronate in multiple myeloma, and with clodronate in prostate cancer.[63,132–135]

Most recently, Paterson et al. reported that, in women with advanced breast cancer without known bone involvement, oral clodronate appeared to reduce the incidence of subsequent development of bone metastases.[136] The rates of vertebral deformities and episodes of hypercalcemia were also decreased. These findings raise the possibility that the bisphosphonates, by their action on normal bone tissue, may be useful in the prevention of metastatic bone disease in certain malignancies.

Although the controlled studies with clodronate and pamidronate support their role in ameliorating pain and in improving mobility in some patients with metastatic bone disease, there are still unanswered questions:

What patients are most likely to benefit?
What is the influence of primary tumor site, location, extent, and nature of bone disease on the analgesic response?

Are there predictive clinical or biochemical markers of response?
What are the optimal doses, routes, and schedules?
Are all bisphosphonates equianalgesic if potency differences are reflected in
dosing schedule?
Are bisphosphonates synergistic with other adjunctive agents, with hormonal
therapy or chemotherapy, or with local radiotherapy?

With the development of potentially more active bisphosphonates, the need
for well designed, controlled studies using validated endpoints of response is
evident. At present, analgesic studies support the use of bisphosphonates in
patients with refractory metastatic bone pain. Responses will be variable and both
dose and dosing schedule should be individualized in accordance with the pain
experience of each patient. Parenteral bisphosphonates are safe and well tolerated and will more likely lead to an early assessment of response. Long-term use
for pain control has not been adequately addressed and represents one challenge
in conducting clinical trials in this population of cancer patients. Often, patients
develop other complications and end-organ dysfunction in the trajectory of the
underlying malignant disease. Pain control measures must be frequently modified
in accordance with each patient's changing clinical status.

Conclusion

The management of bone pain in patients with osseous metastases continues to
be a clinical challenge. The establishment of the underlying pathogenic mechanisms in each patient should be attempted. In all patients, a stepwise analgesic
approach should be implemented. Simple therapeutic maneuvers, such as the use
of opioid analgesics, NSAIDs, and local radiotherapy, may be adequate in achiev-
ing optimal pain relief. In some patients, particularly those who have significant
incident pain, BRI may help to acheive pain control. Calcitonin and gallium
nitrate can be used to treat hypercalcemia of malignancy, but appear to have
limited efficacy in the management of refractory bone pain. Alternatively, the
bisphosphonates can be effective in the acute management of hypercalcemia, in
the reduction of osteolysis and associated complications, and in the treatment of
metastatic bone pain. The agents clodronate and pamidronate have been evaluated most thoroughly in these contexts and both appear to provide similar clinical
effect. Their optimal analgesic use requires further evaluation. Future use may
also be in the prevention of bone metastases.

References

1. Lote K, Walloe A, Bjersand A. Bone metastases. Prognosis, diagnosis and treatment.
   Acta Radiol Oncol 1986; 25:227–232.

2. Paterson AHG. Bone metastases in breast cancer, prostate cancer and myeloma. *Bone* 1987; 8(suppl.):17–22.

3. Nielsen OS, Munro AJ, Tannock IF. Bone metastases: pathophysiology and management policy. *J Clin Oncol* 1991; 9(3):509–524.

4. Abrams HL, Spiro R, Goldstein N. Metastases in carcinoma. Analysis of 1000 autopsied cases. *Cancer* 1950; 23:74–85.

5. Miller F, Whitehill R. Carcinoma of the breast metastatic to the skeleton. *Clin Orthop* 1984; 184:121–127.

6. Patanaphan V, Salazar OM, Risco R. Breast cancer: metastatic patterns and their prognosis. *South Med J* 1988; 81:1109–1112.

7. Jacobs SC. Spread of prostatic cancer to bone. *Urology* 1983; 21:337–344.

8. Campa JA, Payne R. The management of intractable bone pain: a clinician's perspective. *Semin Nucl Med* 1992; 22:3–10.

9. Twycross RG. Management of pain in skeletal mets. *Clin Orthop* 1995; 312:187–196.

10. Averbach SD. New bisphosphonates in treatment of bone metastases. *Cancer* 1993; 72(11):3443–3452.

11. Wagner G. Frequency of pain in patients with cancer. *Recent Results Cancer Res* 1984; 89:64–71.

12. Portenoy RK. Cancer pain: epidemiology and syndromes. *Cancer* 1989; 63:2298–2307.

13. Coleman RE. Assessment of response to treatment. In: Rubens RD, Fogelman I, eds. *Bone Metastases: Diagnosis and Treatment*. London:Springer-Verlag, 1991:99–120.

14. Carter RL. Patterns and mechanisms of bone metastases. *J R Soc Med* 1985; 78(suppl 9):2–6.

15. Galasko CSB. Mechanisms of lytic and blastic metastatic disease of bone. *Clin Orthop* 1982; 169:20–27.

16. Mundy GR. Cytokines and local factors which affect osteoclast function. *Int J Cell Cloning* 1992; 10:215–222.

17. Dodwell DS. Malignant bone resorption, cellular and biochemical mechanisms. *Ann Oncol* 1992; 3:257–267.

18. Scher HI, Yagoda A. Bone metastases: pathogenesis, treatment rationale for use of resorption inhibitors. *Am J Med* 1987; 82(suppl 2A):6–28.

19. Ferreira SH. Prostaglandins: peripheral and central analgesia. *Adv Pain Res Ther* 1983; 5:627–634.

20. Bonica JJ. Control of bone cancer pain. In: Garattinis S, ed. *Bone Resorption, Metastasis and Diphosphonates*. New York:Raven Press, 1985:137–180.

21. Foley KM. The management of cancer pain. *N Engl J Med* 1986; 313:84–95.

22. Albright JA, Gillespie TE, Butaud TR. Treatment of bone metastases. *Semin Oncol* 1980; 7:418–433.

23. Gilbert RN, Kim JH, Posner JB. Epidural spinal cord compression from metastatic tumor. Diagnosis and treatment. *Ann Neurol* 1978; 3:40–45.

24. Sorensen PS, Borgensen SE, Rohde K, et al. Metastatic epidural spinal cord compression: results of treatment and survival. *Cancer* 1990; 65:1502–1506.

25. Portenoy RK, Lipton RB, Foley KM. Back pain in the cancer patient: an algorithm for evaluation and management. *Neurology* 1987; 37:134–142.

26. Peteet J, Tay V, Cohen G, et al. Pain characteristics and treatment in an outpatient cancer population. *Cancer* 1986; 57:1259–1265.

27. Portenoy RK, Hagen NA. Breakthrough pain: definition, prevalence, characteristics. *Pain* 1990; 41:273–282.

28. Hanks GW, Portenoy RK, MacDonald N, O'Neill WM. Difficult pain problems. In: Doyle D, Hanks GW, MacDonald N, eds. *Oxford Textbook of Palliative Medicine.* New York: Oxford University Press, 1994:262–264.

29. Bruera E, Schoeller T, Wenk R, et al. A prospective multicenter assessment of the Edmonton Staging System for cancer pain. *J Pain Symptom Manage* 1995; 10:348–355.

30. Hanks GW. The pharmacological treatment of bone pain. *Cancer Surv* 1988; 7(1):87–101.

31. World Health Organization: *Cancer Pain Relief.* Geneva: World Health Organization, 1986.

32. Ferreira SH. Prostaglandins, aspirin-like drugs and analgesics. *Nature [New Biol]* 1992; 240:200–203.

33. Smith IE, Macaulay V. Comparison of different endocrine therapies in management of bone metastases from breast carcinoma. *J R Soc Med* 1985; 78(suppl 9):15–21.

34. MacDonald N. Principles governing the use of cancer chemotherapy in palliative medicine. In: Doyle D, Hanks GW, MacDonald N, eds. *Oxford Textbook of Palliative Medicine.* New York: Oxford University Press, 1994:105–117.

35. Miller RJ. The role of chemotherapy in the hospice patient. *Am J Hosp Care* 1989; 6:19–26.

36. Poulsen HS, Nielsen OS, Klee M, et al. Palliative irradiation of bone metastases. *Cancer Treat Rev* 1989; 16:41–48.

37. Hoskin PJ. Scientific and clinical aspects of radiotherapy in the relief of bone pain. *Cancer Surv* 1988; 7:69–86.

38. Tong D, Gillick L, Hendrickson FR. The palliation of symptomatic osseous metastases. Final results of the study by the Radiation Therapy Oncology Group. *Cancer* 1982; 50:893–899.

39. Price P, Hoskin PJ, Easton D, et al. Low dose single fraction radiotherapy in the treatment of metastatic bone pain. *Radiother Oncol* 1988; 12:297–300.

40. Okawa T, Kita M, Goto M, et al. Randomized prospective clinical study of small, large and twice daily fraction radiotherapy for painful bone metastases. *Radiother Oncol* 1988; 13:99–104.

41. Cole DJ. A randomized trial of a single treatment versus conventional fractionation in the palliative radiotherapy of painful bone metastases. *Clin Oncol* 1989; 1:59–62.

42. Lodwick GS. Reactive responses to local injury in bone. *Radiol Clin North Am* 1964; 2:209–219.

43. Mirels H. Metastatic disease to long bones. A proposed scoring system for diagnosing impending pathological fractures. *Clin Orthop* 1989; 249:256–264.

44. Bouma WH, Mulder JH, Hop WCJ. The influence of intramedullary nailing upon the development of metastases in the treatment of an impending pathological fracture: an experimental study. *Clin Exp Metastasis* 1983; 1:205–212.

45. Dewald RL, Bridwell KH, Prodromas C, Rodts MF. Reconstructive spinal surgery as palliation for metastatic malignancies of the spine. *Spine* 1985; 10:21–26.

46. Cybulski GR. Methods of surgical stabilization for metastatic disease of the spine. *Neurosurgery* 1989; 25:240–252.

47. Robinson A. Physiotherapy in oncology. *Association of chartered physiotherapists in oncology and palliative care newsletter* 1990:2.

48. Librach SL, Rapson LM. The use of transcutaneous electrical nerve stimulation for the relief of pain in palliative care. *Palliat Med* 1988; 2:15–20.
49. Boyce BF. Normal bone remodelling and its disruption in metastatic bone disease. In: Rubins RD, Fogelman I, eds. *Bone Metastases—Diagnosis and Treatment*. London: Springer, 1991:11–30.
50. Dodwell DJ. Malignant bone resorption: cellular and biochemical mechanisms. *Ann Oncol* 1992; 3:257–267.
51. Cramer S, Fried L, Carter K. The cellular basis of metastatic bone disease in patients with lung cancer. *Cancer* 1981; 48:2649–2660.
52. Mcdonald DF, Schofield BH, Prezioso EM, et al. Direct bone resorbing activity of murine myeloma cells. *Cancer Lett* 1983; 19:119–124.
53. Khansur T, Yam LT, Tavassoli M. Serum moniters of bone metastasis. In: Stoll BA, Parbhoo S, eds. *Bone Metastases: Monitoring and Treatment*. New York: Raven Press, 1983:165–180.
54. Eyre DR. New biomarkers of bone resorption. *J Clin Endocrinol Metab* 1992; 74:470–478.
55. Colwell A, Russell RGG, Eastell R. Factors affecting the assay of urinary 3-hydroxy pyridinium cross-links of collagen as markers of bone resorption. *Eur J Clin Invest* 1993; 23:341–349.
56. Gennari C., Francini G, Gonnelli S, Begazzi S. Treatment of bone metastases with antiresorptive drugs. In: Garattini S, ed. *Bone Resorption, Metastasis and Diphosphonates*. New York: Raven Press, 1985:127–136.
57. Fleish H. Bisphosphonates. Pharmacology and use in the treatment of tumor-induced hypercalcemia and metastatic bone disease. *Drugs* 1991; 42:919–944.
58. Bilezkian JP. Management of acute hypercalcemia. *N Engl J Med* 1992; 326:1196–1203.
59. Harinck HIJ, Bijvoet OLM, Plantingh AST, et al. Role of bone and kidney in tumor-induced hypercalcemia and its treatment with bisphosphonate and sodium chloride. *Am J Med* 1987; 82:1133–1142.
60. Ralston SH, Gardiner MD, Dryburgh FJ, et al. Comparison of aminohydroxypropylidene diphosphonate, mithramycin and corticosteroids/calcitonin in treatment of cancer-associated hypercalcemia. *Lancet* 1985; 2:907–910.
61. Siris ES, Hyman GA, Canfield RE. Effects of dichloromethylene diphosphonate in women with breast carcinoma metastatic to the skeleton. *Am J Med* 1983; 74:401–406.
62. Elomaa I, Blomqvist C, Grohn P. Long-term controlled trial with diphosphonate in patients with osteolytic bone metastases. *Lancet* 1983; 1:146–149.
63. van Holten-Verzantvoort AT, Bijvoet OLM, Cleton FJ, et al. Reduced morbidity from skeletal metastases in breast cancer patients during long-term bisphosphonate treatment. *Lancet* 1987; 2:983–985.
64. Becker KL, Nylen ES, Cohen R. Calcitonin gene family of peptides. In: Kenneth L Becker, ed. *Principles and Practice of Endocrinology and Metabolism*. Philadelphia: JB Lippincott Co., 1995:474–483.
65. Becker KL, Snider RH, Moore CF, et al. Calcitonin in extrathyroidal tissues of man. *Acta Endocrinol* 1979; 92:746–748
66. Copp DH, Cameron EL, Cheney BA, et al. Evidence for calcitonin—a new hormone from the parathyroid that lowers blood calcium. *Endocrinology* 1962; 70:638–641.

67. Habener JF, Jacobs JW. Biosynthesis and control of secretion of the calcium regulating peptides. In: Parsons JA, ed. *Endocrinology of Calcium Metabolism.* New York: Raven Press, 1982:143–181.

68. Macintyre I. Physiological actions of calcitonin. *Triangle* 1983; 2:69–74.

69. Pecile A, Ferri S, Braga PC, Olgiati UR. Effects of intracerebroventricular calcitonin in the conscious rabbit. *Experientia* 1975; 31:332–334.

70. Fraioli F, Fabbri CB. Neurocalcitonin: analgesic action and autoradiographic distribution of the receptors in rat brain. *J Endocrinol Invest* 1984; 7(suppl 1):177–179.

71. Austin LA, Heath III H. Calcitonin physiology and pathophysiology. *N Engl J Med* 1981; 304:269–78.

72. Ceserani R, Colombo M, Olgiati UR, Pecile A. Calcitonin and prostaglandin system. *Life Sci* 1979; 25:1851–1854.

73. Wisneski LA, Croom WP, Silva OL, Becker KL. Salmon calcitonin in hypercalcemia. *Clin Pharmacol Ther* 1978; 24:219–222.

74. Mundy GR, Martin TJ. The hypercalcemia of malignancy: pathogenesis and management. *Metabolism* 1982; 31:1247–1277.

75. Binstock ML, Mundy GR. Effect of calcitonin and glucocorticoids in combination on the hypercalcemia of malignancy. *Ann Intern Med* 1980; 93:269–272.

76. Wener JA, Gorton SJ, Raisz LG. Escape from inhibition of resorption in cultures of fetal bone treated with calcitonin and parathyroid hormone. *Endocrinology* 1972; 90:752–759.

77. Mundy GR. Hormonal factors which influence calcium homeostasis. In: Mundy GR, ed. *Calcium Homeostasis: Hypercalcemia and Hypocalcemia.* London: Martin Dunitz, 1989:28–50.

78. Serdengecti S, Serdengecti K, Derman U, et al. Salmon calcitonin in the treatment of bone metstases. *Int J Clin Pharmacol Res* 1989; 6(2):151–155.

79. Szanto J, Ady N, Jozsef S. Pain killing with calcitonin nasal spray in patients with malignant tumors. *Oncology* 1992; 49(3):180–182.

80. Schiraldi GF, Soresi E, Locicero S, et al. Salmon calcitonin in cancer pain: comparison between two different treatment schedules. *Int J Clin Pharmacol Ther Toxicol* 1987; 25(4):229–232.

81. Hindley AC, Hill AB, Leyland MJ, Wiles AE. A double-blind controlled trial of salmon calcitonin in pain due to malignancy. *Cancer Chemother Pharmacol* 1982; 9:71–74.

82. Roth A, Kolaric K. Analgesic activity of calcitonin in patients with painful osteolytic metastases of breast cancer. *Oncology* 1986; 43(5):283–287.

83. Blomquist C, Elomaa I, Porkka L, et al. Evaluation of salmon calcitonin treatment in bone metastases from breast cancer - a controlled trial. *Bone* 1988; 9:45–51.

84. Hughes TE, Hansen LA. Gallium nitrate (review). *Ann Pharmacother* 1992; 26(3):354–362.

85. Warrell RP, Bockman RS, Coonley CS, et al. Gallium nitrate inhibits calcium resorption from bone and is effective treatment for cancer-related hypercalcemia. *J Clin Invest* 1984; 73:1487–1490.

86. Warrell RP, Bockman RS. Gallium in the treatment of hypercalcemia and bone metastasis. *Important Adv Oncol* 1989; 2:205–220.

87. Bockman RS, Boskey AL, Blumenthal NC, et al. Gallium increases bone calcium and crystallite perfection of hydroxyapatite. *Calcif Tissue Int* 1986; 39:376–381.

88. Hall TJ, Chambers TJ. Gallium inhibits bone resorption by a direct effect on osteo-clasts. *Bone Miner* 1990; 8:211–216.

89. Hall SN, Yeung K, Benjamin RS, et al. Kinetics of gallium nitrate, a new anticancer agent. *Clin Pharmacol Ther* 1979; 25:82–87.

90. Warrell RP, Skezos A, Accock NN, Bockman RS. Gallium nitrate for acute treatment of cancer-related hypercalcemia: clinicopharmacological and dose response analy-sis. *Cancer Res* 1986; 46:4208–4212.

91. Warrell RP, Murphy WK, Schulman P, et al. A randomized double-blind study of gallium nitrate compared to etidronate for acute control of cancer related hyper-calcemia. *J Clin Oncol* 1991; 9(8):1467–1475.

92. Scher HI, Curley T, Geller N, et al. Gallium nitrate in prostatic cancer: Evaluation of antitumor activity and effects on bone turn-over. *Cancer Treat Rep* 1987; 71:887–893.

93. Jung A, Bisaz S, Fleisch H. The binding of pyrophosphate and two diphosphonates on hydroxyapatite crystals. *Calcif Tissue Res* 1973; 11:269–280.

94. Patel S, Lyons AR, Hosking DJ. Drugs used in the treatment of metabolic bone disease. Clinical pharmacology and therapeutic use. *Drugs* 1993; 46:594–617.

95. Yakatan GJ, Poynor WJ, Talbert RL, et al. Clodronate kinetics and bioavailability. *Clin Pharmacol Ther* 1982; 31:402–410.

96. Plosker GL, Goa KL. Clodronate: a review of its pharmacological properties and theraputic efficacy in resorption bone disease. *Drugs* 1994; 47(6):945–982.

97. Fitton A, Mctavish D. Pamidronate: A review. *Drugs* 1991; 41:289–318.

98. Pentikainen PG, Ezomaa J, Nurmi AK, et al. Pharmacokinetics of Clodronate in pa-tients with metastatic breast cancer. *Int J Clin Pharmacol Ther* 1989; 27:222–228.

99. Bounameaux HM, Sheifferli J, Montani JP, et al. Renal failure associated with intravenous bisphosphonates. *Lancet* 1983; 1:471–474.

100. Kanis JA, Preston CJ, Yates AJP, et al. Effects of intravenous diphosphonates on renal function. [Letter] *Lancet* 1983; 1:1328.

101. Fleisch H. Bisphosphonates: A new class of drugs in diseases of bone and calcium metabolism. *Recent Results Cancer Res* 1989; 116:1–28.

102. Mundy, GR, Ibbotson KJ, D'Souza SM, et al. The hypercalcemia of cancer—clinical implications and pathogenic mechansims. *N Engl J Med* 1984; 30:1718–1727.

103. Gallacher ST, Ralston SH, Patel U, Boyle IT. Side-effects of pamidronate. *Lancet* 1989; 2:42–43.

104. Adami S, Bhalla AK, Dorizzi R, et al. The acute phase response after bisphosphonate administration. *Calcif Tissue Int* 1987; 41:326–331.

105. Miller SC, Jee WSS. The effect of dichloromethylene diphosphonate, a pyrophos-phate analogue, on bone and bone cell structure in the growing rat. *Anat Rec* 1979; 193:439–462.

106. Stutzer A, Trezhsez U, Fleisch H, Schenk R. Effect of bisphosphonates on osteoclast number and bone resorption in the rat. (Abstract) *Calcif Tissue Int* 1987; 41(suppl 2):50.

107. Sato M, Grasser N. Effects of bisphosphonates on isolated rat osteoclasts as examined by reflected light microscopy. *J Bone Miner Res* 1990; 5:31–40.

108. Sietsema WK, Ebetino FH, Salvagno AM, Bevan JA. Antiresorptive dose-response relationship across three generations of bisphosphonates. *Drugs Exp Clin Res* 1989; 15:389–396.

109. Shinoda H, Adamek G, Felix R, Fleisch H, Schenk R, Hagan P. Structure–activity relationships of various bisphosphonates. *Calcif Tissue Int* 1988; 25:87–99.

110. Miller SC, Jee NSS. Effects of clodronate and etidronate on growing rat tibia. *Calcif Tissue Res* 1977; 23:207–214.

111. De Vries HR, Bijvoet OLM. Results of prolonged treatment of Paget's disease of bone with disodium ethane-1-hydroxy-1,1 diphosphonate (EHDP). *Neth J Med* 1974; 17:281–298.

112. Rizzoli R, Buchs B, Bonjour JP. Effect of a single infusion of alendronate in malignant hypercalcaemia: dose dependency and comparison with clodronate. *Int J Cancer* 1992; 50:706–712.

113. Delmas PD, Charhon S, Chapuy MC, et al. Long-term effects of dichloromethylene diphosphonate (CI_2MDP) on skeletal lesions in multiple myeloma. *Metab Bone Dis Relat Res* 1982; 4:163–168.

114. Adami S, Milan M. Clodronate therapy of metastatic bone disease in patients with prostatic cancer. *Recent Results Cancer Res* 1989; 116:67–72.

115. Ernst DS, MacDonald N, Paterson AHG, et al. Double-blind, crossover trial of IV clodronate in metastatic bone pain. *J Pain Symptom Manage* 1992; 7:4–11.

116. Ernst DS, Brasher P, Hagen N, et al. A randomized, controlled trial of intravenous clodronate in patients with metastatic bone disease and pain. *J Pain Symptom Manage* 1997; 13:319–326.

117. Glover D, Lipton A, Keller A, et al. IV pamidronate disodium treatment of bone metastases in patients with breast cancer. *Cancer* 1994; 74:2949–2955.

118. Thurlimann B, Morant R, Jungi WF, Radziwill A. Pamidronate for pain control in patients with malignant osteolytic bone disease: a prospective dose-effect study. *Support Care Cancer* 1994; 2(1):61–65.

119. Purohit OP, Anthony C, Radstone CR, et al. High dose IV pamidronate for metastatic bone pain. *Br J Cancer* 1994; 70(3):554–558.

120. van Holten-Verzantvoort ATM, Zwinderman AH, Aaronson NK, et al. The effect of supportive pamidronate treatment on aspects of quality of life of patients with advanced breast cancer. *Eur J Cancer* 1991; 27(5):544–549.

121. Robertson AG, Reed NS, Ralston SH. Effect of oral clodronate on metastatic bone pain: a double blind, placebo controlled study. *J Clin Oncol* 1995; 13(9):2427–2430.

122. Coleman RE, Vinholes J, Abbey ME, Purhit OP. Double-blind randomized trial of pamidronate for the palliative treatment of metastatic bone disease. *ASCO Proceedings* 1996; 15:528 (Abstract #1706).

123. Rizzoli R, Buchs B, Bonjour JP. Effect of a single infusion of alendronate in malignant hypercalcemia: dose-dependency and comparison with clodronate. *Int J Cancer* 1992; 50:706–712.

124. Nussbaum SR, Warrell RP, Rude R, et al. Dose-response study of alendronate sodium for the treatment of cancer-associated hypercalcemia. *J Clin Oncol* 1993; 11:1618–1623.

125. Zysset E, Ammann P, Jenzer A, et al. Comparison of a rapid (2-h) versus a slow (24-h) infusion of alendronate in the treatment of hypercalcemia of malignancy. *Bone Miner* 1992; 18:237–249.

126. O'Rourke NP, McCloskey EV, Rosini S, Coleman RE, Kanis JA. Treatment of malignant hypercalcemia with neridronate. *Br J Cancer* 1994; 96(5):914–917.

127. Pecherstorfer M, Herrmann Z, Body JJ, et al. Randomized phase 2 trial comparing different doses of the bisphosphonate ibandronate in the treatment of hypercalcemia of malignancy. *J Clin Oncol* 1996; 14:268–276.

128. Scher HI, Curley T, Yeh S, et al. Hormone refractory prostatic cancer: the role of radiolabelled diphophonates and growth factor inhibitors. In: Yamanaka H., ed. *Prostate Cancer and Bone Metastases.* New York: Plenum Press, 1992:115–129.

129. Curley T, Scher H, Thaler H, et al. Phase 2 trial of 186-rhenium hydroxyethylidene diphosphonate as treatment of painful bone metastases from prostatic cancer. *ASCO Proceedings* 1992; 11:214 (Abstract #672).

130. Maxon HR, Thomas SR, Hertzberg VS, et al. Rhenium-186 hydroxyethylidene diphosphonate for the treatment of painful ossesous metstases. *Semin Nucl Med* 1992; 22(1):33–40.

131. Paterson AHG, Powles TJ, Kanis J, et al. Double-blind controlled trial of oral clodronate in patients with bone metastases from breast cancer. *J Clin Oncol* 1993; 11:59–65.

132. Hortobagyi GN, Proter L, Blayney D, et al. Reduction of skeletal related complications in breast cancer patients with osteolytic bone metastases receiving chemotherapy by monthly pamidronate sodium infusion. *ASCO Proceedings* 1996; 15:103 (Abstract #99).

133. Berenson JR, Lichtenstein A, Porter L, et al. Effcacy of pamidronate in reducing skeletal events in patients with advanced multiple myeloma. *N Engl J Med* 1996; 334:488–493.

134. Lahtinen R, Laakso M, Palva I, et al. Randomised, placebo-controlled multicentre trial of clodronate in multiple myeloma. *Lancet* 1992; 340:1049–1052.

135. Elomaa I, Kylmala T, Tammela T. Effect of oral clodronate on bone pain: a controlled study in patients with metastatic prostatic cancer. *Int Urol Nephrol* 1992; 42(2):159–166.

136. Paterson AHG, McCloskey EV, Ashley S, et al. Reduction of skeletal morbidity and prevention of bone metastase with oral clodronate in women with recurrent breast cancer in the absence of skeletal metastases. *ASCO Proceedings* 1996; 15:104 (Abstract #83).

137. Siris ES, Sherman WH, Baquiran DC, et al. Effects of dichloromethylene diphosphonate on skeletal mobilization of calcium in multiple myeloma. *N Engl J Med* 1980; 302:310–315.

138. Van Holten-Verzantvoort ATM, Kroon HM, Bijvoet OLM, et al. Palliative pamidronate treatment in patients with bone metastases from breast cancer. *J Clin Oncol* 1993; 11:491–498.

6

Surgical Palliation of Malignant Bone Pain

FRANK J. FRASSICA, DEBORAH ANNE FRASSICA,
STEVEN A. LIETMAN, CAMERON A. HUCKELL, JOHN P.
KOSTUIK, EDMUND Y.S. CHAO, AND FRANKLIN H. SIM

Bone metastases are the third most common site of metastases.[1] Although lung and liver metastases are more common, destructive lesions of the skeleton often cause more problems for the patient than do visceral metastases. A marked reduction in the quality of life can occur when bone metastases are not managed in an aggressive fashion to prevent fractures, pain and neurologic deficits. Patients may despair when they lose their independence as a result of uncontrolled bone metastases.

Surgery is an important adjunct to maintain the independence of the patient with bone metastases. Surgical treatment is centered on three principal areas: prevention and treatment of long bone fractures, reconstruction of major joints, and reconstruction of the spine (with or without decompression) to restore structural stability. Patients must be carefully evaluated prior to surgery and during the perioperative period to minimize the risk of complications.

Preoperative Evaluation

Prior to surgery, patients should be questioned to identify sites of bone destruction that may interfere with subsequent rehabilitation. For instance, it is important to ensure that a patient undergoing intramedullary nail fixation in the lower extremity does not have an impending fracture in the upper extremity. Otherwise, the patient may sustain a fracture in the upper extremity when using crutches or a walker during rehabilitation. Specific queries should include: (1) upper extremity pain over the shoulders and arm, (2) pelvic and hip pain, (3) pain over the thighs, and (4) pain in the cervical spine.

The general medical status of the patient must also be ascertained.[2] Many patients with metastatic bone disease have significant anemia. The anemia is usually the result of a combination of marrow replacement by tumor cells, chemotherapy, radiation therapy to control bone metastases (especially in the pelvis and spine), and anemia of chronic disease. If the hematocrit level is below 30%, we usually transfuse the patient to achieve a level between 30% and 35% prior to surgery. Neutropenia often occurs after cytotoxic chemotherapy regimens. When the absolute neutrophil count is below 500 per cubic centimeter, we avoid invasive procedures. We prefer to let the leukocyte count recover to 2000–3000 per cubic centimeter prior to surgery. Thrombocytopenia can also be a significant problem. If the platelet count is below 30,000 and a trend toward recovery is not present, we avoid surgery. If the count is between 30,000 and 50,000 and the trend is toward recovery, we transfuse the patient with platelets on the morning of surgery.

The serum calcium level should be checked prior to surgery.[3,4] Hypercalcemia is common in patients with lung cancer, breast carcinoma, lymphoma, and myeloma. An elevated calcium level must be corrected before surgery. Hydration, saline diuresis, and intravenous bisphosphonate therapy are the mainstay approaches. A nutritional assessment should also be performed. When necessary, oral or parenteral nutrition supplements are used postoperatively.

Surgery in the Lower Extremity

The pelvis, hip joint, and long bones of the lower extremities are common sites of metastatic bone disease. Bone destruction in these sites can result in pain, the inability to ambulate or get out of bed, and pathologic fractures. Common sites of bone destruction include the ilium and para-acetabular region, femoral neck and head, intertrochanteric and subtrochanteric regions, and the diaphysis of the femur. The distal femoral and proximal tibial metaphyses may also be involved.

The goal of surgery in lower extremity sites is to allow the patient to bear full weight without the fear of fracture or pain. This can be accomplished with both internal fixation devices and prosthetic devices. Internal fixation devices can be augmented with methyl methacrylate to fill gaps and restore missing cortical segments.[5] The cement must be judiciously placed, as bone healing will not occur in areas where there is cement. Periosteal new bone formation will not occur if the bone cement is placed outside of the medullary cavity.

The indications for surgery are individualized for each patient. Factors to be considered include the histology of the lesion, the pattern of bone destruction, the site and size of the lesion, and the general condition of the patient. We do not use arbitrary estimates of life expectancy (such as three month survival) in deciding to offer surgical intervention. If the patient is strong enough to withstand the surgical procedure and the early perioperative period, we prefer to stabilize impending or frank fractures. Even if life expectancy is short, quality of life is much better without fear of fracture or the disabling pain of a pathologic fracture. Many patients outlive estimates of survival.

Variations in the aggressiveness of tumors and the response of bone, as well as the degree of cortical destruction, make it difficult to predict the fracture risk for femoral metastases. We employ guidelines based on the characteristics of the lesion (Table 6.1).

Purely lytic lesions that encompass 50% of the cortical diameter and are in high stress areas carry the greatest risk of fracture. Fracture is especially imminent when these purely lytic lesions exceed 5 cm in length. The presence of pain on weight-bearing is an important symptom to elicit, as it is often a harbinger of fracture. We generally prefer to proceed with prophylactic fixation whenever lytic lesions exceed 50% of the shaft diameter. Lesions that are purely blastic have a much lower risk of fracture and seldom require prophylactic fixation, even when large in size.

Lesions of the pelvis

Destructive lesions in the pelvis and hip are also common. Pelvic lesions may involve all the structures in the pelvic ring: sacrum, ilium, para-acetabular region, pubic rami and ischium, and ischial rami. Most pelvic lesions can be successfully managed with external beam irradiation, and few cases need surgical management. Para-acetabular lesions may threaten the structural integrity of the hip

Table 6.1. Characteristics of metastatic bone lesions

Pattern of bone destruction
  Purely lytic
  Mixed lytic-blastic
  Purely blastic

Location (High stress areas)
  Subtrochanteric femur
  Mid-diaphysis femur
  Femoral neck
  Distal dia-metaphyseal

Degree of cortical involvement
  <25% shaft diameter
  25%–50% shaft diameter
  >50% shaft diameter

Length of lesion
  <2 cm
  2–5 cm
  >5 cm

Pattern of pain
  Weight-bearing
  Non-weight-bearing

joint, and require stabilization. In the absence of intra-articular involvement, however, most patients can be managed without surgery. When the articular cartilage has been compromised, there is often significant mechanical pain and, in this instance, radiotherapy alone will not improve the pain and resulting disability.

Computerized tomographic (CT) scans are useful in characterizing the extent of bone destruction. Other metastatic sites in the pelvic ring can also be identified. The clinician should exclude sacral lesions with nerve root impingement and lumber spine lesions as a source of the patient's pain.

Harrington[6] has classified acetabular lesions into three types: Type I lesions have minimal bone destruction with no compromise of the medial wall or acetabular rims; Type II defects are larger and have compromise of the medial wall; Type III lesions are extensive and have loss of the medial wall and acetabular rims.

Most pelvic and acetabular lesions can be managed without surgery, using external beam irradiation and protected ambulation. CT scans help to quantitate the degree of bone destruction and to define the condition of the subchondral bone and articular cartilage. If the subchondral bone is intact (there are no fratures or incongruities of the joint surface), external beam irradiation and protected weight-bearing can be used. Protected weight-bearing with a walker is usually carried out for eight weeks after the completion of irradiation. Patients then progress to a cane. If pain continues, a repeat CT scan of the pelvis is performed to assess the integrity of the subchondral bone and articular cartilage. When compromised, total hip arthroplasty is indicated.

Type I lesions can be treated successfully with standard cemented acetabular components. Defects in the para-acetabular regions are filled with methyl methacrylate. Type II lesions require augmentation of the medial wall with a composite of methyl methacrylate and wire mesh or other cement–restriction devices. Type III lesions, which have insufficient remaining bone stock to support the acetabular component, present the greatest challenge. The surgeon must reconstruct the acetabulum with fixation into the remaining ilium or sacrum, to prevent superior migration of the component. This is usually accomplished with cement, Steinmann pins, and acetabular reinforcement rings.

Lesions of the proximal femur

Proximal femoral lesions are extremely common. These lesions may involve the femoral head, neck, and intertrochanteric regions either singly or in combination. Small lesions in the femoral head (<50% bone involvement and no destruction of the subchondral or femoral neck cortices) can be managed without surgery. Lesions in the femoral neck with destruction of either the medial or lateral cortices generally require fixation. Although small lesions (<25% cortical destruction) may be managed without surgery, the risk of fracture is high in this region. Bipolar hemiarthroplasty is an effective procedure which has a low morbidity and can address lesions of the femoral neck, head, and limited lesions of the trochanteric region. Patients are allowed immediate full weight-bearing. Pain relief is excellent and patients can return to their homes if their medical condition permits. If the proximal femoral lesion is more extensive, with significant destruction of the femoral neck and intertrochanteric regions, head and neck replacement prostheses are used to reconstruct the deficient bone. Custom proximal femoral replacements are useful when large areas have been destroyed.[7] We generally use the proximal femoral replacement to reconstruct the proximal femur after internal fixation devices fail (Fig 6.1).

Lesions of the femoral shaft

Destructive lesions in the shaft of the femur are common. Interlocking intramedullary nails are extremely effective devices for providing rigid fixation. We prefer to stabilize the lesions before fracture, as rehabilitation is much easier. Before the development of the interlocking nail device, we opened the lesion, curetted out most of the lesion, and supplemented the nail fixation with methyl methacrylate. With the ability to statically lock the nail, it is seldom necessary to open the fracture. If the lesion is large and so destructive (>90% cortical bone destruction) that there is concern that the bone will not share any of the load and the nail will be subject to fatigue failure, we will supplement the fixation by filling the lesion with methyl methacrylate. If the lesion is in the mid-shaft of the diaphysis, we employ a standard intramedullary nail; if the lesion is in the subtrochanteric region, we employ a reconstruction nail (Fig. 6.2).

Lesions in the distal femur or proximal tibia

Distal femoral metaphyseal lesions are less common than more proximal lesions. Plate fixation is commonly used for destructive lesions in the distal metaphyseal region. Intramedullary nails may not achieve rigid fixation for distal lesions that extend to the articular cartilage. The lesions are curetted and the defects filled with methyl methacrylate. The reconstruction is then a composite of the remaining bone, methyl methacrylate, and the internal fixation device. Occasionally, it is necessary to resect the lesion and reconstruct the defect with a custom total knee replacement. In this scenario, there are three indications for resection/reconstruction: *(1)* destruction of the articular cartilage so that a painless articulation would not be feasible with an internal fixation device, *(2)* destruction of the metaphyseal bone such that rigid internal fixation is not attainable, and *(3)* progressive lesion after irradiation (especially when progression occurs after maximum irradiation, when further irradiation would exceed normal tissue tolerances).

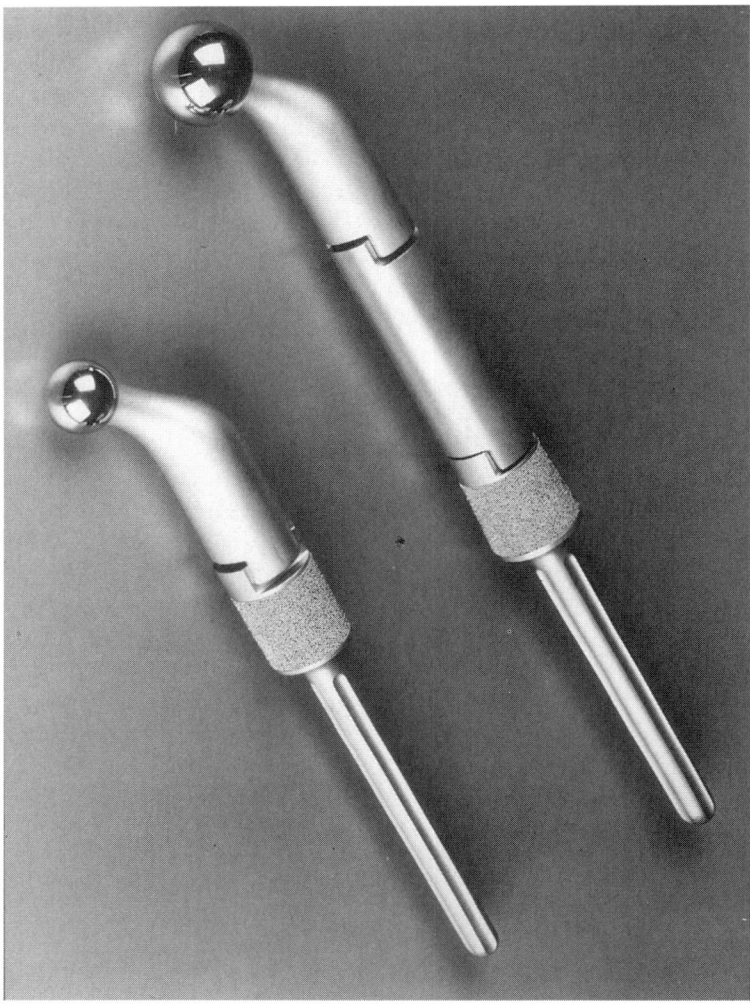

Figure 6.1. Custom proximal femoral replacement prosthesis used to reconstruct large defects where rigid internal fixation is not feasible, or to reconstruct defects when internal fixation devises.

Surgery in the Upper Extremity

Lesions of the proximal humerus

Lesions in the proximal humerus are very common. The bone destruction may occur in the head/anatomic neck of the humerus, metaphyseal area, or the surgical neck, either as isolated lesions or in combination. Standard proximal

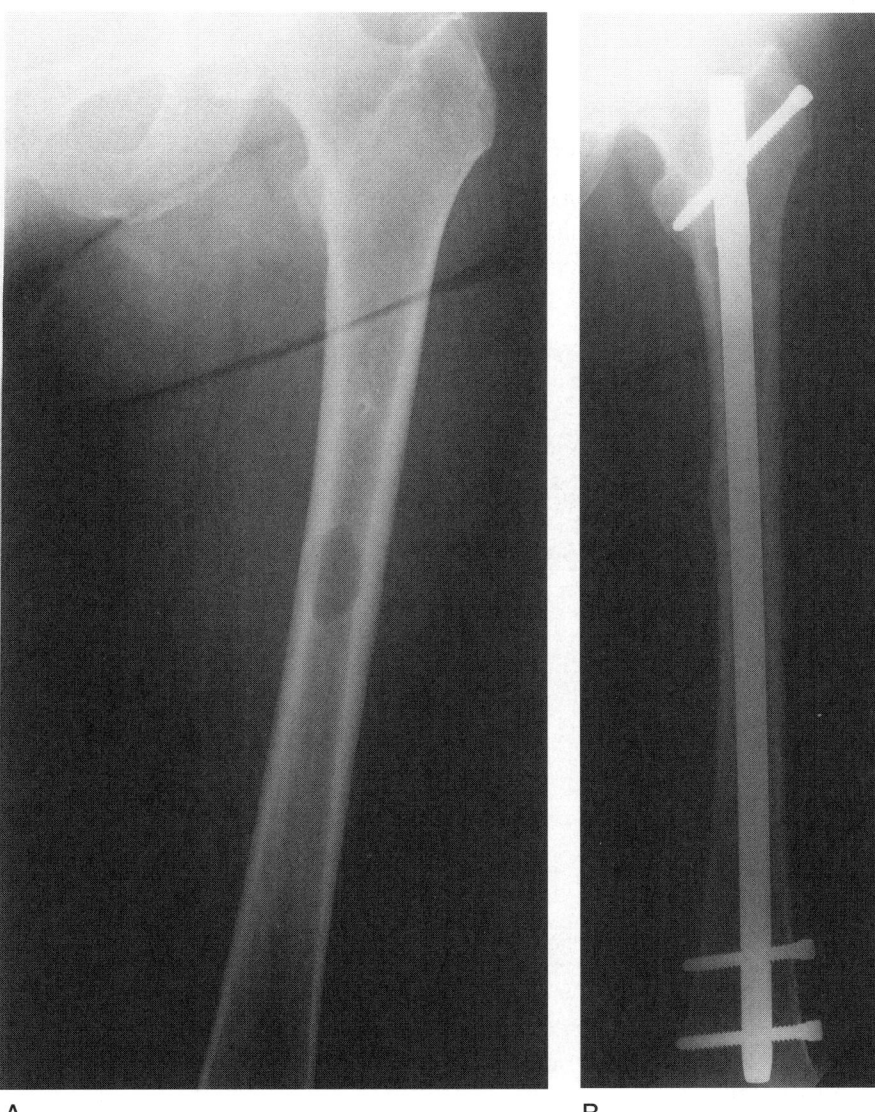

A   B

Figure 6.2. *A.* Anteroposterior radiograph revealing a lytic lesion in the mid-shaft of the diaphysis. *B.* Anteroposterior radiograph showing rigid internal fixation with an intramedullary rod with proximal and distal interlocking.

humeral endoprostheses are used when the articular surface has been destroyed, when fracture occurs through the anatomic neck, or when rigid fixation cannot be achieved with an internal fixation device and cement (Fig. 6.3). Metaphyseal lesions with intact articular cartilage can be treated with Rush rods and methyl methacrylate supplementation (Fig. 6.4). On very proximal lesions it is often not feasible to use standard intramedullary rods, as the working distance in the proximal fragment is so small that rigid fixation cannot be achieved.

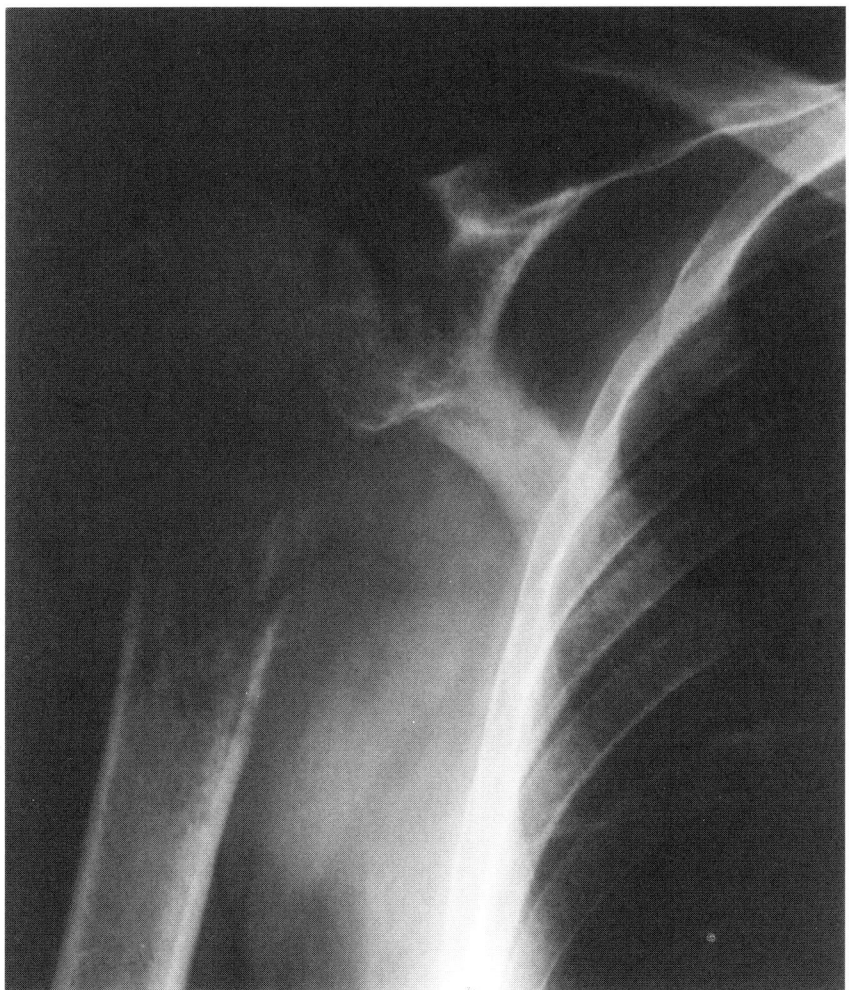

Figure 6.3. *A.* Anteroposterior radiograph revealing a large destructive lesion of the proximal humerus with a pathologic fracture.

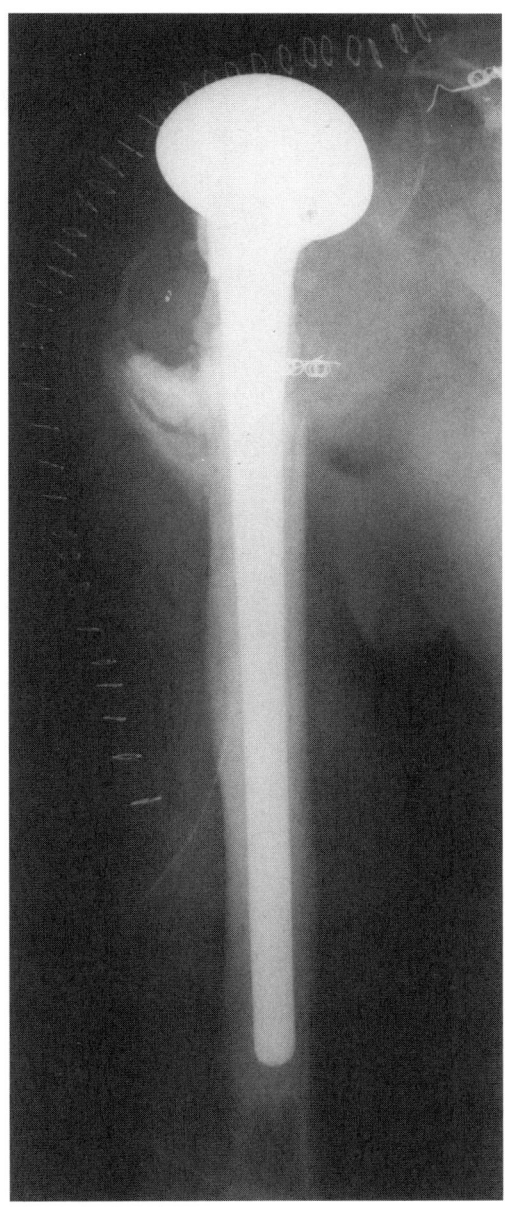

Figure 6.3. *B.* Anteroposterior radiograph showing reconstruction with a standard humeral prosthesis. [Reproduced with permission from Yazawa et al., ref. 13.]

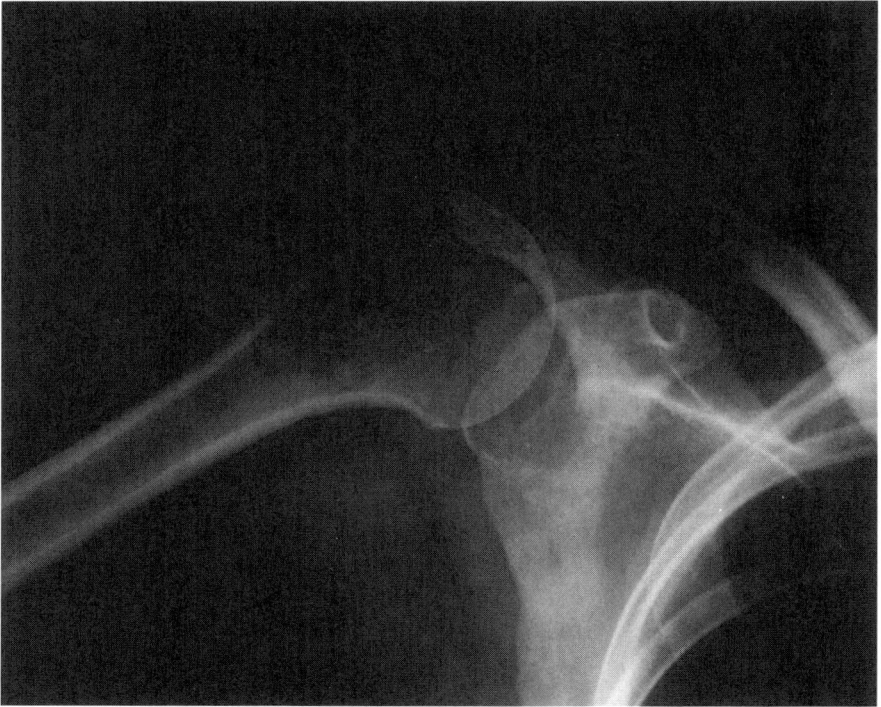

Figure 6.4. A. Anteroposterior radiograph of the shoulder revealing a destructive lesion in the proximal humerus.

Lesions of the mid-shaft humerus

Mid-shaft lesions may be treated with standard interlocking nails or with other intramedullary devices. When intramedullary devices such as Rush rods or En-der's nails are used, the fixation is supplemented with methyl methacrylate to achieve rigid fixation (similar to a locked device). When we use a locked nail, we always lock the nail proximally. Distal interlocking may not provide fixation as rigid as can be achieved in the femur. Distal interlocking is performed when it will significantly add to the rigidity of the fixation. If there is significant bone destruction at the involved site, such that rigid fixation cannot be achieved by the nail alone, we tend to open the fracture site and supplement the fixation with methyl methacrylate. If the diaphyseal bone destruction is so extensive that rigid internal fixation cannot be achieved, we resect the lesion and use a segmental defect prosthesis to reconstruct the bone.[8]

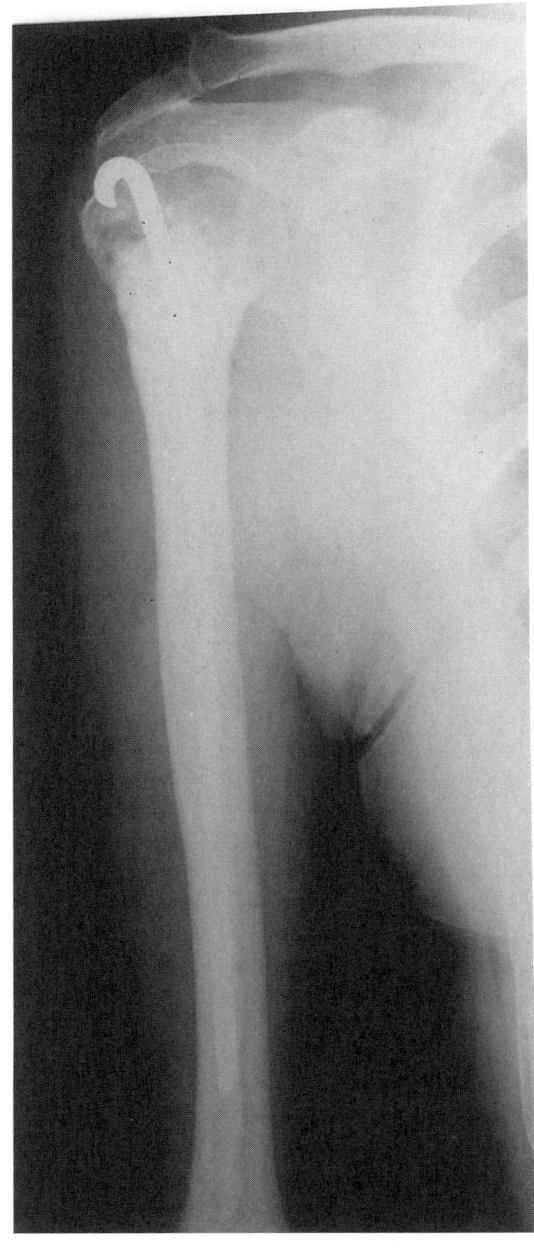

Figure 6.4. *B.* Anteroposterior radiograph showing reconstruction with a Rush rod supplemented with methyl methacrylate.

Surgery in the Spine

Metastatic involvement of the spine is common and occurs in virtually all patients with metastatic bone disease. Involvement of the vertebral column can cause significant clinical problems including pain, pathologic fractures, mechanical instability, and neurologic compromise. Early diagnosis and appropriate nonsurgical and surgical management can effectively control pain, minimize the risk of neurologic injury, and maintain the patient's quality of life.

Metastases to the spine occur in all vertebral segments, either singly or in combination. The clinician must obtain a careful history and physical examination to identify the level of vertebral dysfunction. Plain radiographs and magnetic resonance imaging (MRI) scans are used to define the anatomic features of the metastatic deposits. To plan effective treatment, the clinician must identify the

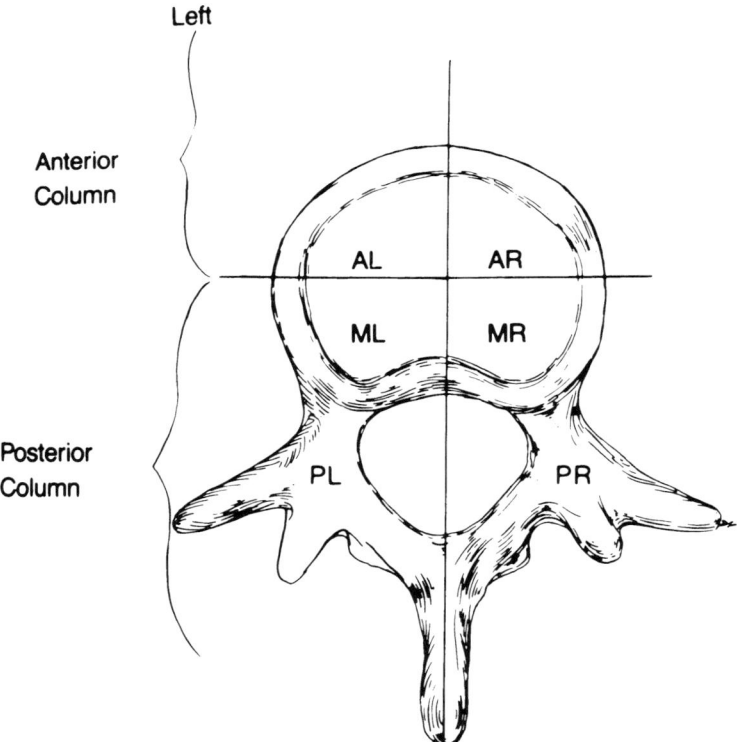

Figure 6.5. An axial CT scan of the lesion is divided into six columns. The lesion is stable if only two columns are destroyed, unstable if three or four columns are destroyed, and markedly unstable if five or six columns are affected. The columns are abbreviated as AR = anterior right; AL = anterior left; MR = medial right; ML = medial left; PR = posterior right; PL = posterior left.

areas of symptomatic bone destruction, determine the etiology of the patient's pain, and estimate the stability of the spine.

With a careful history, the clinician can usually localize the pain to specific areas of the cervical, thoracic, or lumbar spine. There may be tenderness to palpation and percussion over symptomatic areas. Careful neurologic examination is necessary to elicit weakness, reflex changes, and areas of sensory loss. Anteroposterior and lateral radiographs of the involved areas should be obtained. The radiographs should be studied carefully to identify compression fractures, sagittal angular deformity, and posterior element involvement. MRI is an excellent modality to identify multilevel involvement and soft tissue involvement; it is the most sensitive test for identifying spinal metastasis and can precisely localize areas of nerve root and spinal cord compression. In addition, MRI can determine if the neurologic compression is secondary to tumor alone or a combination of tumor, bone, and disk fragments.

Stability of the spine can be estimated by quantitating the amount and location of bone destruction and the status of the ligamentous stabilizers. We employ the Kostuik classification system (Fig. 6.5) to assess stability[9,10] and to diagnose impending vertebral fracture. If greater than three out of six columns are affected, impending fracture is likely. This is best assessed on the axial views of the CT scan. In the assessment of bone destruction, the CT scan is preferable to MRI.

Treatment is based on several factors. The patient's pain may be due to bone destruction, mechanical instability, or neural compression. If neural compression is present, it is important to determine if the compression is secondary to tumor alone or a combination of tumor and debris such as bone, disk, and ligamentous structures. If the patient's pain is secondary to compression from tumor alone, and the spine is stable, then external beam irradiation alone will often be effective. If the particular tumor is radioresistant then nonsurgical treatment may not be feasible even if the above conditions are met. If the patient's pain is due to bone destruction alone and the spine is stable, external beam irradiation alone is a reasonable treatment plan.

Surgical management can control pain and maintain the structural integrity of the spine. With improvements in surgical technique and advances in internal fixation devices, the surgeon can plan reconstructive procedures that have a low morbidity and are quite durable. The current situation reflects great advances over the past, when many surgeons employed laminectomy alone to decompress the spine, a procedure often resulting in inadequate decompression, continued pain, and worsening of mechanical instability (Fig. 6.6). The indications for surgical decompression and reconstruction are: *(1)* mechanical instability; *(2)* neural compression secondary to tumor growth, and debris such as bone ligament and disk material; *(3)* progressing neurologic deficit during or after radiotherapy; and *(4)* sufficient life expectancy to benefit from the procedure. Usually the tumor starts at the pedicle and spreads into the body, and its growth is limited by the disk space. Because most tumors are predominantly anterior, the surgical treatment involves anterior surgical approaches to the spine. Multiple level in-

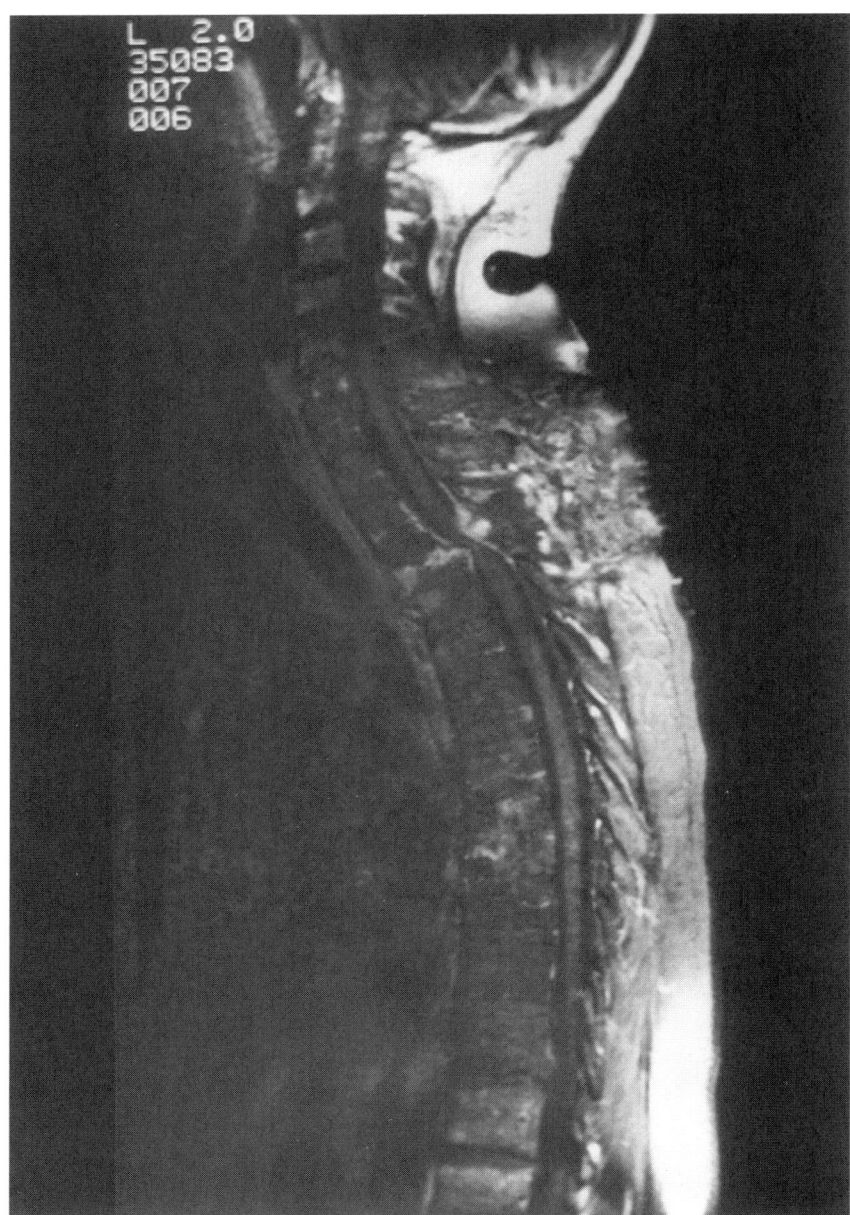

Figure 6.6. A 45-year-old man had a spontaneous pathologic fracture in the thoracic spine (T3) and no known primary lesion. He was treated at another center with a laminectomy and biopsy because of acute paraparesis. Despite the laminectomy, his neurologic condition continued to worsen. After transfer, an urgent anterior thoracotomy and anterior reconstruction with titanium-reinforced methyl methacrylate was performed. The patient's neurologic condition improved and he was ambulatory with a walker two months after decompression and reconstruction. *A*. Mid-sagittal T1-weighted and (*B*) mid-sagittal T2-weighted image following laminectomy revealing little relief from cord decompression and probable increased spinal instability.

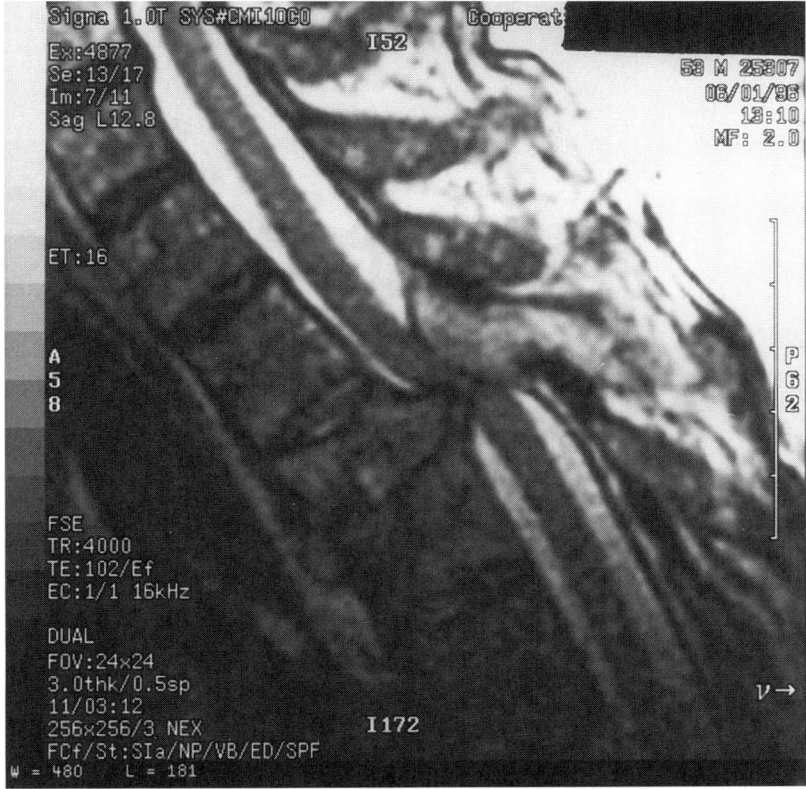

Figure 6.6. *B*. Mid-sagittal T2-weighted image.

volvement is most amenable to a posterior approach. Preoperatively, embolization can reduce blood loss with vascular tumors such as renal cell carcinoma.

Lesions in the cervical spine

Cervical spine lesions usually involve the anterior vertebral body. Progressive
bone destruction results in kyphosis and compression of both the involved nerve
roots and the spinal cord. Decompression and reconstruction are usually performed through an anterior approach. The involved vertebral body is resected.
The surgeon can then remove any debris or tumor that may be compressing the
nerve roots or spinal cord. Frequently, the vertebral artery is surrounded by
tumor and the surgeon must be cognizant of this during decompression. The
superior and inferior vertebral end plates are debrided back to normal bone and
the defect is reconstructed with a composite of methyl methacrylate and Steinmann pins or a threaded rod. At the transitional segment between the cervical
lordosis and the thoracic kyphosis there are increased biomechanical stresses

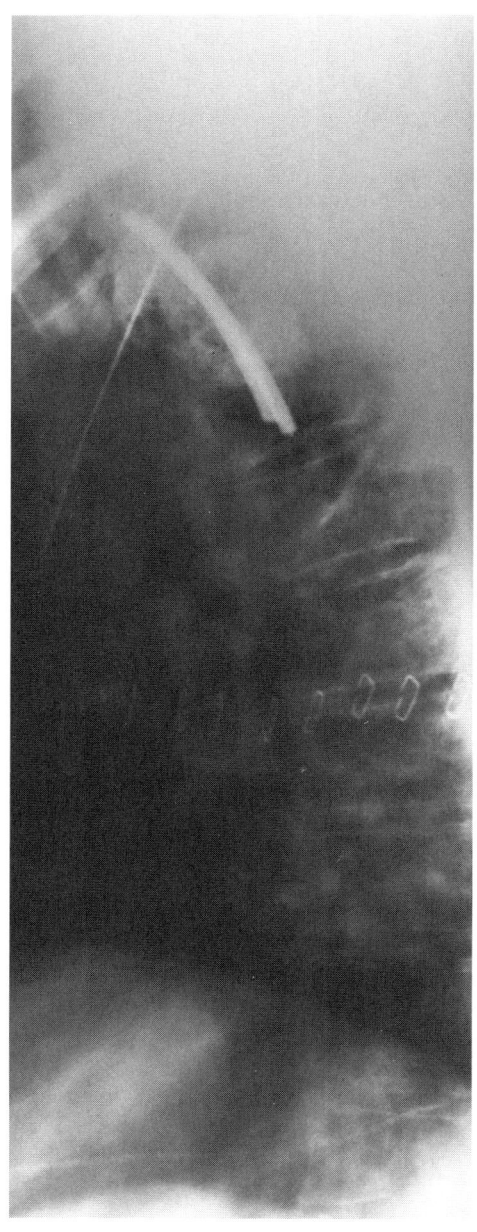

Figure 6.6. *C.* Postoperative lateral radiograph revealing corpectomy and reconstruction with titanium-reinforced methyl methacrylate.

placed on the construct, and a plate may be added for extra rigidity. Rigid fixation is achieved immediately and patients are mobilized quickly after surgery. It is essential to achieve enough initial rigidity to allow the patients to mobilize without bracing, because they have limited life expectancy and generally want an immediate improvement in their quality of life.

Posterior element bone destruction is less common but may occur. In this scenario, the destructive lesion is removed and the spine is stabilized with a standard posterior technique, such as wire fixation or lateral mass plating. The specific procedure depends on the quality of bone, integrity of the laminae, and the number of levels involved.

Lesions in the thoracic spine

As in the cervical spine, most thoracic lesions that require surgery occur in the anterior vertebral bodies. Decompression and reconstruction are usually performed through an anterior approach, which necessitates a thoracotomy. The involved vertebral body is removed and the surgeon is then able to decompress the neural elements under direct vision. Reconstruction is performed with a methyl methacrylate metal composite.[11] Immediate rigid fixation is achieved. Patients are mobilized out of bed quickly and most do not require postoperative bracing.

If multiple levels are involved and progressive kyphotic deformity is the major problem, then posterior stabilization devices may be used. Harrington or Luque rods are usually selected if there are cost considerations. Some patients may require the more modern adaptable and universal systems, which can be used for more challenging reconstructive problems. If a titanium system is used, postoperative imaging can be performed using MRI–metal suppression sequences. This may avoid the need for CT–myelography if there is deterioration at other levels.

Lesions in the lumbosacral spine

Lumbar spine lesions usually occur in the lower lumbar vertebral bodies and involve the anterior elements (Fig. 6.7A,B). Although decompression and stabilization can be performed through a posterolateral approach or an anterior approach, depending on the surgeon's experience, we find that the decompression is technically less difficult via the anterior approach. Reconstruction is usually accomplished with methyl methacrylate/metal composites (Fig. 6.7C,D). Patients with isolated lesions and extremely favorable prognoses (life expectancy greater than two years) can undergo reconstruction using an allograft (such as an allograft tibial shaft fashioned to fit into the defect). If the surgeon underestimates the life expectancy of a patient who was treated with a metal-reinforced anterior methyl methacrylate construct, a protective posterior instrumented fusion across the affected levels can be performed approximately one year after the anterior procedure.

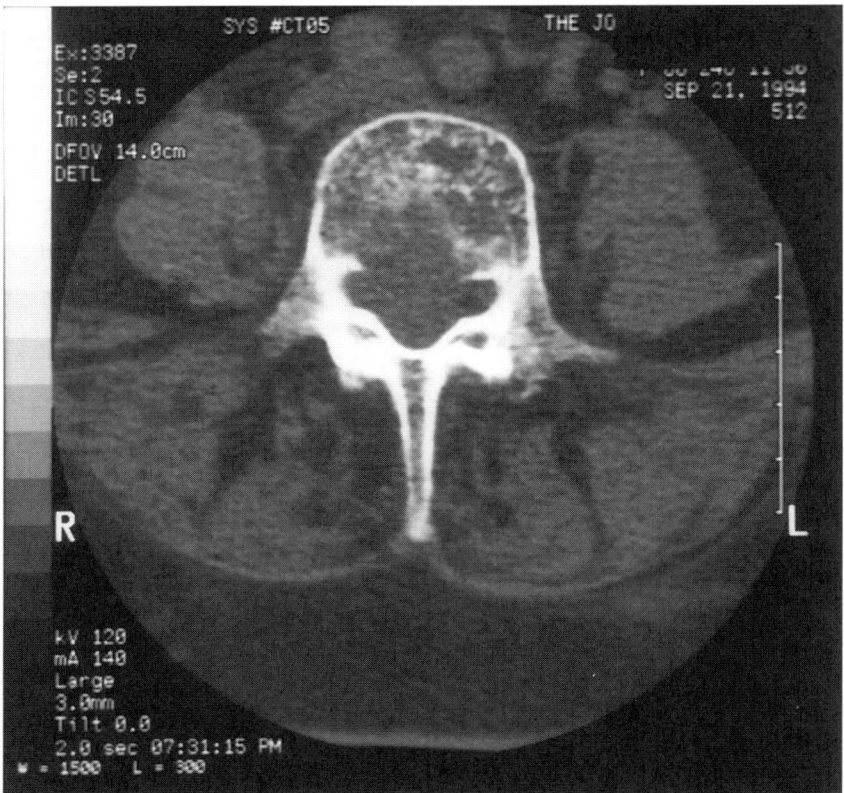

Figure 6.7. A. Axial CT scan shows loss of the posterior cortex in a patient with intractable L4 nerve root radiculopathy after pathologic fracture. (Compare Fig. 6.7B, on next page.)

Postoperative management

The major goals of surgical management of metastatic lesions are pain relief, full weight-bearing without any bracing, and maintenance of independence. When these three goals can be met, the quality of remaining life for the patient is optimized.

During the perioperative period, aggressive management is necessary to prevent complications. Many cancer patients suffer from immunosuppression, poor nutrition, fatigue, and depression; most are prone to thromboembolic disease. In patients who are immunosuppressed, we employ both a cephalosporin and an amino glycoside antibiotic for 48 hours after surgery and at least one antibiotic (usually the cephalosporin) is continued until all the drains have been removed. Patients are encouraged to use nutritional supplements and to get out of bed the day after surgery. They are allowed full-weight bearing during physical

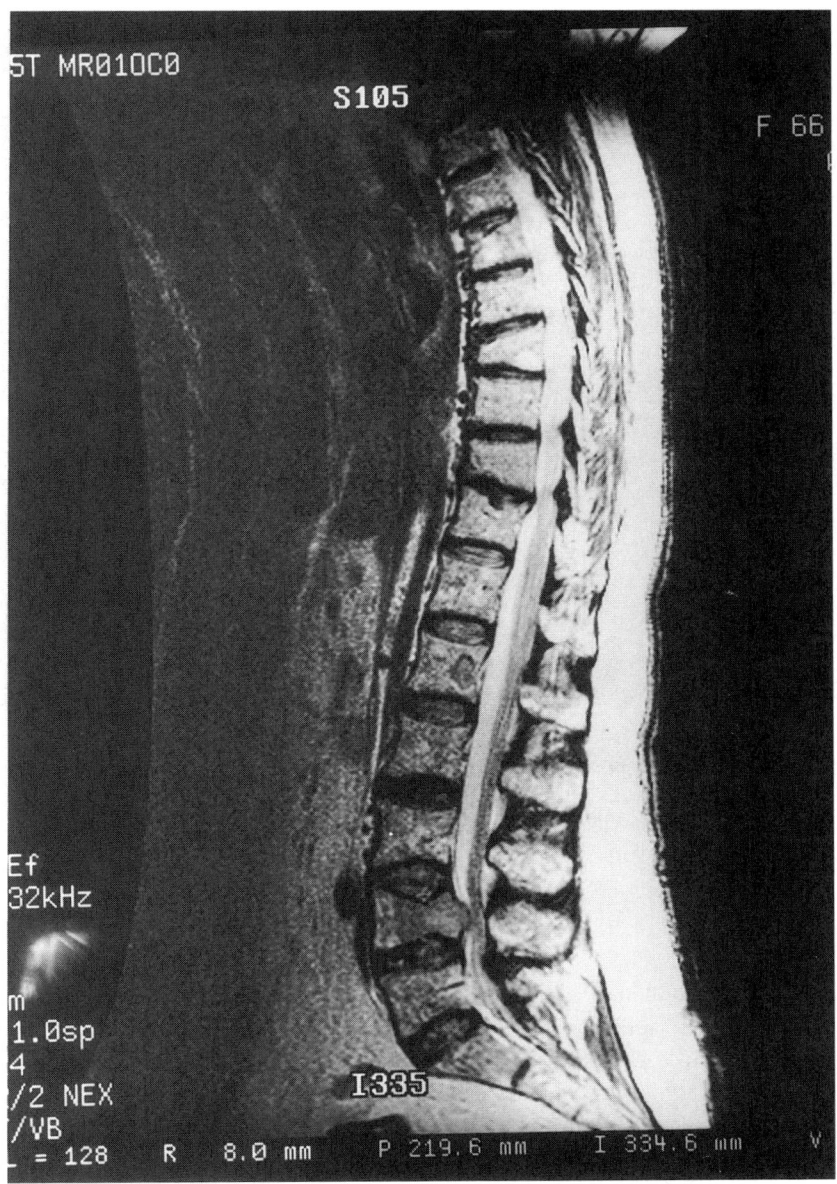

Figure 6.7. *B*. The mid-sagittal T2-weighted MRI image shows the compression of the neural structures in better detail than the CT scan.

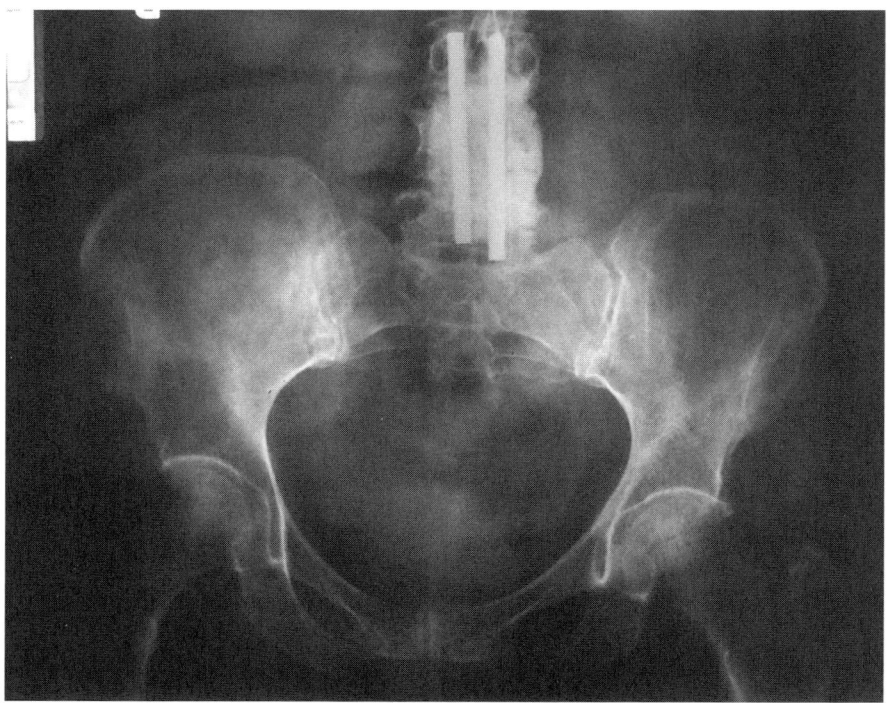

Figure 6.7. *C.* Anteroposterior radiograph after embolization and corpectomy. Reconstruction was performed with titanium-reinforced methyl methacrylate. Postoperatively, full weight-bearing was allowed immediately. Opioid drugs were not necessary after recovery from the surgery.

therapy. Anticoagulation with warfarin is used routinely in patients who have undergone either spine or lower extremity surgery. The warfarin is continued while they are in the hospital and they are given aspirin (325 mg twice daily) on discharge. Patients who have a history of prior thrombosis are continued on warfarin for three months after surgery.

Hypercalcemia may occur after surgery. Tumors commonly associated with this problem include breast and lung carcinomas, lymphoma, and multiple myeloma. The serum calcium level should be checked at least once after surgery. Early symptoms of hypercalcemia include anorexia, fatigue, and nausea or vomiting. As noted previously, hypercalcemia can be treated with saline diuresis, hydration, or an intravenous bisphosphonate such as pamidronate.

External beam irradiation is given to virtually all patients after surgery to prevent progression and to achieve pain control.[14] Radiotherapy may be omitted if the patient's prognosis is especially grave (<4–6 week survival).

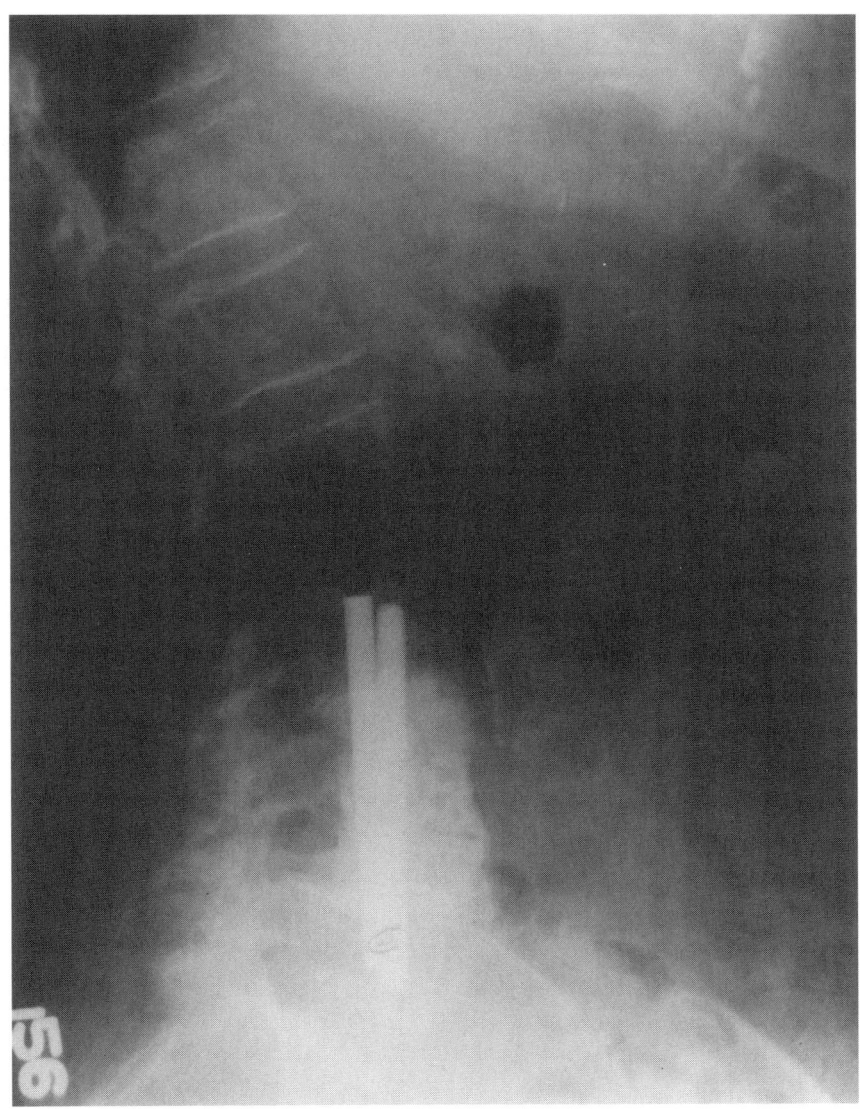

Figure 6.7. *D*. Lateral radiograph after reconstruction.

We generally begin external beam irradiation two weeks after surgery. Treatment is delayed if the wound has not completely healed and there is persistent drainage or evidence of superficial wound infection. We use minimally irritating skin sutures, such as monofilament nylon sutures, and leave them in for three to four weeks to deal with the possibility of delayed wound healing from the radiation. The dose of radiation varies, depending on the histologic type of the tumor, the presence or absence of other skeletal or visceral metastases, and the life expectancy of the patient. For patients with multiple lesions and favorable histologies (e.g., breast, lung, prostate) the usual dose is 3000 cGy in 10 fractions. For patients with relatively radioresistant lesions (such as renal cell tumor) or a single lesion and a long life expectancy, a larger dose is used (4000–5000 cGy over 20 to 25 fractions). Whenever possible, the entire internal fixation device or prosthesis is covered in the treatment fields. The use of strontium-89 as an adjunct to external beam treatment should be considered in patients with multiple bone lesions that are positive on technetium bone scintigram.

Failure rates at five years may be as high as 40% for internal fixation or prosthetic reconstruction of the femur and 20% for humeral lesions (Fig. 6-8). Most failures are secondary to disease progression and inadequate fixation devices. As survival continues to improve, the surgeon must carefully plan reconstruction so that the resulting composite will be both rigid and durable.

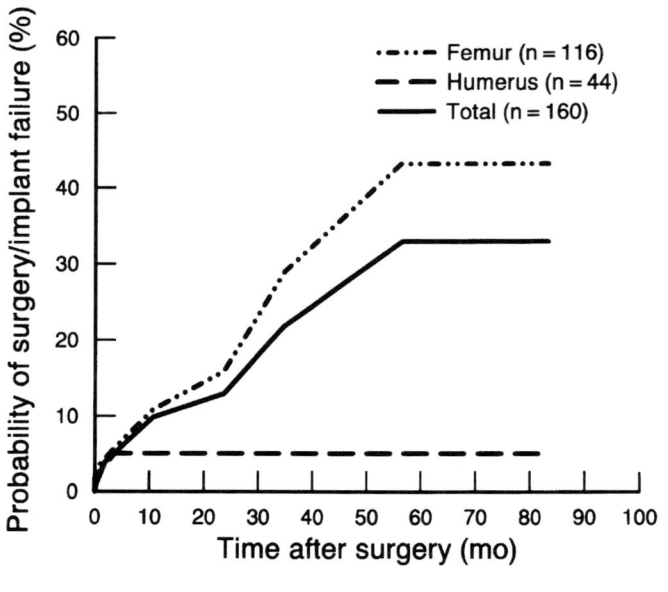

Figure 6.8. Kaplan-Meier curve demonstrating failure rates at 60 months following reconstruction of the humerus or femur.

Summary

Metastatic lesions may cause pain, functional compromise, and fractures. Although the great majority of lesions may be treated successfully with external beam irradiation, surgery plays a major role in maintaining a good quality of life for selected cancer patients. Prophylactic internal fixation should be considered whenever more than 50% of the cortical bone has been destroyed. Methyl methacrylate is used to supplement internal fixation and prosthetic devices when necessary. Prosthetic replacement is employed when rigid internal fixation is not feasible, the articular surface has been destroyed, or the patient has progressive disease despite irradiation. Decompression and reconstruction of the spine are necessary when mechanical instability or progressive neurologic deficits occur, or neurologic compromise is secondary to both tumor and debris such as bone, ligament, and disk fragments. External beam irradiation is used to halt tumor progression after surgery and reduce the need for additional surgical intervention.

References

1. Frassica FJ, Sim FH. Pathogenesis and prognosis of metastatic bone disease. In: Sim FH, ed. *Diagnosis and Management of Metastatic Bone Disease* New York: Raven Press; 1988; 1–6.
2. Frassica FJ, Sim FH. Pathophysiology of Metastatic Bone Disease. In: Sim FH, ed. *Diagnosis and Management of Metastatic Bone Disease* New York: Raven Press; 1988;7–14.
3. Frassica FJ, Gitelis SG, and Sim FH. Metastatic bone disease: general principles, pathogenesis, pathophysiology, and biopsy. *Instruc Course Lect* 1992; 41:293–300.
4. Frassica FJ, Sim FH. General considerations, spinal involvement and treatment of hypercalcemia in metastatic bone disease. *Curr Opin in Ortho* 1992; 3:784–791.
5. Harrington KD, Johnston JO, Turner RH, et al. The use of methyl methacrylate as an adjunct in the internal fixation of malignant pathologic fractures. *J Bone Joint Surg* 1972; 54A:1665–1676.
6. Harrington KD. The management of acetabular insufficiency secondary to metastatic malignant disease. *J Bone Joint Surg* 1981; 63A:653–664.
7. Sim FH, Frassica FJ, and Chaos EYS. Metastatic bone disease: orthopaedic management using new devices and prostheses. *Clin Orthop Rel Res* 1995; 312:160–172.
8. Chin HC, Frassica FJ, Shives TC, Pritchard DJ, and Chao EYS. Diaphyseal fractures of the humerus: the structural evaluation of a new method of treatment with a segmental defect prosthesis. *Clin Orthop Rel Res* 1989; 248:231–239.
9. Kostuik JP, Errico TJ, Gleason TF, et al. Spinal stabilization of vertebral column tumors. *Spine* 1988; 13:250–256.
10. Kostuik JP. Differential diagnosis and surgical treatment of metastatic spine tumors. In: *Advances in Operative Orthopaedics, Vol. 2.* St. Louis: Mosby-Yearbook; 1994:171–203.

11. Harrington KD: The use of methyl methacrylate for vertebral body replacement and anterior stabilization of pathologic fracture dislocations of the spine due to metastatic malignant disease. *J Bone Joint Surg* 1981; 63A:36–46.

12. King GJ, Kostuik JP, McBrom RJ, et al. Surgical management of metastatic renal cell carcinoma of the spine. *Spine* 1991; 16:265–271.

13. Yazawa Y, Frassica FJ, Chao EYS, Pritchard DJ, Sim FH, and Shives TC. metastatic bone disease: a study of the surgical treatment of 166 pathological humeral and femoral shaft fractures. *Clin Orthop* 1990; 251:213–219.

14. Schray MF, Gunderson LL. Principles of Radiation Therapy. In: Sim FH, ed. *Diagnosis and Management of Metastatic Bone Disease* New York: Raven Press; 1988: 141–146.

III

Psychopathology in
Patients with Cancer

Introduction

Psychiatric Disorders in Patients with Progressive Medical Disease: The Importance of Diagnosis

WILLIAM BREITBART

When the doctors
fail to heal you.
When no medicine chest
can make you well.
When no counsel
leads to comfort.
When there are no more lies
we can fake.
No more useless
information,
and the compass spins
between Heaven and Hell.
Let your soul
be your pilot.
Let your soul guide you,
guide your way.

Sting, 1996, "Let Your Soul Be Your Pilot"

The British singer–composer Sting wrote the above lyrics, which are from his album *Mercury Falling*, shortly after visiting a friend who was dying of AIDS in a New York City hospital. Sting reflected a nascent and growing realization in our society that medical technology does in fact have limitations, and that ultimately, perhaps, we must embrace a more spiritual perspective in life, and especially, in the face of death. Much of the re-awakening to the importance of the spiritual components of care is indeed welcome, essential, and healing for individuals with terminal illness and their families. However, I believe that part of what we are experiencing as a renaissance of spirituality in palliative care is in fact a backlash against the "over-medicalization of dying" and the invasion of often unwanted high technology interventions into end-of-life care. Clearly, modern academic palliative medicine must find a proper balance between the medical and spiritual aspects of care of the terminally ill. This balance is best achieved by incorporating into palliative care both patient preferences and values, and recommendations for medical therapeutics that are evidence based and empirically derived.

Perhaps one of the greatest challenges in palliative medicine will be to find the proper balance of the medical and the spiritual as it pertains to the assessment and management of psychiatric symptoms and disorders in the terminally ill. Psychiatric symptoms in patients who are dying seem to be perilously perched along a high wire that marks an illusory boundary between their medical/biological and spiritual/existential aspects. For instance, how one might understand desire for hastened death in a terminally ill patient may vary based on perspective and ideology. The expression of suicidal ideation or desire for death by a patient with progressive medical illness can be alternatively viewed as a rational communication of a socially accepted right to control the processes of dying, or as a sign of a clinical depression or undiagnosed delirium. The danger lies in the abandonment of clinical management based on sound diagnostic and assessment practices, in favor of management guided by ideology, philosophy, or anecdote. Therefore, skills in diagnostic assessment of psychiatric disorders (and neuropsychiatric symptoms), in patients with advanced cancer, AIDS, or other progressive medical illnesses, are of increasing importance to palliative care practitioners. They provide a sound basis for devising and instituting effective interventions in end-of-life care that allow for the proper balance between the medical and spiritual aspects of palliative care.

The Matrix of Physical and Psychological Symptoms

Recent evidence suggests that as patients with cancer or AIDS become progressively ill, entering advanced stages of illness, the burden of both physical and psychological symptoms becomes quite staggering.[1,2] Perhaps most compelling is the newly appreciated fact that physical symptoms such as pain, dyspnea, and constipation are in fact not the most prevalent symptoms of patients with advanced cancer or AIDS. In fact, psychological symptoms such as "worrying," "nervousness," "lack of energy," "insomnia," and "sadness" are among the most prevalent and distressing symptoms encountered in these populations.[2] Symptoms and syndromes of a neuropsychiatric nature, such as mood disorders (depression), cognitive impairment disorders (delirium), anxiety, insomnia, and suicidal ideation have a critically important role in symptom management in patients with advanced disease. Neuropsychiatric symptoms and syndromes coexist with many other physical and psychological symptoms and interact with each other, impacting negatively on quality of life. Psychological symptoms and psychiatric disorders must be understood in the context of the patient and family as the unit of concern. Therefore, the prompt recognition and effective treatment of both psychiatric and physical symptoms becomes critically important to the well-being of the patient with advanced disease, as well as his/her family. In general, palliative care specialists are quite expert at managing a broad spectrum of difficult and complex physical symptoms. It is critically important for the practitioners of palliative medicine to develop their skills in assessment and management of psychiatric symptoms and disorders in patients with progressive medical illness to the same high standard that has been maintained for pain and physical symptom control.

Symptoms, Syndromes, and Disorders

Psychiatric symptom control in patients with advanced disease can be understood and approached in a fashion similar to physical symptom control. That is to say, just as physical symptoms can be approached, from the perspective of management, either as a nonspecific symptom (e.g., pain) or as a specific syndrome (e.g., HIV–related peripheral neuropathy), so can psychological/psychiatric symptoms be understood.[3] One can take the tack of treating fatigue as a symptom and use psychostimulants, or treat insomnia with a benzodiazepine or low-dose sedating antidepressant. Such as approach can be quite reasonable, particularly if the collection of symptoms does not conform to (or meet DSM-IV criteria for) a specific and well-recognized psychiatric syndrome or disorder.[4] Psychiatrists are limited to making diagnoses of psychiatric disorders based on phenomenology, with little confirmation from laboratory or radiographic testing. A diagnosis of Major Depressive Syndrome or Delirium is based on the presence of a threshold number of specific criteria symptoms, which reliably identify a specific syndrome or disorder, and distinguish one psychiatric disorder from others that are phenomenologically similar. The veracity of the diagnosis is often supported by pathophysiologic underpinnings and response to specific pharmacologic/psychotherapeutic interventions. As with the treatment of a physical symptom such as pain, a management approach focusing on psychological symptoms as opposed to syndromes often uses nonspecific treatments (e.g., opioids for pain; benzodiazepines for insomnia) for a *symptom*, but more specific treatments for an identifiable *syndrome* (e.g., adjuvant analgesics for neuropathic pain, or antidepressants for major depression). Purists usually prefer to treat specific syndromes with specific interventions (e.g., an antidepressant for Major Depression). In the context of end-of-life care, however, it is often difficult to be a purist, particularly in the management of psychiatric complications of advanced disease.

As will be described in more detail below, diagnostic assessment of psychiatric symptoms in patients with advanced disease is extraordinarily challenging, partly because of the often unclear origin of these symptoms (i.e., are the symptoms due to advanced medical illness, medical treatments, or a psychiatric syndrome).[1,3,4] Therefore, I find it useful to be flexible in my approach to treatment of psychiatric complications in the terminally ill, and to move fluidly from a symptom–based to a syndrome/disorder–based approach, as the clinical presentation evolves. Nonetheless, one must establish a psychiatric diagnosis when it is present, because the effectiveness of intervention can undoubtedly be maximized.

Prevalence of Psychiatric Disorders in the Terminally Ill

Patients with advanced disease, such as cancer, are particularly vulnerable to the development of psychiatric disorders and complications.[1,3] The incidence of pain, depression, and delirium all increase with higher levels of physical debilitation and advanced illness. Approximately 25% of all cancer patients experience severe depressive symptoms, with the prevalence increasing to 77% in those with advanced illness. The prevalence of organic mental disorder (e.g., delirium) among cancer patients ranges from 25% to 40% and is as high as 85% during the terminal stages of illness. In a recent study,[5] Minagawa and colleagues used the Structured Clinical Interview for DSM-III-R (SCID) to evaluate the incidence of psychiatric disorders in a sample of 109 terminally ill cancer patients admitted to a palliative care unit (90% died within six months of admission; mean survival after admission was 54.7 days). In this sample of cancer patients approaching death, 53.7% met criteria for a specific psychiatric disorder (this incidence rate is similar to the rate of 47% found in a much earlier study of psychiatric disorders in a general cancer population). The most common psychiatric disorders among terminally ill cancer patients were: delirium (28%), dementia (10.7%), adjustment disorders (7.5%), amnestic disorder (3.2%), major depression (3.2%), and generalized anxiety disorder (1.1%). This most recent study dramatically underestimates the prevalence of depression in patients with advanced disease. The sample studied consisted of patients who were admitted to hospice and were only days or weeks away from death. Organic mental disorders were therefore over-represented in the skewed sample of patients with advanced disease requiring palliative care. The palliative care literature is almost completely lacking in data regarding the prevalence of psychiatric disorders in patients with end-stage heart, lung, liver, or other degenerative disorders.

Diagnosing Depression in the Terminally Ill

Only a few studies have examined the prevalence of depression in cancer patients with far-advanced disease, and these suggest that depression is more common in later stages of disease, ranging in prevalence from 23% to 58%.[3] The broad variation in the reported prevalence of depression in this population is due, in part, to the problems of terminology, methodology, and the application of diagnostic systems not originally intended for use in medically ill populations. These problems present a general obstacle to the treatment of depression in patients with advanced disease. The symptom of sadness or depressed mood is not equivalent to the syndrome of Major Depression. Several studies on the prevalence of depression examined levels of severity of depressive symptoms (often as reported by patients on self-report measures such as the Beck Depression Inventory) and do not reflect rates of diagnosis of the specific syndrome of Major Depression (although they are highly correlated). Distinguishing between normal sadness and the syndrome of Major Depression in patients with advanced disease has important treatment implications. Table 1 lists the criteria for a diagnosis of Major Depressive Syndrome according to the *Diagnostic and Statistical Manual of Mental Disorders*, 4th Edition (DSM-IV)[4]. The DSM-IV classification system for psychiatric disorders is the most widely used diagnostic system in North America. When different diagnostic classification systems are used (i.e., DSM-III, DSM-IV, and Research Diagnostic Criteria [RDC]), the rates of detection of depression in patients with life threatening illness may vary greatly. A critical problem associated with diagnosing depression in patients with advanced disease lies with the issue of how best to interpret the physical/somatic symptoms of depression.

Four different approaches to the diagnosis of major depression in the terminally ill patient have been described:[1,3] (*1*) an inclusive approach, which includes all symptoms whether or not they may be secondary to illness or treatment; (*2*) an exclusive approach, which deletes and disregards all physical symptoms from consideration, not allowing them to contribute to a diagnosis of Major Depressive Syndrome; (*3*) an etiologic approach, in which the clinician attempts to determine if the physical symptom is due to cancer illness or treatment (and so does not include it) or to a depressive disorder (in which case it is included as a criterion symptom); and (*4*) a substitutive approach, where physical symptoms of an uncertain etiology are replaced by other nonsomatic symptoms. The last approach is best exemplified by the Endicott Substitution Criteria, employed in studies by Chochinov and colleagues.[6,7] Endicott Substitution Criteria include replacing: change in appetite or weight *with* tearfulness, depressed appearance; sleep disturbance *with* social withdrawal, decreased talkativeness; fatigue or loss of energy *with* brooding, self-pity, pessimism; and diminished ability to think or concentrate, or indecisiveness *with* lack of reactivity. Chochinov and colleagues[6] studied

Table 1 DSM-IV criteria for major depressive syndrome

At least five of the following symptoms have been persistent for two weeks or more:
Depressed mood, dysphoria, loss of interest or pleasure, or anhedonia (at least one symptom must be from this group)
Physical/somatic symptoms: sleep disorder, appetite or weight change, or fatigue or loss of energy
Psychological/cognitive symptoms: worthlessness/guilt, indecisiveness/poor concentration, or thoughts of death/suicidal ideation

Table 2 Diagnostic assessment methods for depression
in patients with progressive medical disease

Diagnostic classification systems
   Diagnostic and Statistical Manual (DSM) III, III-R, IV
   Endicott Substitution Criteria
   Research Diagnostic Criteria
Structured diagnostic interviews
   Schedule for Affective Disorders and Schizophrenia (SADS)
   Diagnostic Interview Schedule (DIS)
   Structured Clinical Interview for DSM-III-R (SCID)
Screening instruments - self-report
   General Health Questionnaire −30 (GHQ)
   Hospital Anxiety and Depression Scale (HADS)
   Beck Depression Inventory (BDI)

---

the prevalence of depression in a terminally ill cancer population and compared
low and high diagnostic thresholds, as well as Endicott Substitution Criteria.
Interestingly, identical prevalence rates of 9.2% for major depression and 3.8%
for minor depression (total=13%) were found using RDC high threshold criteria
and high threshold Endicott criteria. Most recently, Chochinov and colleagues[7]
also reported that a single item screening measure (i.e., asking, in effect, "Are you
depressed?") was as accurate a diagnostic strategy as the use of a structured
clinical interview for depression. Table 2 lists some of the diagnostic assessment
methods commonly used for evaluating depression.

Diagnosing Delirium in the Terminally Ill

Cognitive disorders, and delirium in particular, have enormous relevance to
symptom control and supportive care.[1,3,8–10] In patients with advanced disease,
particularly in the last weeks of life, delirium is highly prevalent with rates ranging
from 25% to 85%. Delirium is associated with increased morbidity in the terminally ill, causing distress in patients, family, and staff. Delirium can interfere
dramatically with the recognition and control of other physical and psychological
symptoms, such as pain, in later stages of illness. Often a preterminal delirium has
multiple etiologies in the patient with advanced disease, including infection,
organ failure, chemotherapy, side effects from other medications (including
opioids), and rare paraneoplastic syndromes. Unfortunately, delirium is under-
recognized and under-treated. It is an area under-researched in palliative medicine. Impediments to progress in treatment and research in delirium have included confusion about terminology and lack of consistency in using diagnostic

Table 3 DSM-IV criteria for delirium

293.00 Delirium due to a general medical condition

A. Disturbance of consciousness (that is, reduced clarity of awareness of the environment) with reduced ability to focus, sustain, or shift attention.

B. Change in cognition (such as memory deficit, disorientation, language disturbance, or perceptual disturbance) that is not better accounted for by a pre-established or evolving dementia.

C. The disturbance develops over a short period of time (usually hours to days) and tends to *fluctuate* during the course of the day.

D. There is *evidence* from the history, physical examination, or laboratory findings *of a general medical condition* judged to be *etiologically related* to the disturbance.

classification systems. Multiple terms are often used to refer to similar cognitive disorders: delirium, reversible dementia, acute confusional states, cognitive failure, encephalopathy, organic brain syndrome, and an organic mental disorder. Clinical case studies or research reports that use varied or idiosyncratic terminology are less helpful contributions to the literature than those that use standard, uniform terminology or diagnostic classification systems. The use of a uniform diagnostic classification system would increase the consistency and reliability of both prevalence and intervention studies in the area of delirium and other cognitive disorders.

Despite changes in the classification of organic mental disorders or cognitive impairment disorders made in the evolution from DSM-III to DSM-III-R to DSM-IV, the essential nature of delirium as a syndrome has been maintained. Table 3 lists the DSM-IV criteria for delirium. The essential features of acute onset of disordered attention and cognition are retained. Associated phenomena such as psychomotor behavioral changes, perceptual disturbances, hallucinations, or delusions are no longer viewed as essential to the diagnosis of delirium. Diagnostic assessment methods for delirium in patients with advanced disease are listed in Table 4, and have been reviewed extensively elsewhere.[8] Only a limited number of studies of cognitive impairment disorders in palliative care settings have used such research methods.

Influence of Accurate Psychiatric Assessment on Care of the Terminally Ill

Ultimately, the importance of accurate psychiatric diagnostic assessment in end-of-life care lies in its ability to positively influence the care of patients and their families. Patients who express suicidal ideation or a desire for hastened death represent a clinical scenario in which accurate psychiatric diagnosis appears to have dramatic relevance. Several recent studies[1,3] suggest that unrecognized delirium and depression are important factors. Approximately 30% of hospital-

Table 4 Diagnostic assessment methods for delirium in patients with progressive medical disease

Diagnostic classification systems
    DSM-III, DSM-III-R, DSM-IV
    ICD-9, ICD-10

Diagnostic interviews/instruments
    Delirium Symptom Interview (DSI)
    Confusion Assessment Method (CAM)

Delirium rating scales
    Delirium Rating Scale (DRS)
    Confusion Rating Scale (CRS)
    Saskatoon Delirium Checklist (SDC)
    Memorial Delirium Assessment Scale (MDAS)

Cognitive impairment screening instrument
    Mini-Mental State Exam (MMSE)
    Short Portable Mental Status Questionnaire (SPMSQ)
    Cognitive Capacity Screening Examination (CCSE)
    Blessed Orientation Memory Concentration Test (BOMC)

ized cancer patients who express suicidal ideation have an unrecognized, untreated delirium.[1] Chochinov and colleagues[11] found that of 200 terminally ill cancer patients in a palliative care unit, 8.5% reported a clinically significant desire for death. Among patients with a desire for death, 60% met criteria for a diagnosis of Major Depression, compared with only 8% in patients without a desire for death.

Conclusion

The psychiatric dimensions of palliative care are being increasingly appreciated as critically important components of care at the end of life. Optimal management of psychiatric symptoms and syndromes in patients with progressive medical illness begins with accurate and sophisticated diagnostic assessment.

References

1. Breitbart W, Chochinov HM, Passik SD. Psychiatric aspects of palliative care. In Doyle D, Hanks GW, MacDonald N, eds. *Oxford Textbook of Palliative Medicine,* Second Edition. Oxford: Oxford University Press, 1997: 933–954.
2. Portenoy RK, Thaler HT, Kornblith AB, et al. The Memorial symptom assessment scale: an instrument for evaluation of symptom prevalence, characteristics and distress. *Eur J Cancer* 1994; 30A:1326–1336.

3. Breitbart W, Bruera E, Chochinov H, Lynch M. Neuropsychiatric syndromes and psychological symptoms in patients with advanced cancer. *J Pain Symptom Manage* 1995; 10:131–141.

4. American Psychiatric Association. *Diagnostic and Statistical Manual of Mental Disorders*. 4th Ed. Washington, D.C.: APA, 1994.

5. Minagawa H, Uchitomi Y, Yamawaki S, Ishitani K. Psychiatric morbidity in terminally ill cancer patients. *Cancer* 1996; 78:1131–1137.

6. Chochinov HM, Wilson KG, Enns M, Lander S. Prevalence of depression in the terminally ill: effects of diagnostic criteria and symptom threshold judgements. *Am J Psychiatry* 1994; 151:537–540.

7. Chochinov HM, Wilson KG, Enns M, Lander S. "Are you depressed?" Screening for depression in the terminally ill. *Am J Psychiatry* 1997; 154:674–676.

8. Smith MJ, Breitbart W, Platt MM. A critique of instruments and methods to detect, diagnose, and rate delirium. *J Pain Symptom Manage* 1995; 10:35–77.

9. Breitbart W, Marotta R, Platt MM, Weisman H, Derevenco M, Grau C, Corbera K, Raymond S, Lund S, Jacobsen P. A double-blind trial of haloperidol, chlorpromazine, and lorazepam in the treatment of delirium in hospitalized AIDS patients. *Am J Psychiatry* 1996; 153:231–237.

10. Breitbart W. Identifying patients at risk for, and treatment of major psychiatric complications of cancer. *Support Care Center* 1995; 3:45–60.

11. Chochinov HM, Wilson KG, Enns M, Mowchua N, Lander S, Levitt M, Clinch JJ. Desire for death in the terminally ill. *Am J Psychiatry* 1995; 152:1185–1191.

7

An Introduction to Psycho-oncology with Special Emphasis on Its Development in the Historical and Cultural Context

FRIEDRICH STIEFEL, PATRICE GUEX, AND OLIVIER REAL DEL SARTE

In many countries around the world, a new speciality, called psycho-oncology, has emerged during recent decades. Psycho-oncology deals with the psychosocial aspects of malignant diseases. As with any other medical speciality, the clinical, scientific, and educational work of psycho-oncology are closely related to its historical and cultural development.

A Short History of Psycho-oncology

Until the late nineteenth century, no curative or palliative treatment was available for cancer. Even the word "cancer" was not mentioned to the patient.[1] However, changes have occurred with the development of treatment modalities and societal shifts in many countries. The psychological and social aspects of cancer have increasingly become the focus of scientific study, education, and clinical care. Although many cancer patients cannot be cured, the achievements of curative and palliative treatments have transformed this once incurable, horrifying, and painful disease to a serious, but treatable and often chronic, disease.[2–4] The development of psycho-oncology is closely related to the development of oncology, which is itself embedded in the development of medicine and society as a whole (see Table 7.1).

While it is impossible to describe the complete history of psycho-oncology, a few important steps in its development can be highlighted. The interest in

Table 7.1 Some developments in medicine, oncology, and psycho-oncology°

	Medicine and oncology	Psycho-oncology
1800s	Anaesthesia (1846) Disease as a cellular disorder (1858) Antisepsis (1867) Radium (1898)	Reverse of fortune, bad socioeconomic conditions, and "mental misery" as source of cancer
1900–1920s	Surgical removal of some cancers Radiation for palliative cancer treatment American Cancer Society (1913) started	First studies on psychodynamics in cancer
1930s	National Cancer Institute (USA) and International Union Against Cancer	Increase of psychiatric wards in general hospitals
1940s	Nitrogen mustards with antitumor action	Psychosomatic movement
1950s	Chemotherapy cure of choriocarcinoma	Cancer personality
1960s	Combined treatment modalities	Consultation/Liaison/Psychiatry, thanatology movement
1970s	Hospice movement Life–sustaining support	Biopsychosocial concept of disease
1980s	Cancer "survivors"	Studies on survivors, quality of life
1990s	Genetic detection, supportive care	Ethical issues, psychotherapeutic interventions and quality of life, survival

°Modified after Holland JC (Reference 1).

psychological aspects of patients with cancer has existed for centuries. Galen, in the second century AD, thought that melancholic women were predisposed to breast cancer.[5] This theme was taken up again in the eighteenth century by Gendron, who found that patients who suffered from depression and anxiety were more subject to cancer, and by Guy, who added a little more detail by observing that nervous and hysterical women developed cancer after existential traumas and bereavements.[6] In the nineteenth century, it was asserted that reversals of fortune, bad socioeconomic conditions, and "mental misery" were the source of carcinomas.[7,8] In 1900, there was a renewed emphasis on the influence of emotional loss, bereavement, and melancholy. Evans[9] was the first to formulate the basis for psychodynamic theories about patients with cancer, after having studied the material from one hundred psychotherapeutic treatments.

The following decades were dominated by the *psychosomatic movement*[10–12] and the search for mind–body interrelationships. Psychoanalytic observations were recorded during the treatment of patients with various diseases, such as duodenal ulcer, ulcerative colitis, neurodermatitis, or essential hypertension.[13] Later hypotheses proposed specific emotional factors in somatic disturbances. According to one theory, physiologic responses to emotional stimuli, both normal and morbid, vary according to the nature of the precipitating emotional state; other non-emotional factors determine the type of physiologic response and ensuing pathology.[13]

Research in psycho-oncology also turned to the investigation of psychological factors in the development of cancer. Initially, isolated cases were described in which there was a striking correlation between emotional traumas and the appearance of cancer.[14-17] Later, longitudinal prospective studies, with more elaborate methodology, aimed to establish links between psychological problems or personality factors and the onset of cancer.[18-27]

A central observation seems to run through all these publications: cancer may be related somehow to the experience of separation, emotional upheavals, or very painful bereavement, often cumulative, and without the possibility of resolution in a favorable environment.[28] However, as Fox has put it: "Evidence both supports and rejects the view that psychological factors and stress are related to increased risk of cancer incidence, relapse and mortality in man. Evidence at hand, including demographic, suggests that if psychosocial factors and stress do have an effect on incidence of cancer in humans, it is small. The relationship of psychosocial factors and stress to cancer prognosis is more likely."[23]

With the development of *consultation–liaison psychiatry*, a broader concept of the psychiatrist's role in the general hospital emerged.[29] Consultation and liaison psychiatry attempted to evaluate and manage medically ill patients who develop psychological problems (consultation) and to serve the treating staff by providing supervision and other means beneficial to the needs of health care providers (liaison).[30,31]

The broader underlying concept derives from a theoretical framework proposed by Engel,[32] the *biopsychosocial model of disease*. This model assumes that disease cannot be sufficiently explained in biomedical terms, but has to include the contributory role of psychological and social dimensions in the disease process and their interrelationship. Clinicians with an interest in psycho-oncology also broadened its concepts by turning away from investigating the role of psychological and social factors in cancer development and the course of the disease and focusing instead on the effects of cancer on the psychological and social dimension of a patient.[33,34] These efforts led to important results in cancer prevention, detection, and clinical care.[35]

From Psychosomatic to Somatopsychic . . . and Back to Psychosomatic

The early practitioners in the psychosomatic movement failed to demonstrate the scientific value and the clinical usefulness of their concepts. One of the reasons may be that their psychiatric and psychoanalytic background led to a concentration on psychological factors while neglecting the somatic factors in the development of disease. Although this work contributed to newer concepts, such as the biopsychosocial model of disease, it also fostered a skeptical attitude among many psychiatrists working with patients with somatic diseases. This attitude rejected any notion of a psychosomatic conceptualization of disease. Some psychiatrists, especially in psycho-oncology, adopted and still adopt a purely somatopsychic conceptualization that attempts to relate all psychological phenomena observed in cancer patients to the cancer and its treatment, without any perception of an interdependence of body and mind in the development and course of malignant neoplastic disease. Similar to the representatives of the early psychosomatic movement, these psycho-oncologists have an extreme position with regard to the conceptualization of illness. While they accept that some cancers developed by noxious processes (such as smoking, diet, or alcohol) are modified by psychological factors or by personal habits,[27] they refuse to enter into any discussion of psychogenesis of malignant disease.[36]

There is still no complete understanding of the etiology of neoplastic disease. Changes in the genetic material of the neoplastic cell are important factors, but they do not offer sufficient explanation for the genesis of all cancers.[37] It may, therefore, be a mistake to refuse any notion of a "psychosomatic dimension" of disease solely on the grounds that the psychosomatic movement of the past was too narrow-minded in its approach.

Newer theories that have tried to re-integrate the Cartesian duality of body and mind have not only become more complex, but also have been supported by neurohormonal and psychoimmunological research.[38] Neurohormonal studies[39] reveal possible actions of stress hormones and central nervous system–effects on targets (such as estrogen and progesterone receptors) that could be linked to cancer initiation or progression. Research in psychoimmunology has been able to trace links between mind and body. For example, scores on mood and social support scales predict natural killer cell activity after treatment in patients with breast cancer[40]—a finding that may not only be scientifically interesting, but is also clinically useful. According to Bovbjerg,[41] the plausibility of psychoimmune involvement in cancer is based on research into the following critical hypotheses: (1) cancer incidence and progression are affected by psychosocial variables; (2) cancer incidence and progression are influenced by the activities of the immune system; and (3) the kinds of immune responses that influence cancer incidence and progression are themselves affected by psychosocial variables. Finally, psychotherapeutic interventions have had beneficial effects on survival of cancer patients.[42–45]

Although these neurohormonal and psychoimmunological findings may be promising, they have to be considered as preliminary. Differences between *in vitro* and *in vivo* findings, as well as differences between the *statistical significance* and the *clinical significance* of these findings, have to be taken into account when evaluating their impact. It is also too early to understand fully the effects of psychotherapeutic interventions on survival of cancer patients. While psychoimunological factors may be responsible for these outcomes, psychotherapy may also contribute to a patient's autonomy, leading to a more active role and a more comprehensive somatic treatment. Fox[46] has noted the inconsistency between the survival curve obtained in a psychotherapeutic intervention study and one based on normative data in a local population. Confidence in this research may therefore be diminished by confounding variables which include physical, sociodemographic, and psychosocial factors.

A theoretical reintegration of mind and body cannot be conceptualized with classic hierarchical systems, but has to simultaneously consider different systems, such as the biological, social, psychological, and cultural context of the individual. The emergence of the cognitive sciences may provide a historical opportunity to develop such a theoretical framework. The theses of McCulloch and others[47-49] suggest that the relationship of body, brain, and psyche cannot be conceptualized in terms of causality, but requires instead a "coding process." Contrary to the genetic code, the code relating body, brain, and psyche remains unknown. Yet, it may be that a disease, is actually an expression of body, brain, and psyche, which must first be coded among the three before it emerges. A clinical application of such ideas would imply acceptance of the idea that body, brain, and psyche represent different agendas that must be taken into account. Depending on the symptomatology, one of the agendas might outweight the others, but all must be considered by the members of an interdisciplinary team. Although, such interdisciplinary models of medical care are now accepted, there is still a considerable gap between theory and reality.

Culture and Psycho-oncology

The developments described above mainly reflect the situation in the United States, a leading country in the speciality of psycho-oncology. However, psycho-oncology does not have a unified theoretical framework and a general clinical agenda. Its guiding concepts vary from country to country. Some general impressions may help to illustrate the directions psycho-oncology has taken in different countries.

Viewing only the published material on psychotherapy in psycho-oncology,[50] gives the impression that psycho-oncology is mainly based on counseling,[51,52] family therapy,[53] cognitive–behavioral[54] and psychoeducative approaches,[55] and psychopharmacology combined with psychotherapy. According to the chapter on psychotherapeutic interventions of the most comprehensive textbook of psycho-oncology,[57] psychosocial interventions for cancer patients include individual and group interventions based on educational approaches, supportive psychotherapy, crisis intervention, psychodynamic therapy, and combinations of these approaches. This picture is valid for the United States, and there is no doubt that most of the studies on psychotherapeutic interventions in cancer patients employed counseling, supportive therapy, and psychoeducative group therapy. The best known studies of these approaches have used quantitative approaches to evaluate group therapies based on a cognitive–educative and time–limited approach. Most of these studies have been published in the leading medical language, English. These facts raise some questions:[58] Are current scientific methods adequate for investigating such a complex topic as psychotherapy? Are there psychotherapeutic approaches that are difficult to assess, but still of clinical value? Is quantitative research in psychotherapy the only way to prove its efficacy and are the end-points used to measure "success" reasonable? Are group therapies transferable to all cultures? Do cognitive–educative models benefit the majority of psycho-oncological problems, or were these approaches chosen because they were best suited for the standardized conditions of the intervention? Is the choice of time–limited therapies influenced by financial restrictions, and would this be reason enough to promote their implementation? Are there successful psycho-oncologists who use different approaches but do not publish, and what role does the use of the English language have in spreading the word? Who dominates the "market" in the medical literature and what consequences will this have on the dissemination and acceptance of a given psychotherapeutic approach?

Whatever the answers to these questions may be, the fact is that the clinical models of psychotherapeutic interventions differ among and within countries. Whereas the crisis intervention model, counseling, and cognitive–behavioral approaches are predominant in North America, in large parts of South America, and Central and Eastern Europe, a psychoanalytically-oriented and individual approach is the most common type of intervention.[59–64]

There are also particular approaches, such as the *psychosomatic approach*, which takes into consideration the interactions among biological, psychological, and social factors independent of the primary somatic pathology. Training the physician to integrate psychosocial aspects in everyday work is the prime objective of this approach, which is practiced in Germany.[65]

In developing countries, psycho-oncologists are often confronted with other tasks, such as the facilitation and implementation of palliative treatments or education about lay-representations and religious beliefs concerning illness.[66,67] It is therefore important to state that some publications on psycho-oncology neither reflect the "state of the art" nor demonstrate the most effective interventions.

Most of the publications on psycho-oncology come from the United States and reflect American thinking, which, according to Cassidy,[68] is based on "activism," "teleology," and "positivism." This paradigm argues that we can and should mold the future, that humans are constantly improving, and that the future will be better than the present. However, in large parts of the world, completely opposite paradigms are accepted, leading to another attitude toward cancer and the goals of psycho-oncology. Non-positivist thinkers pay attention to accumulated wisdom of the elders and are likely to question new knowledge as possibly being insufficiently tested.[68] Psycho-oncology is therefore a speciality with a large variety of possible approaches, depending on medical and psychiatric developments and cultural context. While some biomedical procedures may be internationally uniform, psycho-oncology will and should differ according to local circumstances.

Recent Developments in Psycho-oncology

Three recent concepts have had major influences on psycho-oncology in developed countries:[69] First, physicians now widely accept the view that cancer and its treatments constitute a stress imposed on a previously healthy individual, involving adjustment efforts and possibly adjustment disorders. This concept treats psychological disturbances as the consequence of a sustained stressful situation. Several recent articles have evaluated the psychosocial disorders associated with cancers in terms of adaptation[70] or adjustment.[71]

Second, improvement in cancer treatment and prognosis means that a diagnosis of cancer can no longer be equated with a death sentence. Survivorship, especially in patients with cured hematological malignancies,[72] has increased, and with it the need to achieve and maintain an optimal quality of life for these patients. Consequently, oncologists are increasingly aware of the patient's needs regarding the return to a normal and useful life, and they therefore are more concerned not only about the short-term psychological effects of their treatments[73] but also about the long-term quality of life[74–77] and rehabilitation.

Third, rehabilitation of the cancer patient, which seems to be the current leading concept, includes specific support by a multidisciplinary team.[78,79] From this perspective, psychosocial interventions will become part of large programs oriented toward the rehabilitation and quality of life of cancer patients.

Although most recent articles are related to these promising topics, only a minority describe ways to make them operational. These have largely explored two types of interventions known to be effective for common psychiatric disorders: psychological support and psychotropic medication.[69] Psycho-oncology has also become important to the multidisciplinary teams treating the patient with advanced disease. An increasing number of psycho-oncologists have experiences in palliative care settings, and the increasing number of articles on this topic reflect this development.[78–80]

Common Psychiatric Disorders in Cancer Patients

While the role of psycho-oncology extends beyond clinical work with patients, and includes research, education, cancer prevention, ethics, and palliative care, we can only present here a short summary of the most common disorders observed in cancer patients, to illustrate the nature of the clinical work.

Among the investigations on the prevalence of psychiatric disorders in cancer patients, the study by the Psychosocial Collaborative Oncology Group[82] is the most widely cited. This group observed in a mixed oncological patient population (inpatients and outpatients in three cancer centers) a prevalence rate of 47% for psychiatric disorders as defined in the Diagnostic and Statistical Manual of Mental Disorders III (DSM-III).[83] This prevalence has been confirmed in other studies[84-86] and is approximately twice that reported for psychiatric disorders in medical patients and three times the modal estimate for the general population.[69] Only one investigation[87] has reported a lower prevalence of depression among women with cancer than all other studies. In the Psychosocial Collaborative Oncology Group study, adjustment disorders accounted for 68% of all diagnoses. Other diagnoses were major affective disorders (13%), organic mental disorders (8%), personality disorders (7%), and anxiety disorders (4%). The proportion of these diagnoses may vary with the stage of disease (e.g., an increased incidence of acute confusional states [delirium] is observed in advanced cancer[88]), the type of cancer (e.g., increased incidence of depression in head and neck cancer[89] or pancreatic cancer[90]), or other factors, such as physical condition.[91] Most importantly, the majority of these psychiatric disorders are treatable, but often are not detected or are misdiagnosed by the treating physicians.[92,93]

Adjustment disorders are thought to arise as a direct consequence of stress or trauma. It is therefore assumed that adjustment disorders would not occur without the impact of the stress that cancer represents. Unlike acute stress reactions, which are transient disorders of significant severity that appear within minutes and subside within hours or days, adjustment disorders usually arise within one month after the occurrence of a stressful event and have a duration that usually does not exceed six months. These disorders are characterized by distress and emotional disturbances (anxious and/or depressive symptoms) that interfere with social functioning and performance. Adjustment disorders have to be differentiated from grief, acute stress reactions, anxiety disorders, depression, or posttraumatic stress disorders.

The diagnosis of an adjustment disorder can be difficult for a clinician who is not experienced with cancer patients. Although adjustment disorders are common in patients with cancer, relatively little is known about screening procedures, vulnerability factors to predict patients at risk, or the most successful psychotherapeutic approaches. Adjustment disorders can be screened with self-administered questionnaires (with a reported sensitivity of 84% and specificity of 66%[94]). Treatment usually consists of supportive psychotherapy.

The use of psychotropic drugs (benzodiazepines or antidepressants) in the treatment of adjustment disorders is still controversial. No studies clearly support combined treatment, but there may be theoretical reasons to proceed in this way. In one study of alprazolam and relaxation for cancer–related anxiety and depression (mostly adjustment disorders[95]) both treatment arms were effective, but patients receiving alprazolam showed a slightly more rapid decrease in anxiety and greater reduction in depressive symptoms. In contrast, a recent randomized, double-blind, placebo-controlled trial of alprazolam for anxiety associated with cancer[96] found no significant difference in response between patients receiving alprazolam and patients receiving placebo. The later result suggests that non-drug factors or spontaneous improvement may play a greater role than pharmacotherapy in the treatment of anxiety associated with cancer.

Based on clinical observation, it is likely that a person with an adjustment disorder who is suffering from significant symptoms of anxiety and/or depression could benefit (especially in the case of anxious mood) from transient treatment with a benzodiazepine. Drug therapy should be considered if supportive psychotherapy does not decrease symptomatology within a few days. Although there may be theoretical reasons to avoid psychotropic treatment, the reality is that few cancer centers have enough psychiatric staff to offer adequate treatment using psychotherapy alone. Psychotropics cannot replace psychotherapeutic support in such conditions, but they can at least alleviate some of the emotional suffering.

Major affective disorders (unipolar and bipolar depression, atypical depression, and dysthymic depression) accounted for 13% of the observed psychiatric disorders in the prevalence study mentioned above.[82] The prevalence of major depression is thought to vary: a higher prevalence is observed in patients with pancreatic cancer, with head and neck cancer, a history of alcohol abuse, patients with pain, or patients with a family or personal history of depression.[97] Organic factors related to cancer (brain metastases, hypercalcemia[98]) or its treatment (corticosteroids, vincristine, interferon, or cimetidine)[99] can also cause depression. Treatment usually combines supportive psychotherapeutic approaches with antidepressant medication. Very few psychotropics have been tested in oncology,[100–104] and there is a great need for the investigation of the effectiveness of antidepressants in patients with cancer.

Acute confusional states (delirium) are common in patients with cancer and their prevalence increases with advanced disease.[105] Delirium (especially hypoactive–hypoalert delirium) often remains undetected[106] and may in fact be the most commonly neglected psychiatric syndrome, partly because it is often seen by non-psychiatric physicians.[107] Since Engel and Romano's classic studies on delirium,[108] there has been little research on the management of this uncomfortable condition, and only recently has a new interest in delirium been observed.[109,110]

Personality disorders were found in 7% of patients evaluated in the Psychosocial Collaborative Oncology Group study.[82] In our experience, the patient with a personality disorder is often misunderstood by non-psychiatrists and provokes time-consuming discussions and arguments among the staff. The role of the consulting psychiatrist is often focused on explanations of the psychopathology and the development of beneficial management strategies.[111]

Anxiety appears frequently in cancer patients as a symptom of adjustment disorders or anxiety disorders. However, anxiety can also be a normal reaction to a threatening situation, a symptom of an acute stress reaction, a psychiatric disorder (e.g., panic disorder, delirium), an underlying somatic process (e.g., pain, hypoxia), a treatment side effect (e.g., corticosteroids), or an expression of a spiritual and existential dimension. To assess anxiety, the main diagnostic tool remains the dialogue with the cancer patient and/or significant others. Possible misconceptions, unrealistic fears, psychiatric disorders, and somatic complaints can be discussed, and if an organic cause is suspected as the source of anxiety, additional medical examinations and laboratory work-up, as well as chart review for side effects of administered drugs, are required. Repeated examinations of cognitive functions in anxious cancer patients is also mandatory to detect delirium. To assume that an anxious cancer patient "has the right to be anxious, since he or she has cancer" is probably the most common obstacle to diagnosis and appropriate treatment. Any therapeutic approach includes a discussion with the patient to understand possible reasons for anxiety. A discussion focused on the patient's understanding about the illness and the future, how he or she copes with the situation, and what physical symptoms he or she suffers is necessary for proper treatment. This discussion may in itself be therapeutic. A dialogue, in which a patient is allowed to express feelings and possible misconceptions and unrealistic fears, is the best therapeutic procedure. If organic causes or psychiatric disturbances as a source of anxiety are ruled out, and psychotherapeutic intervention and spiritual support are not successful, symptomatic treatment with psychotropic medication (e.g., low doses of benzodiazepines or neuroleptics) is indicated.

References

1. Holland JC. Historical Overview. In: Holland JC, Rowland JH, eds. *Handbook of Psychooncology*. New York: Oxford University Press, 1989:3–12
2. Fainsinger R, MacEachern T, Hanson J, Miller M, Bruera E. Symptom control during the last week of life on a palliative care unit. *J Palliat Care* 1991; 7:5–11.
3. Portenoy RK, Coyle N. Controversies in the long-term management of analgesic therapy in patients with advanced cancer. *J Palliat Care* 1991; 7(2):13–24.
4. Klastersky J, Schimpff SC, Senn HJ. Preface. In: Klastersky J, Schimpff SC, Senn HJ, eds. *Handbook of Supportive Care in Cancer*. New York: Marcel Dekker, Inc., 1995.
5. Stiefel F, Guex P. Cancer and the mind—do we still believe Galen? *Eur J Cancer* 1996; 32A(12):2041
6. Guex P. Psychosomatics and cancer. In: Guex P, ed. *An Introduction to Psycho-Oncology*. London: Routledge, 1994:1–10.
7. Walshe WH. *The Nature and Treatment of Cancer*. London: Taylor and Walton, 1846.
8. Patterson JJ. *The Dread Disease: Cancer and Modern American Culture*. Cambridge, Mass.: Harvard University Press, 1987.
9. Evans E. *A Psychological Study of Cancer*. New York: Dodd, Mead and Co., 1926.
10. Wolff HG. Personality features and reactions of subjects with migraine. *Arch Neurol Psychiat* 1937; 37:895.
11. Dunbar F. *Emotions and Bodily Changes*. New York: Columbia University Press, 1947.
12. Alexander F. *Psychosomatic Medicine*, 2nd ed. New York: W.W. Norton and Company, Inc., 1987.

13. Pollock G. Foreword to the 1987 Edition. In: Alexander F, ed. *Psychosomatic Medicine*. New York: W.W. Norton and Company, Inc., 1987:3–6.
14. Abse AW, Wilkins MM, Buxton WA, et al. Personality and Behavioral characteristics of 23 lung cancer patients. Psychosomatic Res 1973; 18:101–109
15. Booth G. General and organ-specific object relationships in cancer *Ann N Y Acad Sci* 1969; 164:568–574.
16. Baltrusch HJF. Ergebnisse klinisch-psychosomatischer Krebsforschung. *Psychosom Med* 1975; 5:175–208.
17. Bahnson CB. Emotional and personality characteristics of cancer patients. In: Sutnick AI, Engstrom PF, eds. *Oncology Medicine*. Baltimore: University Park Press, 1976:
18. Thomas CB, Greenstreet RL. Psychobiological characteristics in youth as predictors of five disease states: suicide, mental illness, hypertension, coronary heart disease and tumor. *Hopkins Med J* 1973; 16:132–144.
19. Greer S, Morris T, Psychological attributes of women who develop breast cancer: a controlled study. *J Psychosomatic Res* 1975; 19:147–153.
20. Fox BH. Premorbid psychological factors as related to cancer incidence. *J Behav Med* 1978; 1:45–65.
21. Greer S, Morris T, Pettingale KW. Psychological response to breast cancer: effect on outcome. *Lancet* 1979; II:785–787.
22. Shekelle RB, Raynor WJ, Ostfeld A, et al. Psychological depression and 17-year risk of death from cancer. *Psychosom Med* 1981; 43(2):117–125.
23. Fox BH. Current theory of psychogenic effects on cancer incidence and prognosis. *J Psychosoc Oncol* 1983; 1(1):17–31.
24. Kneier AW, Temoshok L. Repressive coping reactions in patients with malignant melanoma as compared to cardiovascular disease patients. *J Psychosom Res* 1984; 28(2):145–155.
25. Cassileth BR, Walsh WP, Lusk EJ. Psychosocial correlates of cancer survival: A subsequent report 3 to 8 years after cancer diagnosis. *J Clin Oncol* 1988; 6(11):1753–1759.
26. Hahn RC, Petitti DB. Minnesota Multiphasic Personality Inventory-rated depression and the incidence of breast cancer. *Cancer* 1988; 61:845–848.
27. Redd WH, Jacobsen PB. Emotions and cancer. *Cancer* 1988; 62:1871–1879.
28. LeShan LL. Untersuchugen zur Persönlichkeit der Krebskranken. *Zeitschrift für Psychosomatische Medizin und Psychoanalyse* 1963; 9:246–253.
29. Stiefel F. Psychosocial aspects of cancer pain. *Support Care Cancer* 1993; 1:130–134.
30. Hackett TP, Cassem NH, Stern TA, Murray GB. Beginnings: Consultation psychiatry in a general hospital. In: Cassem NH, ed. *Massachusetts General Hospital Handbook of General Hospital Psychiatry*. St. Louis: Mosby Year Book, 1991:1–8.
31. Schwarz R. Die Bedeutung der psychosozialen Onkologie in der Behandlung von Krebskranken. *Zsch Psychosom Med* 1993; 39:14–25.
32. Engel GL. The need for a new medical model: a challenge for biomedicine. *Science* 1977; 196:129–136.
33. Sutherland AM. Psychological impact of cancer and its therapy. In: Holleb AI, Braun M, eds. *Classics in Oncology*. New York: American Cancer Society, Inc., 1987:449–463.
34. Weisman AD. Vulnerability and the psychological disturbance of cancer patients. Psychosomatics 1989; 30(1):80–85.

35. Breitbart W, Holland JC. Psychiatric complications of cancer. In: Brain MC, Carbone PP, eds. *Current Therapy in Hematology Oncology* − 3. Toronto: B.C. Decker, Inc., 1988:268–274.

36. Cassileth BR. History of psychotherapeutic intervention in cancer patients. *Support Care Cancer* 1995, 3:264–266.

37. Greer S, Watson M. Towards a psychobiological model of cancer: psychological considerations. *Soc Sci Med* 1985; 20:773–777.

38. Van der Pompe G, Antoni MH, Mulder CL, Heijnen C, Goodkin K, De Graeff A, Garssen B, De Vries MJ. Psychoneuroimmunology and the course of breast cancer: An overview. *Psychooncology* 1994; 3:271–288.

39. Razavi D, Farvacques C, Delvaux N, et al. Psychosocial correlates of oestrogen and progesterone receptors in breast cancer. *Lancet* 1990; 335:931–933.

40. Levy S, Herberman R, Lippman M, d'Angelo T. Correlation of stress factors with sustained depression of natural killer cell activity and predicted prognosis in patients with breast cancer. *J Clin Oncol* 1987; 5(3):348–353.

41. Bovbjerg D. Psychoneuroimmunology and cancer. In: Holland JC, Rowland JH, eds. *Handbook of Psychooncology*. New York: Oxford University Press, 1989:727–734.

42. Spiegel D, Bloom J, Kraemer HC, et al. Effect of psychosocial treatment on survival of patients with metastatic breast cancer. *Lancet* 1989; II:888–891.

43. Fawzy FI, Fawzy NW, Hyun CS, Elashoff R, Guthrie D, Fahey JL, Morton D. Malignant melanoma: effects of an early structured psychiatric intervention, coping, and affective state on recurrence and survival 6 years later. *Arch Gen Psychiatry* 1993; 50:681–689.

44. Fawzy IF. A short-term psychoeducational intervention for patients newly diagnosed with cancer. *Support Care Cancer* 1995; 3:235–238.

45. Spiegel D. Essentials of psychotherapeutic intervention for cancer patients. *Support Care Cancer* 1995; 3:252–256.

46. Fox BH. Some problems and some solutions in research on psychotherapeutic intervention in cancer patients. *Support Care Cancer* 1995; 3:257–263.

47. McCulloch W. *Embodiment of Mind.* Cambridge, Mass.: The M.I.T. Press, 1975.

48. Minsky M. *The Society Theory of Mind.* New York: Simon and Schuster, 1986.

49. Cellérier G. La psychologie génétique et le cognitivisme. *Le Débat* 1987; 47:116–129.

50. Linn MW. Psychotherapy with cancer patients. *Adv Psychosom Med* 1988; 18:54–65.

51. Fallowfield LJ. Counselling for patients with cancer. *BMJ* 1988; 297:727–728.

52. Payne S. Anxiety and depression in women with advanced cancer: implications for counselling. *Counselling Psychology Quarterly* 1989; 2(3):337–344.

53. Friedman LC, Baer PE, Nelson DV, Lane M, Smith FE, Dworkin RJ. Women with breast cancer: perception of family functioning and adjustment to illness. *Psychosom Med* 1988; 50:529–540.

54. Moorey S, Greer S, Watson M, et al. Adjuvant psychological therapy for patients with cancer: Outcome at one year. *Psycho-oncology* 1994; 3:39–46.

55. Fawzy IF, Fawzy NW. A structured psychoeducational intervention for cancer patients. *Gen Hosp Psychiatry* 1994; 16:149–192.

56. Massie MJ, Lesko LM. Psychopharmacological management. In: Holland JC, Rowland JH, eds. *Handbook of Psychooncology*. New York: Oxford University Press, 1989:470–491.

57. Massie MJ, Holland JC, Straker N. Psychotherapeutic interventions. In: Holland JC, Rowland JH, eds. *Handbook of Psychooncology*. New York: Oxford University Press, 1989:455–469.

58. Stiefel F. Flims 95: The united psychotherapeutic interventions of psycho-oncology. *Support Care Cancer* 1995; 3:215–216.

59. Jenner C. Zur Frage einer persönlichkeitsspezifischen Disposition zum Magen-Carcinom. *Zschr Psychosom Med* 1981; 27:73–83.

60. Wirsching M, Stierlin H, Weber G, Wirsching B, Hoffmann F. Brustkrebs im Kontext - Ergebnisse einer Vorhersagestudie und Konsequenzen für die Therapie. *Zschr Psychosom Med* 1981; 27:239–252.

61. Glicenstein M, Lehmann A. Cancer et histoire: comment le sujet ré-écrit son histoire. *Psychosomatique* 1987; 9:27–32.

62. Meerwein F. Liaison psychiatry on an oncology ward. *Recent Results Cancer Res* 1988; 108:239–242.

63. Guex P. Psychosomatique et cancer. In: Guex P, ed. *Psychologie et Cancer*. Lausanne: Payot, 1989:13–21.

64. Risko A, Fleischmann T, Molnar Z, Schneider T, Varady E. Influence of the pathological psychological state of cancer patients on their decisions. *Support Care Cancer* 1996; 4:51–55.

65. Uexküll von T. Was ist und was will "Integrierte Psychosomatische Medizin"?. In: Adler R, Bertram W, Haag A, Herrmann JM, Köhle K, von Uexküll T, eds. *Psychosomatische Medizin*. Stuttgart - New York: Schattauer, 1994:17–34.

66. Chaturvedi SK. What's important for quality of life for Indians in relation to cancer? *Soc Sci Med* 1991; 33:91–94.

67. Ibudeh MNJ. Culture and illness. The Nigerian experience. *Newsletter of the International Psycho-Oncology Society* 1994: 8–12.

68. Cassidy C. Social science theory and methods in the study of alternative and complementary medicine. *J Altern Complement Med* 1995; 1(1):19–40.

69. Razavi D, and Stiefel F. Psychiatric and emotional problems of cancer patients. In: Klastersky J, Schimpff SC, Senn HJ eds. *Handbook of Supportive Care in Cancer*. New York: Marcel Dekker, Inc., 1995:221–243.

70. Eil K, Nishimoto R, Morvay T, Mantell J, Hamovitch M. A longitudinal analysis of psychological adaptation among survivors of cancer. *Cancer* 1989; 63:406–413.

71. Vinokur A, Threatt B, Caplan R, Zimmerman B. Physical and psychosocial functioning and adjustment to breast cancer: long-term follow-up of a screening population. *Cancer* 1989; 66:394–405.

72. Lesko L, Holland J. Psychological issues in patients with hematological malignancies. *Recent Results Cancer Res* 1988; 108:243–270.

73. Love R, Leventhal H, Easterling D, Nerenz D. Side effects and emotional distress during cancer chemotherapy. *Cancer* 1989; 66:604–612.

74. Ochs J, Mulheim R, Kun L. Quality-of-life assessment in cancer patients. *Am J Clin Oncol* 1988; 11:415–421.

75. Bernhard J, Gusset H, Hürny C. Quality-of-life assessment in cancer clinical trials: an intervention by itself? *Support Care Cancer* 1995; 3:66–71.

76. Feld R. Endpoints in cancer clinical trials: is there a need for measuring quality of life? *Support Care Cancer* 1995; 3:23–27.

77. Wolberg W, Romsaas E, Tanner M, Malec J. Psychosexual adaptation to breast cancer surgery. *Cancer* 1989; 66:1645–1655.
78. Holland JC, Rowland JH. Psychological reactions to breast cancer and its treatment. In: Harris JR, Hellman S, Henderson IC, Kinne DW, eds. *Breast Diseases. Patient Rehabilitation and Support.* Philadelphia: J.B. Lippincott, 1987:632–647.
79. Kurtzman S, Gardner B, Kellner W. Rehabilitation of the cancer patient. *Am J Surg* 1988; 155:791–801.
80. Miller RD, Walsh DT. Psychosocial aspects of palliative care in advanced cancer. *J Pain Symptom Manage* 1991; 6(1):24–29.
81. Stiefel F, Guex P. Palliative and supportive care: at the frontier of medical omnipotence. *Ann Oncol* 1996; 7:135–138.
82. Derogatis LR, Morrow G, Fetting J, et al. The prevalence and severity of psychiatric disorders among cancer patients. *JAMA* 1983; 249(6):751–757.
83. American Psychiatric Association. *Diagnostic and Statistical Manual of Mental Disorders*, Third Edition. Washington, D.C.: American Psychiatric Association, 1980.
84. Craig TJ, Abeloff MD. Psychiatric symptomatology among hospitalized cancer patients. *Am J Psychiatry* 1974; 131(12):1323–1327.
85. Bukberg J, Penman D, Holland JC. Depression in hospitalized cancer patients. *Psychosom Med* 1984; 46(3):199–212.
86. Stephanek ME, Derogatis LP, Shaw A. Psychological distress among oncology outpatients. *Psychosomatics* 1987; 28:530–539.
87. Lansky SB, List MA, Herrmann CA, et al. Absence of major depressive disorder in female cancer patients. *J Clin Oncol* 1985; 3(11):1553–1560.
88. Massie MJ, Holland J, Glass E. Delirium in terminally ill cancer patients. *Am J Psychiatry* 1983; 140:1048–1050.
89. Baile WF, Gibertini M, Scott L, Endicott J. Depression and tumor stage in cancer of the head and neck. *Psychooncology* 1992; 1:15–24.
90. Holland JC, Hughes A, Tross S, et al. Comparative psychological disturbance in patients with pancreatic and gastric cancer. *Am J Psychiatry* 1986; 143(8):982–986.
91. Ahles TA, Blanchard EB, Ruckdeschel JC. The multi-dimensional nature of cancer-related pain. *Pain* 1983; 17:277–288.
92. Levine PM, Silberfarb PM, Lipowski ZJ. Mental disorders in cancer patients - a study of 100 psychiatric referrals. *Cancer* 1978; 42:1385–1391.
93. Stiefel FC, Kornblith AB, Holland JC. Changes in the prescription patterns of psychotropic drugs for cancer patients during a 10-year period. *Cancer* 1990; 65:1048–1053.
94. Razavi D, Delvaux N, Bredart A. Screening for psychiatric disorders in a lymphoma out-patient population. *Eur J Cancer* 1992; 28A(11):1869–1872.
95. Holland JC, Morrow GR, Schmale A, et al. A randomized clinical trial of alprazolam versus progressive muscle relaxation in cancer patients with anxiety and depressive symptoms. *J Clin Oncol* 1991; 9(6):1004–1011.
96. Wald TG, Kathol RG, Noyes R, Carroll BT, Clamon G. Rapid relief of anxiety in cancer patients with both alprazolam and placebo. *Psychosomatics* 1993; 34(4):324–332.
97. Stiefel F, Volkenandt M, Breitbart W. Suizid und Krebserkrankung. *Schweiz Med Wochenschr* 1989; 119:891–895.

98. Massie MJ, Holland JC. Diagnosis and treatment of depression in the cancer patient. *J Clin Psychiatry* 1984; 45:25–28.
99. Breitbart W, Stiefel F, Kornblith AB, Pannullo S. Neuropsychiatric disturbance in cancer patients with epidural spinal cord compression receiving high dose corticosteroids: a prospective comparison study. *Psychooncology* 1993; 2:233–245.
100. Greenspoon J, Leuchter RS, Semrad N. Lorazepam for chemotherapy–induced emesis. *Arch Intern Med* 1984; 144:2432–2433.
101. Costa D, Mogos I, Toma T. Efficacy and safety of mianserin in the treatment of depression of women with cancer. *Acta Psychiatr Scand* 1985; 72:85–92.
102. Fernandez F, Adams F, Holmes VF. Methylphenidate for depressive disorders in cancer patients. *Psychosomatics* 1987; 28:455–461.
103. Greenberg DB, Surman OS, Clarke J, Baer L. Alprazolam for phobic nausea and vomiting related to cancer chemotherapy. *Cancer Treat Rep* 1987; 71(5):549–550.
104. Holland JC, Morrow GR, Schmale A, et al. A randomized clinical trial of alprazolam versus progressive muscle relaxation in cancer patients with anxiety and depressive symptoms. *J Clin Oncol* 1991; 9(6):1004–1011.
105. Stiefel F, Holland J. Delirium in cancer patients. *Int Psychogeriatr* 1991; 3(2):333–336.
106. Stiefel F, Bruera E. Psychostimulants for hypoactive–hypoalert delirium? *J Palliat Care* 1991; 7(3):25–26.
107. Lipowski ZJ. *Delirium: Acute Confusional States.* New York: Oxford University Press, 1990.
108. Engel GL, Romano G. Delirium, a syndrome of cerebral insufficiency. *J Chron Dis* 1959; 9:260–277.
109. Stiefel F. Opening new doors: Second International Congress of Psycho-Oncology in Kobe (Japan). *Support Care Cancer* 1996; 4:64–66.
110. De Stoutz ND, Stiefel F. Reversible delirium (acute confusional states) in cancer patients: a clinical perspective with special emphasis on etiology, assessment and management. In: Portenoy RK, Bruera E, eds. *Topics in Palliative Care.* New York: Oxford University Press, 1997:21–43.
111. Groves JE. Patients with borderline personality disorders. In: Cassem NH, ed. *Massachusetts General Hospital Handbook of General Hospital Psychiatry.* St. Louis: Mosby Year Book, 1991:191–215.

8

From Sadness to Major Depression: Assessment and Management in Patients with Cancer

MARYFRANCES R. PORTER,
DOMINIQUE L. MUSSELMAN,
J. STEPHEN McDANIEL,
AND CHARLES B. NEMEROFF

Mental health professionals face the challenge of differentiating expected emotional distress associated with a cancer diagnosis (such as sadness, grief, and bereavement) from the disabling psychiatric disorder of major depression. To manage patients appropriately, professionals must contend with patients' hurried schedules and sudden hospitalizations, educate family members, negotiate complex medication regimens, and interact with a multidisciplinary treatment team. Skillful diagnosis and careful attention to management strategies are needed to optimize care.

Prevalence of Depression in Patients with Cancer

For most patients, an initial diagnosis of cancer, or a recurrence, typically provokes a brief reactive period of disbelief and shock followed by a period of adjustment and bereavement lasting for seven to ten days.[1] Bereavement, which is often identified by the individual as a "normal reaction," is characterized by sadness (tearfulness/grief), insomnia, poor appetite, and weight loss.[2] Emotional support from the patient's family, friends, community/church, and physician are important in alleviating this distress.[1] For some patients, distress is sufficiently complicated, severe, or prolonged to warrant a diagnosis of *major depression*. For example, bereavement may be complicated by inappropriate and excessive guilt (such as guilt about surviving), thoughts of death (feeling one would be better off dead), psychomotor retardation, prolonged functional impairment, and/or hallucinations (other than auditory or visual hallucinations of the deceased).[2] When such complications arise, psychiatric consultation is indicated.

Major depressive disorder is a well-characterized psychiatric syndrome defined by the *Diagnostic and Statistical Manual of Mental Disorders*, version IV (DSM-IV)[2] as the presence of depressed mood (dysphoria) and/or the loss of interest or pleasure (anhedonia) for at least two weeks, and the presence of at least four of the following symptoms (or three symptoms if the patient is experiencing both dysphoria and anhedonia): weight gain or loss of at least 5% of body weight in one month; insomnia or hypersomnia; psychomotor agitation or retardation (observable by others); fatigue or loss of energy; feelings of worthlessness or inappropriate/excessive guilt; difficulty concentrating or inability to make decisions; and recurrent thoughts of death.

Major depression is exceedingly common, with a lifetime prevalence rate of 13% within the general population of the United States.[3] Although major depression is the most common psychiatric disorder encountered in the primary care setting,[3] it remains under-recognized and under-treated.[4] McDaniel et al.[5] reported that prevalence rates of major depression in patients with cancer vary dramatically from 1.5% in patients with acute leukemia awaiting bone marrow transplantation to 50% in patients with pancreatic cancer (see Table 8.1). Studies also reveal that depression becomes more prevalent as the severity of the medical illness increases.[25-27]

Which Patients with Cancer are at the Highest Risk for Major Depression?

The recent explosion of psycho-oncologic literature has afforded investigators and clinicians an opportunity to explore the relationship between emotional distress and the course and treatment of cancer in growing detail. Although research that examines psychiatric morbidity varies with regard to sampling techniques, cancer types, disease stage, hospitalization status, and diagnostic methods, there are recent comprehensive reviews of the literature that point out specific guidelines for assessment and treatment of psychiatric disorders, as well as directions for future research (Table 8.2). These articles provide detailed information about the spectrum of psychiatric morbidity among patients with cancer, as well as a more comprehensive grasp of the wealth and variety of the current research.

The identification of major depression in patients with and without cancer is assisted by understanding the risk factors for this disorder (Table 8.3). Significant pain doubles the prevalence of depressive disorders.[35] As cancer metastasizes and treatment becomes increasingly aggressive, pain often increases and causes other physical limitations such as lethargy, fatigue, and loss of libido. In addition, medications administered to patients with cancer to control pain, nausea, anxiety, and

Table 8.1. Prevalence of depression by cancer site

Cancer site Source, year	No. of subjects	Diagnostic method	Prevalence
Pancreas			
Fras et al., 1967[6]	46	Interview, MMPI[a], DRS	50% mean prevalence
Joffe et al., 1986[7]	12	SAD-L, HSC, BDI	50% mean prevalence
Kelsen, et al., 1995[8]	130	BDI	38% mean prevalence
Oropharynx			
Morton et al., 1984[9]	48	Interview	40% mean prevalence
Davies, et al., 1986[10]	72	GHQ, LSSD	22% mean prevalence
Baile et al., 1992[11]	45	Interview, MCMI	40% mean prevalence
Breast			
Maguire et al., 1978[12]	201	Interview	26% mean prevalence
Silberfarb et al., 1980[13]	146	Interview	10% primary cancer, 15% recurrent cancer, 4.5% advanced cancer, 10% mean prevalence
Farber et al., 1984[14]	141	HSC	18% severe depression, 21% moderate depression, 19.5% mean prevalence
Grandi et al., 1987[15]	18	Interview	22%
Fallowfield et al., 1990[16]	269	Interview	21% mastectomy, 19% lumpectomy, 20% mean prevalence[b]
Hopwood et al., 1991a[17]	81	HADS, RSCL	20%
Hopwood et al., 1991b[18]	222	HADS, RSCL	21% HADS, 22% RSCL, 24.5% mean prevalence
Goldberg et al., 1992[19]	320	RSCL	32%
Pinder et al., 1993[20]	139	HADS, interview	13%
Colon			
Fras et al., 1967[6]	64	Interview, MMPI, DRS	13%
Koenig et al., 1967[21]	36	MMPI	25%
Gynecological[c]			
Evans et al., 1986[22]	83	Interview, HDRS, CRSD	23% major depression
Lymphoma[d]			
Devlen et al., 1987[23]	90	Interview	17%
Gastric			
Joffe et al., 1986[7]	9	SADS-L, HSC, BDI	11%
Acute leukemia[e]			
Colon et al., 1991[24]	100	Interview	1% major depression, 2% organic affective syndrome, 1.5% mean prevalence

[a]MMPI indicates Minnesota Multiphase Personality Inventory; DRS, Depression Rating Scale; SADS-L, Schedule for Affective Disorders and Schizophrenia-Lifetime Version; HSC, Hopkins Symptoms Checklist; BDI, Beck Depression Inventory; GHQ, General Health Questionnaire; LSSD, Leeds Scale for Self-Assessment of Depression; MCMI, Million Clinical Multiaxial Inventory; HADS, Hamilton Anxiety and Depression Scale; RSCL, Rotter Symptom Checklist; HDRS, Hamilton Depression Rating Scale; CRSD, Carroll Rating Scale for Depression.
[b]For the purposes of this review, a mean prevalence was determined for those individual studies that reported more than one prevalence depending on cancer disease stage, depression symptom severity, cancer treatment, diagnostic method, and definition.
[c]Gynecological refers to cervical, endometrial, or vaginal.
[d]Hodgkin's and non-Hodgkin's lymphoma
[e]Before bone marrow transplantation
Source: Modified from McDaniel et al.[5]

Table 8.2. Review articles on the diagnosis and treatment of depression in patients with cancer

---

Holland JC. ed. *Psycho-oncology* New York: Oxford University Press, 1998.
Examines the available research on several individual cancer sites including specific psychiatric diagnostic issues and treatment modalities

Razavi D, Stiefel F. Common psychiatric disorders in cancer patients, I. adjustment disorders and depressive disorders. *Support Care Cancer* 1994; 2:223–232.
Explores the risk factors, diagnosis, and treatment of major depression and related psychiatric disorders across cancer populations

Lynch ME. The assessment and prevalence of affective disorders in advanced cancer. *J Palliat Care* 1995; 11:10–18.
Reviews the prevalence and assessment of psychiatric disorders in patients with cancer with special attention to screening instruments

Valente SM, Saunder JM, Cohen MZ. Evaluating depression among patients with cancer. *Cancer Practice* 1994; 2:65–71.
Explores the risk factors and diagnosis of major depression and related psychiatric disorders across cancer populations

Holland JC. Anxiety and cancer: the patient and the family. *J Clin Psychiatry* 1989; 50(suppl):20–25.
Explores anxiety in patients with cancer with a particular focus on the family unit

Fawzy IF, Fawzy NW, Arndt LA, Pasnau RO. Critical review of psychosocial interventions in cancer care. *Arch Gen Psychiatry* 1995; 52:100–113.
Examines the efficacy of several psychological and behavioral treatment options for patients with cancer

McDaniel JS, Nemeroff CB. Depression in the cancer patient: diagnostic, biological, and treatment aspects. In: Chapman CR, Foley KM, eds. *Current and Emerging Issues in Cancer Pain: Research and Practice*. New York: Raven Press, Ltd., 1993:1–19.
Reviews literature with specific focus upon the underlying pathophysiology and pharmacological management of patients with cancer and depressive disorders

McDaniel JS, Musselman DL, Porter MR, Reed DA, Nemeroff CB. Depression in patients with cancer: diagnosis, biology, and treatment. *Arch Gen Psychiatry* 1995; 52:89–99.
Reviews literature with specific focus to the underlying pathophysiology and pharmacological management of patients with cancer and depressive disorders

Mermelstein HT, Lesko L. Depression in patients with cancer. *Psychooncology* 1992; 1:199–215.
Examines the prevalence of psychiatric disorders, their etiology, and pharmacological management

Breitbart W. Identifying patients at risk for, and treatment of major psychiatric complications of cancer. *Support Care Cancer* 1995; 3:45–60.
Examines the prevalence of psychiatric disorders, their etiology, and pharmacological management

---

other treatment side effects may create a cluster of symptoms which mirror the symptoms of major depression. Table 8.4 lists some of the most commonly prescribed compounds which should be minimized or eliminated before a diagnosis of major depression is concluded. Careful attention should also be paid to medications prescribed to control the side effects of other agents, such as antinausea medications (see Case Study 1).

Table 8.3. Factors influencing risk of psychiatric morbidity in cancer patients

Cancer-Related Factors	*Cancer Treatment-Related Factors*
Advanced stages	Corticosteroids
Functional limitations	Opiates (analgesics)
Pain	Antivirals
Tumor type, site	Antifungals
Physical symptoms (e.g., pain)	Miscellaneous medications
Psychological symptoms (e.g., prolonged	
bereavement)	Antinausea medications
Nutritional	Antianxiety (dependence forming) medications
Endocrine	
Neurologic	
Paraneoplastic	
Psychiatric History	*Social Factors*
Depression	Concurrent life stresses (e.g., financial, marital,
	occupational)
Bereavement experience	Absence of quality social support
Substance abuse	Family history
Prescription or illicit drugs	Cancer history
Alcohol	Psychiatric history
Anxiety disorders	
Psychotic disorders	
Childhood trauma/Post-traumatic stress	
disorder	

Source: Adapted from Breitbart.[35]

The location and type of tumor may also have a significant impact on mood in patients. Certain types of malignancies are associated with higher rates of depression. For example, patients with pancreatic cancer, which is especially difficult to detect and is often fatal, exhibit the highest prevalence of major depression (approaching 50%).[6,7] As might be expected, patients with cancer of the central nervous system are also especially vulnerable to emotional disorders.[36]

Personal and familial psychiatric histories of depression and other psychiatric disorders may also place the cancer patient at increased risk for major depression. Our research group has found that the first degree relatives of depressed patients with cancer have a higher rate of psychiatric disorders than those of nondepressed patients with cancer (unpublished data). The patient's history of adjustment to adverse life changes, coping ability prior to cancer diagnosis, and current or past alcoholism, substance abuse, or suicide attempts offer crucial information about adjustment and coping with the cancer diagnosis.[34,37–39]

Patient denial often "masks" depressive disorders. Patients may either ignore their symptoms of depression, dismissing them as "normal" reactions to life-threatening illness, or exhibit atypical symptoms of depression.[2] Although not specified by the DSM-IV, forgetfulness, irritability, excessive silence in the presence of supportive caregivers, particularly passive participation in treatment, missed chemotherapy appointments, complaints of "excessive" pain, or preoccu-

Table 8.4. Commonly prescribed medications reported to induce depression

Generic name	Trade name	Generic name	Trade name
Antihypertensive Agents		*Anti-inflammatory or Pain Medications*	
clonidine	Catapress	corticosteroids	Deltasone,
diltiazem	Cardizem	e.g., prednisone,	Hydrocortone,
propranolol	Inderal	hydrocortisone	Decadron
methyldopa	Aldomet		
spironolactone	Aldactone	opiates	
nifedipine	Procardia	e.g., codeine,	Codeine,
chlorothiazide	Dilril	morphine,	MS Contin,
		hydromorphone,	Dilaudid,
Antimicrobial and Antiviral Agents		meperidine	Demerol
acyclovir	Zovirax	pentazocine	Talwin
ampicillin	Unasyn		
isoniazid	INH	*Antinausea Medications*	
metronidazole	Flagyl	inapsone	Droperidol
norfloxacin	Noroxin	metaclopromide	Reglan
trimethoprim-	Bactrim	prochlorperazine	Compazine
sulfamethoxazole		dronabinol	Marinol
Antiparkinsonian Agents		*Antipsychotic Medications*	
amantadine	Symmetrel	haloperidol	Haldol
levodopa	Dopar	fluphenazine	Prolixin
Anticonvulsants		*Heart Medications*	
phenytoin	Dilantin	lanoxin	Digoxin
		isosorbide dinitrate	Isordil
Sedative-Hypnotics/Tranquilizers			
diazepam	Valium	*Antineoplastic Agents*	
lorazepam	Ativan	asparaginase	Elspar
flurazepam	Dalmane	interferon alfa	Intron-A
alprazolam	Xanax		
triazolam	Halcion	*Commonly Abused Substances*	
		alcohol	
		cocaine	
		amphetamines	

pation with physical discomfort despite adequate evaluation and treatment measures are often observed in patients likely to be experiencing unacknowledged major depression severe enough to warrant psychiatric consultation.

Diagnostic Considerations in Patients with Cancer

Table 8.5 addresses basic principles in the diagnosis of major depression in patients with cancer. These factors must be reviewed and considered to diagnose

Table 8.5. Basic principles in the diagnosis of major depression in patients with cancer

Review of medical history and treatment

Review cancer site, course of disease, and treatment

Investigate comorbid medical conditions (treated and untreated)

Review medication regimen for mood-altering or addicting substances

Consider complicating diagnoses of bereavement, post-traumatic stress syndrome, dementia, dysthymia

Consider possible atypical symptoms of depression

Review of social support systems

Determine accessibility of social support

Assess quality of relationships

and treat major depression accurately. The aims of these guidelines are to minimize risk factors, manage external stressors, and ensure effective pharmacological management of the patient.

Numerous diagnostic systems have been proposed to diagnose major depression in the medically ill. These systems have been developed because: (*1*) some depressive symptoms are appropriate and expected in the context of the stress of adjusting to and coping with a serious medical illness, and (2) the physical manifestations of depression, that is, the vegetative signs and symptoms, are sometimes similar to those of the medical illness itself.[40,41]

Cohen-Cole et al.[42] reviewed the conceptual approaches to the diagnosis of major depression in such patients and proposed the use of two diagnostic systems. The first system, the *exclusive approach*, is recommended for use in research settings. Initially proposed by researchers at the Memorial Sloan-Kettering Cancer Center in New York City,[43] the exclusive approach eliminates anorexia and fatigue from the diagnostic criteria for depression, and requires only four of the remaining DSM-IV symptoms to be present. Anorexia and fatigue are arguably the most difficult symptoms to separate from the course of cancer (and other medical illnesses) and its treatment; their elimination allows for a more definitive diagnosis of major depression, based more on psychological symptoms than the DSM-IV. Mermelstein and Lesko[34] have emphasized focusing on the patient's psychological symptoms of persistent dysphoria, feelings of helplessness or hopelessness, loss of self-esteem, feelings of worthlessness, and wishes to die. When these symptoms overwhelm the patient or interfere with functioning, treatment is indicated.

The second system, the *inclusive approach*, is suggested for use in clinical settings. This approach recommends that clinicians count each relevant depressive symptom regardless of whether the symptom can be attributed to the disease process or its treatment. In clinical settings, the inclusive approach reduces the number of patients who may be under-diagnosed and therefore untreated.

Regardless of the diagnostic criteria used, clinicians should rely on empathic clinical observations and employ a lower threshold of symptom severity for major depression in patients with cancer.[5] This is particularly important in cancer patients, who may fail to fulfill criteria for major depression but experience considerable dysphoria. When treated with antidepressants, cancer patients with subsyndromal or minor depression exhibit significant improvement (see Pharmacological therapy, below).

Approximately 30 years of investigation of the biological alterations associated with unipolar depression have resulted in the discovery of so-called biological markers, measures that presumably reflect the underlying pathophysiologic processes of this disorder. The presence of such markers would ideally aid clinicians in both the diagnostic process and in choice of psychosocial and/or pharmacologic treatment. Of all these markers, the most intensively studied and well characterized have been measures of hypothalamic-pituitary-adrenal (HPA) axis hyperactivity, specifically elevated corticotropin-releasing factor (CRF) concentrations in cerebrospinal fluid (CSF), a blunted corticotropin (ACTH) response to CRF, and dexamethasone (DST) nonsuppression.[44]

Several screening tools have been commonly used to identify symptoms of depression and quality of life (including social support and marital cohesion) when evaluating patients with cancer (Table 8.6).

Table 8.6. Commonly used tools for assessment of depression, anxiety, and quality of life in patients with cancer

Screening Tool	Abbreviation	Method*	Use	Time Required
Unstructured Interview		Administered		Variable
Structured Clinical Interview for the DSM-IV	SCID	Administered	Diagnoses DSM-IV Axis I disorders	1–2 hours
Hamilton Depression Rating Scale	HAMD	Administered	Measures depression severity	15–20 minutes
Symptom Checklist-90-Revision	SCL-90-R	Self-report	Screens for depression, obsessions and compulsions, anxiety, anger, psychosomatic complaints, phobias, and psychotic thinking	15–20 minutes
Beck Depression Inventory	BDI	Self-report	Measures depression severity	5 minutes
Carroll Depression Rating Scale	CDRS	Self-report	Measures depression severity	5 minutes
Inventory of Current Concerns	ICC	Self-report	Assesses quality of life	10 minutes
Cancer Rehabilitation Evaluation System	CARES	Self-report	Assesses quality of life	10–15 minutes

* Screening tools are either administered by trained personnel ("Administered") or self-reported by patients ("Self-report").

Dimensional measures, such as the Beck Depression Inventory (BDI) and Carroll Depression Rating Scale (CDRS), require only a few minutes to complete and score. They offer a reliable and rapid method of assessing the severity of dysphoria, but their usefulness is limited in the cancer population because they do not distinguish physical symptoms (i.e., fatigue, sexual dysfunction, appetite) from the major depression symptom cluster. Other dimensional measures, which take more time to complete and score, such as the Symptom Checklist-90-Revised (SCL-90-R) and the Cancer Rehabilitation Evaluation System (CARES), offer a more detailed and multidimensional profile of the patient's emotional state and quality of life, respectively. The Structured Clinical Interview for the DSM-IV (SCID), which may take up to two hours to administer, requires rater training and input and cooperation from patient and family. Points which may inadvertently be omitted from an open interview are systematically probed in the SCID, allowing the interviewer to make a reproducible, categorical psychiatric diagnosis. Additionally, in contrast to the dimensional measures mentioned above, the SCID gives the clinician the opportunity to record all current symptoms of depression, regardless of etiology, and valuable information about other current and past psychiatric disorders (e.g., psychotic disorders, mania, somatoform disorder).

Issues in the Treatment of Major Depression in Patients with Cancer

Treatment of depression in patients with cancer is crucial because of considerable evidence that depression adversely impacts survival[45–49], length of hospitalization[49], compliance with therapy[50] and self-care, quality of life[51], and overall disability 1989.[52]

Psychological treatment, including individual, group, and family therapy, is effective in alleviating sadness and grief, improving self-concept, improving active treatment compliance, increasing energy, enhancing coping with sexual problems, reducing anxiety, and managing pain and nausea.[33] Several studies have found that patients with cancer receiving psychotherapy exhibit significantly improved survival time,[53] decreased mortality, fewer recurrences,[54] and evidence of increased immune function.[55,56] Furthermore, pharmacological management of major depression in patients with cancer has been shown not only to treat the depression effectively, but also to enhance overall quality of life.[57,58]

Psychosocial therapy

Fawzy et al.[32] reviewed the efficacy of four interventions (education, behavior therapy, individual psychotherapy, and group interventions) in patients with cancer, with and without psychiatric diagnoses, to ascertain the effect of psychosocial therapy on survival. Each of these interventions has a unique goal and diverse measures of success (Table 8.7).

All four interventions had a positive impact on the treatment group with regard to emotional distress (i.e., anxiety, sadness, sense of hopelessness or helplessness, and feelings of isolation). Although the benefits overlapped in some respects, each modality exhibited relatively specific effects. The educational approach, which increased knowledge and understanding of cancer treatment, stood out as the most beneficial method for improving treatment compliance. Behavior therapy proved uniquely advantageous in helping patients control the effects of cancer treatment (decreasing pre-treatment anxiety, nausea, and vomiting) and improving the patients' perception of control of their treatment. Individual psychotherapy, of patients with newly diagnosed cancer, is often short-term supportive therapy focusing on alleviating specific distress and symptoms (e.g., anxiety, pain management, depression)[59] and provides the patient with the emotional tools needed to cope with the disease.[32] Group interventions appeared to have the most all-encompassing benefits, including increased knowledge of cancer and cancer treatment, enhanced physical capabilities, improved effective interpersonal relationships, better coping skills, decreased reported pain, and increased survival. These far-reaching and varied benefits probably result from the inclusion of education, behavior training, and emotional engagement of the patient. According to Spiegel and colleagues, seven participants in a group is optimal in encouraging members to become intimately involved with each other, which results in lessened feelings of alienation, improved coping skills, and personal empowerment and growth (review by Massie).[59]

Family therapy and the caregiver

Time should be taken to consider the patient's family, not only as support for the patient but as "second-order patients" themselves. The term "second-order patient" is not intended in any way to be prejorative or to minimize the importance of the family and its dysfunctions. The family, though clearly not the primary concern of the treatment team, should be considered in the treatment of the patient, and is thus a "patient" in the second-order.[60]

Although most of the available research investigates the impact of childhood cancer on the family, there is increasing interest in other family relationships. Spouses and other family members experience their own cascade of emotional responses to the cancer diagnosis of a loved one.[61] Families, especially the spouse, are often the primary source of social support for patients,[62] and experience the physical and emotional strain resulting from the sudden assumption of additional household responsibilities, such as child care, financial management, transportation, and decision making.

Table 8.7. Review of psychological and educational treatment modalities used in patients with cancer

Intervention	Goals	Desired results
Educational	↓ Helplessness and ↓ inadequacy due to lack of knowledge	↓ Anxiety
• Informational pamphlets	Provide cancer information	↓ Problems associated with treatment
• Educational sessions	Provide treatment information	↓ Depression
• Slide/video presentation	Demonstrate coping/ communication skills	↑ Compliance with treatment
Behavioral Therapy	↓ Psychological stress	↓ Adverse side effects of chemotherapy (i.e., nausea and vomiting)
• Progressive muscle relaxation	↓ Physical complications	
• Hypnosis		↓ Pre-treatment anxiety (psychological arousal)
• Deep breathing		↑ Immune function
• Meditation		↑ Locus of control
• Biofeedback		
• Passive relaxation		
• Guided imagery (visualization)		
Individual Therapy	Crisis intervention	↓ Emotional distress (↓ negative affect)°
• Support: compassion, empathy	↓ Psychological distress	↓ Confusion
• Emotional engagement	↓ Coping skills	↓ Social isolation
		↓ Sexual dysfunction and physical distress
		↑ Return to work
		↑ Coping skills
		↑ Quality of life
		↑ Health perception
Group Interventions	↓ Living with cancer, coping skills	↓ Anxiety, tension, fatigue, depression, phobias
• Support/coping	Issues of death and dying	↑ Vigor, activity (including sexual), body image
• Sharing	Enriching life	↓ Social isolation, ↑ relationship strength
	↑ Family and communication problems	↑ Support, coping, social activities
		↑ Attitude toward treatment
		↑ Purpose in living, satisfaction, quality of life
		↑ Improved perceptions of death
		↑ Cancer knowledge
		↑ Communication skills
		↓ Pain
		↑ Survival
		↑ Immune function

Well, yes I'm depressed. I guess having cancer is depressing for everyone. Am I supposed to be happy? • Before I got sick, I used to work in the garden a lot. I can't garden but read now to kill time, but everything seems gray and dull. • Treatment is making me so nauseated I can't eat. I've lost about 15 pounds this past month. My husband has to force me to eat. • My medications make me feel so groggy. I sleep a lot during the day, but I also wake up a lot in the middle of the night. I never sleep deeply. • I don't have a lot of stamina. • I always knew I would get breast cancer. • I feel bad for being so unhappy when all the other people in my support group have it so much worse than I do. • It's difficult for me to think things through. There's so much information for me to absorb. I have my wife take notes for me at appointments. • This disease has had me incapacitated for so long, when I pass it will be a relief to my family. • No, my wife shouldn't stay with me while I'm coming for treatment, she's trying to keep our business open.

Figure 8.1. Depressive symptoms often reported by patients with cancer.

Although families are often self-reliant for emotional and practical support, each must be evaluated and treated, if necessary, as a component of successful psychiatric and oncologic management of the patient with cancer.[60] This is of paramount importance because clinical experience suggests that a patient's positive cancer treatment response may be reversed if the patient is discharged into an unstable family situation.[63] To foster a positive family environment for the patient, family intervention should be focused on five areas:[60] education about cancer and its treatment, improvement of familial communication, successful incorporation of the family in the treatment of the patient, information regarding cancer resources, and the mobilization of social support (including friends, churches, social clubs, and support groups).

Pharmacological therapy

Only a few research teams have investigated antidepressant drug treatment of patients with cancer in placebo-controlled studies. Most notably, Costa et al.[57] and Evans et al.[58] conducted controlled trials of mianserin in depressed women with cancer and imipramine in women with gynecological cancer, respectively. Both studies reported that antidepressant pharmacotherapy yields a significant reduction in depressive symptoms and improved quality of life when administered in adequate doses. Furthermore, antidepressant treatment has been shown not only to alleviate the symptoms of major depression, such as abnormal sleep, but also to diminish perceived levels of pain in patients with cancer (reviewed in McDaniel and Nemeroff[33]). Our group is currently one of three medical centers in the United States conducting a placebo-controlled, double-blind trial of paroxetine and desipramine in depressed breast cancer patients. Selective serotonin reuptake inhibitors (SSRIs) do not cause the anticholinergic, antihistaminic, antiadrenergic, sedative, and hypotensive side effects of tricyclic antidepressants (such as imipramine) and monoamine oxidase inhibitors (such as phenelzine) and, therefore, offer an effective alternative for the treatment of depression in patients with cancer.

Cancer patients are at increased risk for delirium related to infection, metabolic abnormalities, metastases to the brain, and complex medication regimens. To minimize this risk, antidepressant medications with short half-lives, inactive metabolites, and minimal effects on the hepatic cytochrome P450 system should be used. Such medications reduce the occurrence of drug–drug interactions and drug–induced delirium. Furthermore, analysis of plasma tricyclic antidepressant concentrations can assist the clinician in avoiding adverse side effects. Recent reviews provide an extensive discussion of the psychopharmacologic management of cancer patients.[35,64] Table 8.8 recommends some psychopharmacologic medications for the treatment of anxiety, depression, psychosis, and insomnia.

Table 8.8. Psychotropic medications recommended in the psychiatric treatment of patients with cancer

Generic Name	Trade Name	Comments
Benzodiazepines (Tranquilizers)		*Risk of tolerance, dependence, and withdrawal symptoms with ALL benzodiazepines*
lorazepam	Ativan	Anxiolytic, effective antinauseant
temazepam	Restoril	Sedative hypnotic
clonazepam	Klonopin	High potency tranquilizer; can cause sedation and confusion
Antidepressants		
Selective Serotonin Reuptake Inhibitors (SSRIs)		*Can cause anxiety, insomnia, sedation, and diminished appetite; convenient dosing; safe in overdose; can affect metabolism of other drugs; can cause Serotonin Syndrome*
sertraline	Zoloft	Short half life
paroxetine	Paxil	Short half life, no active metabolites
fluoxetine	Prozac	Long half life
Tricyclics (TCAs)		*ALL TCAs can be fatal in overdose*
nortriptyline	Pamelor	Relatively less sedation, anticholinergic side effects, and hypotension than other TCAs
desipramine	Norpramin	Relatively less sedation, anticholinergic side effects, and hypotension than other TCAs
amitryptiline	Elavil	Use low doses (25–50 mg per day) for reduction of neuropathic pain
Atypical Antidepressants		
venlafaxine	Effexor	Short elimination half-life; does not inhibit any hepatic enzymes; effective in refractory depression
trazodone	Desyrel	Sedating and induces hypotension; in low doses can be used as a sleep aid; effective in the depressed patient with anxiety and insomnia
Antipsychotics		*Can cause Parkinsonian-like side effects as well as neuroleptic malignant syndrome (often fatal)*
haloperidol	Haldol	For agitation due to delirium and psychosis or depression with psychotic features
fluphenazine	Prolixin	Relatively less sedation, hypotension, and anticholinergic side effects compared with other antipsychotics
risperidol	Risperidone	A newer atypical antipsychotic medication with a more favorable side effect profile
Antimania Agents		
lithium	Lithobid	Used in cancer patients with bipolar disorder (manic-depression); drug levels must be closely monitored because cancer patients may experience severe side effects even at usual therapeutic levels (0.6–1.2 mm/L)
Sleep Aids		
zolpidem	Ambien	No known tolerance or dependence

Case Studies: Differential Diagnosis of Depression in Patients with Cancer

Two case studies are presented to illustrate psychiatric diagnostic and treatment considerations in patients with cancer.

Case 1

Medical History: Ms. B was a 48-year-old, married, black woman who, eleven weeks prior to the interview, found a lump in her left breast and was referred for oncological assessment and treatment by her gynecologist. A biopsy revealed that the lump was malignant with 5/14 lymph nodes involved (stage II). A modified radical mastectomy with reconstruction was performed. Four weeks after surgery she received her first of three cycles of Adriamycin and cycloposphamide chemotherapy (at three week intervals). At the time of psychiatric interview, she had finished her second cycle of chemotherapy. She had discovered another mass under her right arm two days prior to interview and was awaiting further diagnostic procedures to determine if this mass was malignant.

As part of the chemotherapy regimen, Ms. B received dexamethasone, 8 mg by mouth twice daily for two days, then 4 mg twice daily for two days. Thereafter, she was offered prochlorperazine, 15 mg by mouth as needed, to control nausea. She also received lorazepam, 1 mg every 4–6 hr (3 mg total daily dose) to control anxiety, as well as oxycodone, 5–10 mg by mouth every 4–6 hr for the control of post-surgical pain. Ms. B's preoperative laboratory tests were normal, other than a mildly elevated thyroid stimulating hormone (TSH) level.

After the onset of chemotherapy, Ms. B was referred for psychiatric consultation when her oncology nurse noticed Ms. B's diminished emotional responsiveness, increased agitation, and decreased motivation.

Developmental and Social History: Ms. B was born in an urban environment and came from a middle-class background. She and her husband saw a marriage counselor for a brief period shortly after the birth of their first child because of financial stress, which occurred when her husband lost his job. On the recommendation of her oncologist, she attended three breast cancer support group meetings to help her with initial feelings of sadness, grief, and shock from her diagnosis of breast cancer.

Family History: Review of her family's psychiatric history revealed that her grandmother had a "nervous breakdown" when her mother was a young child and that her father was briefly "addicted" to prescription pain medication but never received psychiatric assessment or treatment. Ms. B also reported a history of breast cancer in her maternal grandmother.

Psychiatric Interview: Ms. B presented as a petite woman who was casually dressed and fully oriented. Ms. B's husband reported that since her surgery she had become increasingly emotionally detached and disconnected from family activities. Mr. B further reported that his wife was unable to pay attention to her oncologist's instructions during appointments and that he took notes for her. She was visibly nervous and fidgety during the interview. She reported hypersomnia, sleeping up to 12 hours a night and taking afternoon naps (1–2 hours per day). Her mood was depressed, although she was not tearful. She stated that "I just don't know what's wrong" and that "I should be able to handle this." On the self-rated Carroll Depression Rating Scale (CDRS), she scored a 15 (>10 indicates significant dysphoria). She scored 50 and 30, respectively, on the State-Trait Anxiety Scales (STAS). The state portion of the STAS measures current anxiety levels and the trait portion measures usual levels; scores greater than 48 indicate significant symptoms of anxiety. Using the inclusive diagnostic approach, the Structured Clinical Interview for the DSM-IV (SCID) revealed a categorical diagnosis of an initial episode of major depression with moderate severity. Ms. B was asked to rate her pain on a scale of 1 (mild) – 10 (extreme). She rated her current pain as 5 and indicated that her pain was currently at its worst.

Psychiatric Recommendations: Although categorical and symptom severity measures indicated an initial episode of major depression of moderate severity, a definitive diagnosis was delayed pending the discontinuation of prochlorperazine and lorazepam. The following recommendations were made: (1) discontinuation of prochlorperazine (which can cause an internal restless feeling called akathisia); (2) continuation of lorazepam, 0.5 mg by mouth every 8 hr, with a gradual downward taper until nausea and akathisia resolve; (3) continuation of oxycodone with a change to acetaminophen 500 mg, 1–2 tablets every 6 hr two weeks after the completion of her final cycle of chemotherapy; (4) referral to endocrinology for evaluation and treatment of possible subclinical hypothyroidism; and (5) psychiatric re-evaluation in three weeks.

Follow-up: At the three-week follow-up, Ms. B's symptoms of anxiety and depression were diminished. Her CDRS score was 5 and her STAS scores were 46 and 29. She reported feeling more "with it" and appeared visibly less anxious. Her husband also reported that she was "becoming her old self again." Orders were written to have Ms. B complete a CDRS at each subsequent oncology visit to screen for any recurrence of depressive symptoms.

Case 2

Medical History: Mr. M was a 36-year-old, divorced, white male who was diagnosed with Clark's stage V melanoma two years prior to interview. The tumor was removed from his right shoulder by wide excision; there was positive lymph node involvement. He completed a full course of chemotherapy. Two weeks prior to the interview, Mr. M had a grand mal seizure at work and was admitted to the hospital. Magnetic resonance imaging (MRI) indicated that there were four metastatic brain lesions. He began his first cycle of BCNU (carmustine) and cisplatin chemotherapy after being informed by his oncology team that his life expectancy was 6–12 months. Mr. M said he had no significant nausea and/or vomiting. He reported periodic headaches, which were managed by dexamethasone, up to 16 mg per day. Mr. M was free of seizures while hospitalized. His blood chemistries were within normal limits when admitted to the hospital. After hospitalization, the staff noticed increasing lethargy, evidence of significant weight loss, uncontrollable tearfulness, minimal appetite, and excessive sleeping. A psychiatric consultation was recommended, but Mr. M refused. He later agreed to a psychiatric consultation at discharge and was seen by the Consultation–Liaison Psychiatry team the following day as an outpatient. On discharge, Mr. M was receiving lorazepam 1 mg every 4–6 hr (3 mg total daily dose) for nausea and vomiting, dexamethasone 8 mg per day (increased to 12 mg per day) for headache pain, phenytoin 100 mg in the morning and 200 mg in the evening, for control of seizures, and amitriptyline, 25 mg per day for depressed mood.

Developmental and Social History: Mr. M reported that he came from a lower middle class background and had worked as a contractor since graduation from high school. He had been divorced for 10 years and had three teenage children who lived with their mother.

Family History: He had four younger siblings, two of whom were alcoholic. His paternal aunt committed suicide when she was 21 years old. One of Mr. M's children was undergoing psychological treatment for depression. He reported no family history of cancer.

Psychiatric Interview: Mr. M was an extremely thin, fully oriented, casually dressed male who appeared older than his stated age. He was very still and intermittently tearful during the interview. Mr. M had no close friends or relatives who were available to provide further information. He related that "I have never *really* been happy" but attributed this to a life of "bad luck." He reported that his diagnosis of melanoma was just more "bad luck" but than he "couldn't handle" the possibility of the cancer's spread to his brain, that he "wasn't ready to die," and was feeling desperate and increasing "overwhelmed and low." The oncology nurse reported that Mr. M had a history of being "moody." Prior to each appointment, he would call to ask for his appointment time because he "forgets." He scored a 36 on the CDRS and a 45 and 39, respectively, on the STAS. The SCID, using the inclusive diagnostic approach, indicated that Mr. M was experiencing a double depression: a current severe major depression (six weeks in duration) superimposed on dysthymia beginning at age 12. Mr. M rated his current headache pain as 5 on a scale of 1 (mild)–10 (extreme). At its worst, he rated his pain at 8.

Psychiatric Recommendations: Given the severity of Mr. M's major depressive episode, history of pre-existing dysthymia, family history of psychiatric disorders, lack of social support, and poor prognosis, the following recommendations were made: (1) discontinuation of amitriptyline (increasing the dose to attain therapeutic blood plasma concentration would likely produce anticholinergic side effects); (2) initiation of paroxetine 20 mg per day; (3) continuation of dexamethasone to control headache pain; (4) weekly to twice-monthly appointments with the oncology social worker to help him reduce his anxiety, obtain increased support from his family, and apply for disability; and (5) referral to a cancer support group and/or church for additional emotional encouragement and support.

Follow-up: Mr. M missed his next scheduled appointment with the oncology social worker, but called and rescheduled. He reported feeling "somewhat relieved" after having been able to talk about his fears in his last appointment. He was going to a support group meeting that same evening. He was less tearful, but continued to exhibit slowed speech and movement. His emotional and psychiatric progress was monitored closely by the oncology staff and social workers, and he met with the oncology social worker for six sessions over six months. After four weeks, he exhibited marked reduction of depressive symptoms and reported increased contact with his family before being transferred to a hospice care facility.

Conclusion

Adequate diagnosis and treatment of major depression in patients with cancer is a complex and multifaceted task which is vital to optimize the patient's successful completion of cancer treatment and reduce medical and psychiatric morbidity. Symptoms of major depression are often masked by complicated bereavement, the side effects of medication and cancer treatment, the course and site of the tumor itself, and/or patient denial. Therefore, diagnosis is aided by the inclusion of many sources of information, including the course of illness, medication regimens, personal and family psychiatric history, and observations by medical staff and family members. Questionnaires (self-rating scales) are also often helpful in obtaining a brief, dimensional screening of symptom severity in patients at risk for major depression. Similarly, successful treatment always includes one or more categorical psychiatric diagnoses, simplification of medication regimens, and the introduction of appropriate combinations of somatic and psychological therapy. Social support and the family system should not be overlooked as vital components of successful oncologic and psychiatric treatment, because an absent or ineffective social support system can thwart the patient's recovery. As research into the pathophysiology of depression in patients with cancer expands, the details of the complex interplay of psychotherapy, antidepressant treatment, and immune and neuroendocrine function will be clarified, and diagnostic and treatment modalities will undoubtedly be enhanced.

Acknowledgments

The authors greatly appreciate the assistance of Barbara Rock, MD, Assistant Professor of Dermatology at Emory University School of Medicine, Karen Shires, RN, of the Division of Hematology-Oncology in the Department of Internal Medicine at The Emory Clinic, and Cynthia Osowski, PharmD at the Pharmacy at Emory University Hospital. This work was supported by grant NIMH-1-RO1-MH49523-01 from the National Institute of Mental Health.

References

1. Holland JC. Anxiety and cancer: the patient and the family. *J Clin Psychiatry* 1989; 50(suppl):20–25.
2. American Psychiatric Association. *Diagnostic and Statistical Manual of Mental Disorders*, 4th ed. Washington, DC: American Psychiatric Association, 1994.

3. Kessler RC, McGonagle KA, Zhao S, Nelson CB, Hughes M, Eshleman S, Wittchen HU, Kendler KS. Lifetime and 12-month prevalence of DSM-111-R psychiatric disorders in the United States: Results from the National Comorbidity Survey. *Arch Gen Psychiatry* 1994, 51:8–19.

4. Gregory RJ, Jimerson DC, Walton BE, Daley J, Paulsen RH. Pharmacology of depression in the medically ill: prevalence by self-report questionnaire and recognition by nonpsychiatric physicians. *Gen Hosp Psychiatry* 1992; 14:36–42.

5. McDaniel JS, Musselman DL, Porter MR, Reed DA, Nemeroff CB. Depression in patients with cancer: diagnosis, biology, and treatment. *Arch Gen Psychiatry* 1995; 52:89–99.

6. Fras I, Litin EM, Pearson JS. Comparison of psychiatric symptoms in carcinoma of the pancreas with those in some other intra-abdominal neoplasms. *Am J Psychiatry* 1967; 123:1553–1562.

7. Joffe RT, Rubinow DR, Denicoff KD, Maher M, Sindelar WF. Depression and carcinoma of the pancreas. *Gen Hosp Psychiatry* 1986; 8:241–245.

8. Kelsen DP, Portenoy RK, Thaler HT, Niedzwiecki D, Passik SD, Tao Y, Bauks W, Brennan MF, Foley KM. Pain and depression in patients with newly diagnosed pancreatic cancer. *J Clin Oncol* 1995; 13:748–755.

9. Morton RP, Davies ADM, Baker J, Baker GA, Stell PM. Quality of life in treated head and neck cancer patients: a preliminary report. *Clin Otolarnygol* 1984; 9:181–185.

10. Davies ADM, Davies C, Delpo MC. Depression and anxiety in patients undergoing diagnostic investigations for head and neck cancers. *Br J Psychiatry* 1986; 149:491–493.

11. Baile WF, Bilbertini M, Scott L, Endicott J. Depression and tumor stage in cancer of the head and neck. *Psychooncology* 1992; 1:15–24.

12. Maguire GP, Lee EG, Bevington DJ, Kuchemann CS, Crabtree RJ, Cornell CE. Psychiatric problems in the first year after mastectomy. *Br Med J* 1978; 1:963–965.

13. Silberfarb PM, Maurer LH, Crouthamel CS. Psychological aspects of neoplastic disease, I: functional status of breast cancer patients during different treatment regimens. *Am J Psychiatry* 1980; 137:450–455.

14. Farber JM, Weinerman BH, Kuypers JA. Psychosocial distress in oncology outpatients. *J Psychosoc Oncol* 1984; 2:109–118.

15. Grandi S, Fava GA, Cunsolo A, Ranieri G, Gozzetti G, Trombini G, Major depression associated with mastectomy. *Med Sci Res* 1987; 15:283–284.

16. Fallowfield LJ, Hall A, Maguire GP, Baum M. Psychological outcomes of different treatment policies in women with early breast cancer outside of a clinical trial. 1990; 301:575–580.

17. Hopwood P, Howell A, Maguire P. Screening for psychiatric morbidity in patients with advanced breast cancer: validation of two self-report questionnaires. *Br J Cancer* 1991a; 64:353–356.

18. Hopwood P, Howell A, Maguire P. Psychiatric morbidity in patients with advanced cancer of the breast: prevalence measured by two self-report questionnaires. *Br J Cancer* 1991b; 64:349–352.

19. Goldberg JA, Scott RN, Davidson PM. Psychological morbidity in the first year after breast surgery. *Eur J Surg Oncol* 1992; 18:327–331.

20. Pinder KL, Ramirez M, Black E, Richard MA, Gregory WM, Rubens RD. Psychiatric disorder in patients with advanced breast cancer: prevalence and associated features. *Eur J Cancer* 1993; 29(suppl):524–527.

21. Koenig R, Levin SM, Brennan MT. The emotional status of cancer patients as measured by a psychological test. *J Chronic Dis* 1967; 20:923–930.
22. Evans DL, McCarney CF, Nemeroff CB, Raft D, Quade D, Golden RN, Haggerty JJ, Holmes V, Simon JS, Droba M, Mason GA, Fowler WC. Depression in women treated for gynecological cancer: clinical and neuroendocrine assessment. *Am J Psychiatry* 1986; 143:447–452.
23. Devlen J, Maguire P, Phillips P, Crowther D, Chamblers H. Psychological problems associated with diagnosis and treatment of lymphomas, I: retrospective study. *Br Med J* 1987; 295:953–954.
24. Colon EA, Callies AL, Popkin MK, McGlave PB. Depressed mood and other variables related to bone marrow transplantation survival in acute leukemia. *Psychosomatics* 1991; 32:420–425.
25. Stewart MS, Drake W, Winokur G. Depression among medically ill patients. *Dis Nerv Syst* 1968; 115:1365–1369.
26. Moffic HS, Paykel ES. Depression in medical inpatients. *Br J Psychiatry* 1975; 126:346–353.
27. Cavanaugh SA. The prevalence of emotional and cognitive dysfunction in a general medical population: using the MMSE, GHQ, and BDI. *Gen Hosp Psychiatry* 1983; 5:15–24.
28. Holland JC. *Psycho-oncology* New York: Oxford University Press, 1998.
29. Razavi D, Stiefel F. Common psychiatric disorders in cancer patients, I. adjustment disorders and depressive disorders. *Support Care Cancer* 1994; 2:223–232.
30. Lynch ME. The assessment and prevalence of affective disorders in advanced cancer. *J Palliat Care* 1995; 11:10–18.
31. Valente SM, Saunder JM, Cohen MZ. Evaluating depression among patients with cancer. *Cancer Practice* 1994; 2:65–71.
32. Fawzy IF, Fawzy NW, Arndt LA, Pasnau RO. Critical review of psychosocial interventions in cancer care. *Arch Gen Psychiatry* 1995; 52:100–113.
33. McDaniel JS, Nemeroff CB. Depression in the cancer patient: diagnostic, biological, and treatment aspects. In: Chapman CR, Foley KM, eds. *Current and Emerging Issues in Cancer Pain: Research and Practice*, New York: Raven Press, Ltd., 1993:1–19.
34. Mermelstein HT, Lesko L. Depression in patients with cancer. *Psychooncology* 1992; 1:199–215.
35. Breitbart W. Identifying patients at risk for, and treatment of major psychiatric complications of cancer. *Support Care Cancer* 1995; 3:45–60.
36. Breitbart W. Psychiatric complications of cancer. In: Brain MC, Carbone PP, eds. *Current Therapy in Hematology Oncology. three*. Toronto/Philadelphia: Decker Press, 1988:268–274.
37. Plumb M, Holland J. Comparative studies of psychological function in patients with advanced cancer, II: interviewer-rated current and past psychological symptoms. *Psychosom Med* 1981; 43:243–254.
38. Massie MJ, Holland JC. The cancer patient with pain: psychiatric complications and their management. *Med Clin North Am* 1987; 71:243–257.
39. Holland JC, Korzun AH, Tross S, Silberfarb P, Perry M, Comis R, Oster M. Comparative psychological disturbances in patients with pancreatic and gastric cancer. *Am J Psychiatry* 1986; 143:982–986.

40. Kathol RG, Mutgi A, Williams J, Clamon G, Noyes R. Diagnosis of major depression in cancer patients according to four sets of criteria. *Am J Psychiatry* 1990a; 147:1021–1024.

41. Kathol RG, Noyes R, Williams J, Mutgi A, Carroll B, Perry P. Diagnosing depression in patients with medical illness. *Psychosomatics* 1990b; 31:434–440.

42. Cohen-Cole SA, Brown FW, McDaniel JS. Diagnostic assessment of depression in the medically ill. In: Stoudemire A, Fogel B, eds. *Psychiatric Care of the Medical Patient.* New York: Oxford University Press, 1993:53–70.

43. Bukberg J, Penman D, Holland JC. Depression in hospitalized cancer patients. *Psychosom Med* 1984; 46:199–212.

44. Musselman DL, McDaniel JS, Anderson G, Porter MR, Nemeroff CB. Depression in patients with cancer. *Directions in Psychiatry* 1996; 16:1–11.

45. Abram HS, Moore GL, Westervelt FB. Suicidal behavior in chronic dialysis patients. *Am J Psychiatry* 1971; 127:1199–1204.

46. Hawton K. The long-term outcome of psychiatric morbidity detected in general medical patients. *J Psychosom Res* 1981; 25:237–243.

47. Rodin GM, Chmara J, Ennis J. Stopping life-sustaining medical treatment: psychiatric considerations in the termination of renal dialysis. *Can J Psychiatry* 1981; 26:540–544.

48. Murphy E, Smith R, Slatter J. Increased mortality rates in late-life depression. *Br J Psychiatry* 1988; 152:347–353.

49. Koenig HG, Shelp F, Goli V, Cohen HJ, Blazer DG. Survival and healthcare utilization in elderly medical inpatients with major depression. *J Am Geriatr Soc* 1989; 37:599–606.

50. Stoudemire A, Thompson TL. Medication noncompliance: systematic approaches to evaluation and intervention. *Gen Hosp Psychiatry* 1983; 5:233–239.

51. Koenig HG, Cohen HJ, Blazer DG, Meador KG, Westlung R. A brief depression scale for use in the medically ill. *Int J Psychiatry Med* 1992; 22:183–195.

52. Wells KB, Hays RD, Burnam MA, Rogers W, Greenfield S, Ware JE. Detection of depressive disorder for patients receiving prepaid or fee-for-service care: results from the medical outcomes study. *JAMA* 1989; 262:3298–3302.

53. Spiegel D, Bloom JR, Kraemer HC, Gottheil E. Effect of psychosocial treatment on survival of patients with metastatic breast cancer. *Lancet* 1989; 2:888–891.

54. Fawzy FI, Fawzy NW, Hyun CS, Elashoff R, Guthrie D, Fahey JL, Morton DL. Malignant melanoma: effects of an early structured psychiatric intervention, coping, and affective state on recurrence and survival 6 years later. *Arch Gen Psychiatry* 1993; 50:681–689.

55. Fawzy FI, Fawzy FI, Kemeny ME, Fawzy NW, Elashoff R, Morton D, Cousins N, Fahey JL. A structured psychiatric intervention for cancer patients, II: Changes over time in immunological measures. *Arch Gen Psychiatry* 1990; 47:729–735.

56. Gruber BL, Hersh SP, Hall NRS, Waletzky LR, Kunz JF, Capenter JK, Kverno KS, Weiss SM. Immunological responses of breast cancer patients to behavioral interventions. *Biofeedback Self Regul* 1993; 18:1–22.

57. Costa E, Mogos I, Toma T. Efficacy and safety of mianserin in the treatment of depression of women with cancer. *Acta Psychiatr Scand* 1985; 72:85–92.

58. Evans DL, McCartney CF, Haggerty JJ, Nemeroff CB, Golden RN, Simon JB, Quade D, Holmes V, Droba M, Mason GA, Fowler WC, Raft D. Treatment of depression

in cancer patients is associated with better life adaptation: a pilot study. *Psychosom Med* 1988; 50:72–76.

59. Massie MJ. Depression, In: Holland JC, Rowland JH, eds. *Handbook of Psychooncology: Psychological Care of the Patient with Cancer.* New York: Oxford University Press, 1990:283–290.

60. Rait D, Lederberg M. The family of the cancer patient. In: Holland JC, Rowland JH, eds. *Handbook of Psychooncology: Psychological Care of the Patient with Cancer.* New York: Oxford University Press, 1990:585–597.

61. Plumb MM, Holland JC. Comparative study of psychological function in patients with advanced cancer: 1. self-reported depressive symptoms. *Psychosom Med* 1977; 39:264–275.

62. Rowland J. Interpersonal resources: social support. In: Holland JC, Rowland JH, eds. *Handbook of Psychooncology: Psychological Care of the Patient with Cancer.* New York: Oxford University Press, 1990:58–75.

63. Lesko LM. Bone marrow transplantation. In: Holland JC, Rowland JH, eds. *Handbook of Psychooncology: Psychological Care of the Patient with Cancer.* New York: Oxford University Press, 1990:163–173.

64. Arana GW, Hyman SE. *Handbook of Psychiatric Drug Therapy,* 3rd Edition. Boston/Toronto/London: Little, Brown and Company, 1995.

9

Symptom Control in Patients with Severe Character Pathology

STEVEN D. PASSIK AND JENNIFER L. HAY

Living with life-threatening illness presents all patients with profound physical and emotional challenges. Physically, they must often adapt to painful, uncomfortable, invasive, or exhausting treatment regimens, and they may experience increasing bodily or cognitive decline. Emotionally, patients must contend with reactions such as shock, fear, anxiety, or sadness upon learning their diagnosis, and then make the necessary changes required to live with it.[1] Such emotional reactions are to be expected, even in the psychologically healthy. Indeed, a prevalence study of psychiatric disorders in cancer patients found that emotional distress was quite common: nearly half (47%) of assessed inpatients and outpatients had levels of emotional disturbance that could be classified as a psychiatric disorder.[2]

Symptom control helps most patients adjust and cope better. However, symptom control is difficult. It requires consistency, communication, and the ability to tolerate distress until improvement is noted—both by patients and palliative care professionals. For a subset of patients, those with severe character pathology, affording symptom control is even more of a challenge. Such patients are often inconsistent, not trusting or trustworthy, impulsive in their medication-taking, and unable to tolerate negative physical and emotional states long enough to allow for palliative care specialists to diagnose and treat their distress.

Illness is emotionally daunting for most people. Those who eventually cope well contain their sadness and fear, and direct their physical and emotional energy toward fighting their disease while maintaining a realistic view of their limitations and prognosis. Those who adjust well also flexibly and fluidly renegotiate their relationships with others to maximize their care—whether toward greater dependency and diminished personal control, or toward reestablishing autonomy as symptoms abate.[3]

Character Pathology in Patients with Life-threatening Illness

In essence, illness requires a person to tolerate dramatic life uncertainty, while maintaining a collaborative relationship with doctors, other caregivers, and family. These tasks may be precisely the most difficult for severely character disordered individuals, particularly those with *borderline personality disorder* (BPD), or borderline traits. Through their regressive and sometimes unrealistic manner of coping with threat, their often distorted perceptions of other people, and their inflexible ways of relating, physically ill borderline patients may be among the most difficult to manage in the medical setting.[4–11] While such individuals may function more or less adequately when they are not stressed, their defensive attempts to maintain equilibrium when faced with illness can become increasingly rigid, counterproductive, or even irrational. Reactions to other people may also become a hindrance. These individuals may veer toward dependent clinging, manipulation, hostile over-entitlement, paranoia, or complete withdrawal.[6,12] Frequent co-morbid substance abuse[13] or a history of early life trauma[14] may further complicate the picture. Illness can lead character disordered patients to decompensate psychiatrically, and consciously or unconsciously sabotage their own treatment. We have noticed that staff often unconsciously react to such patients by becoming "deskilled," or less effective in their normal ability to carry out their caregiving duties. This can lead to staff anger, burnout, or withdrawal.

Long-term psychotherapy with severely character disordered individuals may aspire to bring about lasting change.[15,16] In the medical setting, however, goals of psychiatric management are quite different.[8] These patients require: (*1*) assessment and comprehensive treatment of their multiple psychiatric symptoms or co-morbid disorders; (*2*) decisive restraint, limited setting, and preventive measures if there is potential for impulsivity or self-destructive acts such as suicide, substance abuse, or medical noncompliance, and finally; (*3*), containment of behaviors that disrupt or interfere with the adequate functioning of the medical staff. Often, the psychiatrist's or psychologist's role centers on supporting staff who may come to hate, fear, or reject these exasperating, labile patients. Left unchecked, anger, fear, or avoidance on the part of caregivers can lead to poor staff–patient relations that become a self-fulfilling prophecy for the patient. Coming to illness with a problematic past generally means that patients' most basic sense of self among others[17] is faulty. Thus, they expect poor care, and lack of attention to pain, suffering, and their negative feeling states. These unfortunate patients have a propensity to embroil unsuspecting staff in these very same patterns.

Defining Character Pathology

A character, or personality, disorder involves a severe, stable pattern of experiencing and behaving which generally begins by adolescence or early adulthood.

The disorder has a pervasive effect on important aspects of functioning, such as thinking, emotion, interpersonal relatedness, and impulse control. When extreme, the result is impaired functioning or psychological distress.[18]

Currently accepted diagnostic criteria[18] identify ten specific personality disorders, which are grouped into three broad clusters based on descriptive similarities.[19] Cluster A individuals often appear odd or eccentric, and include paranoid, schizoid, and schizotypal personality disorders. Cluster B individuals are overly reactive or dramatic, and include antisocial, borderline, histrionic, and narcissistic personality disorders. Cluster C patients are anxious or fearful, and include those with avoidant, dependent, and obsessive–compulsive personality disorders. Certainly, character disordered individuals other than those with BPD may present with problems in the medical setting.[12,20] For example, those who are schizoid or avoidant may complicate their medical treatment through their profound social withdrawal and inability to communicate. Schizotypal individuals may perplex the medical staff because they are eccentric or bizarre. Yet it is the defensive maneuvers and interpersonal relationships characteristic of the patient with BPD, as well as those transiently exhibiting such borderline characteristics, that wreak the most havoc in the medical setting.[6]

Psychoanalysts such as Kernberg[21] have discussed borderline as a level of personality or character organization between neurotic (normal) and psychotic levels. Impulsivity, primitive attachments to others, poor affect tolerance, and ineffective defenses characterize all individuals who function predominantly at this level. Other personality disordered individuals may function at this level but have features of dependency (dependent personality disorder [DPD]) or oddness (schizotypal) that imply a specific style of defenses, way of making attachments, and tolerating affects. Their diagnosis is often mixed personality disorder, which implies functioning at a borderline level with a particular dominant style.

Borderline Personality Disorder

Patients with BPD are characteristically unstable. They can be labile and unpredictable in their moods and emotions, and often present with ever-changing combinations of debilitating psychiatric symptoms. Kernberg[21] has referred to their presentation with different Axis I symptoms as a "pan-symptomatic neurosis." Despite these dramatic shifts, borderline patients often feel empty. Many attempt to address chronic boredom or feelings of worthlessness with quick shifts in jobs, goals, or values, or through reckless behavior such as substance abuse, sexual promiscuity, or other impulsive acts. Patients with BPD sometimes exhibit chronically self-injurious behavior, such as multiple suicide attempts or self-mutilation.

Borderline patients have a marked inability to achieve relationships that are lasting and mutual, and they often present with unstable or chaotic relationship histories. These patients tend towards intense, fleeting intimacies where their feelings can oscillate quickly from love to hate. They often perceive the worth of others exclusively in relation to their own desires, directing idealization toward those who satisfy, and rageful retaliation toward those who do not. These dramatically shifting perceptions reflect borderline patients' difficulty in reconciling positive and negative aspects of other people, or tolerating a realistic sense of ambivalence. Their intense dread of abandonment sometimes leads them to seek attention and caretaking through manipulative measures such as self-neglect or self-destructiveness. While they can sometimes be intensely seductive, these patients also alienate others through their unmitigated neediness, wildly shifting emotions, pronouncements of their own entitlement, or tendency toward provocation.[21–23]

Borderline Personality in the Palliative Care Setting

The anxiety, uncertainty, and discomfort associated with severe medical illness or lengthy hospitalization can engender extreme difficulty for borderline patients. Discord in several areas, including the patient's sense of reality, manner of relating to others, and potential for aggression and destructiveness, usually represent the greatest obstacles.[8]

Perceptions of reality

The use of regressed, primitive defense mechanisms by borderline patients is accentuated when they feel threatened. All people attempt to cope with stress by marshaling defenses. Psychologically healthy individuals use "higher level defenses" that allow them to maintain a realistic grasp of reality and an appreciation of their own thoughts and feelings, while providing some shelter from emotional overload. Higher level defenses such as anticipation, humor, and sublimation, allow a person to adjust to, and surmount, difficulty. The "lower level defenses" used by borderline patients lead them to distort reality in the service of emotional protection. Ultimately these coping maneuvers do more harm than good.[9,11,24]

Because of their difficulty reconciling the positive and negative aspects of other people, borderline patients often engage in *unconscious splitting*, where they rigidly separate others, particularly caretakers, into "good ones" and "bad ones." In inpatient settings, the patient's rigid approval of, and cooperation with, "good" caretakers, and disdain toward "bad" caretakers, can lead staff to experience the patient quite differently. Staff may come to disagree on the patient's level of pain, the need for psychotropic medication, or the validity of physical complaints. These distinctions can lead to staff discord, reduced communication, and inconsistent care. It can also lead the staff to engage in "taking sides"—either for or against—a difficult patient.

The patient may also rigidly adhere to one side of the split, demonstrating impervious grandiosity or self-degradation, and projecting the corresponding perceptions onto others. This can increase the staff's difficulty in entering into a cooperative, caretaking alliance with the patient. Through *projective identificat-ion*, of which "deskilling" is an example, the patient can often unconsciously elicit the expected positive or negative response, be it rejection, anger, or idealization. The staff remain unaware that they are "acting out," and thus confirming, the patient's distorted view of the world.

BPD patients can also engage in *denial*, which involves a rigid repudiation of unacceptable aspects of reality, or a belief in powerful, yet fictional, wishes. Such a defense could lead patients to avoid knowledge of their illness, decide precipi-tously that they are cured, or flee from medical treatment altogether.

Recent work also has confirmed that those with BPD are more likely than others to experience transient episodes of dissociation when they are under stress.[25,26] Because an accurate awareness of reality is critical to a patient's ac-knowledgement of illness, ability to comply with treatment and participate in medical decision making, and correctly interpret caregivers' benevolent motives, the borderline patient's assaults on reality testing must always be adequately and efficiently addressed.

Interpersonal relationships

In their adult relationships, those with BPD tend to reenact the same relationship patterns they experienced as children. These patterns often originate in environ-ments characterized by chaotic unpredictability, emotional neglect, and parental hostility.[27,28] Recently, the high frequency of childhood verbal, physical, and sexual abuse in those diagnosed with BPD has been elucidated.[29] Not surpris-ingly, borderline parents tend to raise borderline children, and the etiology is thought to be largely environmental, rather than biological.[30] Psychoanalytic theorists[21–23] see BPD as developing from traumatic, premature autonomy, and parental failure to allow gradual, nontraumatic separation from the soothing maternal or paternal presence. Thus, borderline patients never learn to modulate their own emotions or quell impulses. They remain intensely fearful of being alone. The entire character structure of BPD patients with abusive backgrounds can be viewed as an ongoing response to trauma.

These deficits manifest in the medical setting in two ways. First, those with BPD have trouble negotiating social distance.[8] Medical staff expects patients to be involved, but not overly involved, with their caretakers. Most normal adults, who experienced adequate parenting, can comfortably regress and allow them-selves to be cared for when necessary. Their basic sense of safety in the hands of others allows them to do so. Patients with BPD, on the other hand, have no such basic sense of safety. The "endpoint" of the regression caused by illness evokes their innermost fears of neglect, abandonment, and terror.

In contrast to the psychologically healthy patient, who tolerates greater care-taking and dependency when ill, borderline patients' intense fears of abandon-ment can lead them to become clingy and demanding, withdrawn or rejecting, or manipulative. These distortions of normal social distance represent desperate attempts on the part of the patient to maintain self-control or ward off abandonment. Ultimately they alienate and anger the staff, or lead staff to feel guilty and resentful when they cannot fulfill all the patient's needs. These interpersonal dynamics can lead the staff to feel ineffectual and "deskilled."

Case Example.

> A young female patient with gastric lymphoma was regularly admitted the day before chemotherapy (Dartmouth protocol) for hydration and a 24-hr urine collection for creatinine clearance. In the hospital, she would wear revealing lingerie and sport a tattoo of a rose on her left breast. At each admission, she would arrive already angry at nurses for their "ineptitude," and accuse them of wanting to prolong her admission and keep her from leaving on time to enjoy her weekend. Following a period of sexual provocation and constant insults, one of the nurses absent-mindedly discarded collected urine, thereby delaying the patient's discharge. This produced prolonged and angry entanglements with staff.

Borderline patients tend to enact childhood relationships with their medical caregivers. When patients require help with basic physical needs, these enactments can become vividly realistic. These patients can begin to act like rageful, demanding, impulsive children, and can elicit in a caregiver the sense of being an ineffective, hostile, rejecting parent. As a result, the patient with BPD can initiate oscillating experiences of victimization and abusiveness, with staff members feeling first victimized by the patient's unending demands, and then abusive in the face of the defenseless, needy patient. Dissonant interactions can lead staff to withdraw, or retaliate, in attempts to protect patients and themselves. These experiences may feel alien in caregivers who generally see themselves as caring and skillful.

Control of aggression

Problems arise in the medical setting when patients direct aggression at staff, other patients, or themselves. Hostility directed toward the staff may be mild, and involve sulking, lack of minimal gratitude for care, or repeated complaints. Borderline patients may split the staff, and direct hostility at only certain doctors and nurses. Menacing, threatening behavior is even more distressing and disruptive. Patients' difficulty with social distance may lead them to become overly involved, or actively disruptive, with other patients. Self-destructiveness can take the form of substance abuse, suicidal tendencies, or sabotaging their treatment. Again, these behaviors can be intensely burdensome to staff, as well as destructive to the patient's medical care.

Unnerving peculiarities of the medical setting

It is important to note that certain aspects of medical care and hospitalization may be uniquely difficult for patients with BPD. For instance, painful procedures may re-traumatize patients who have suffered physical abuse as children. The lack of privacy in hospital rooms, particularly at night, can exacerbate boundary problems and cause patients to react strongly to perceived intrusions. This situation can also cause patients to intrude on other patients and disrupt their sleep or care (for example, they may interact inappropriately with family members of roommates, or turn the television up too loud). Finally, patients with BPD, who frequently have difficulty maintaining relationships, are negatively affected by frequent changes in staffing, such as shift or resident rotations.

Assessing the Character Disordered Patient

Diagnosis of a personality disorder in the medical setting presents unique impediments, and may not be necessary for effective treatment.[6] A firm diagnosis requires confirmation of the historical stability of the characterological symptoms, and such a history is often difficult to acquire in a meeting with a medically ill, distressed individual. Interestingly, we have found that the initial diagnosis is sometimes most clear in the social history. Multiple changes in goals, jobs, schools, or relationships, or the lack of substantive social ties, are often clues. Patients who have large families from whom they are estranged, or who are chronically angry, or who receive few visitors even when seriously ill, may have a personality disorder. The damage done to relationships throughout life can leave such patients isolated and alone when disease occurs. In the palliative care setting, a lack of social support may mean that few people will be close to the patient to assist in caregiving or symptom control efforts.

Personality traits must be clearly distinct from characteristics and symptoms that might emerge in response to situational stressors, substance intoxication and withdrawal (including prescribed medications), or co-occurring mood or cognitive disorders such as delirium. This level of clarity is rare when first interviewing medical patients. Often multiple interviews of the patient, as well as interviews of family members or staff, are necessary to reach any diagnostic certainty. The stress and discomfort of severe medical illness can lead many individuals to display rigid, maladaptive coping strategies typical of severely character disordered individuals, even when their psychiatric history does not substantiate long-standing pathology. Importantly, the formal diagnosis of a character disorder is less critical than the recognition and management of lower level defense mechanisms, and enactments of abusive or maladaptive interpersonal relationships.

Palliative care professionals may suspect the presence of character disorder when discussions about the patient are tinged with anger, fear, or confusion.[8] The emotional reactions of staff always provide valuable information concerning such difficult patients. A multi-perspective approach, in which the psychiatrist or psychologist interviews the staff as well as the patient, and conceives of this interaction as an interdependent system, best allows the clinician to formulate an understanding of the patient's predominant defenses and a "flavor" of the interpersonal enactments surrounding his or her medical care.[7] The clinician can also find the rational part of the patient's complaints and act as ombudsman.

In the initial meeting, the psychiatric clinician should structure the interview by introducing the patient to the clinician's role, and to the rationale and reasonable outcome of the interview. This will allay some of the patient's anxiety, provide a basis for a positive and genuine alliance, and give the patient a sense of the clinician's potential to help. At the outset, the clinician must assess the patient's view of any problems or misunderstandings, as well as his or her ideas for solutions.[6] The clinician should clarify the patient's sense of what role the clinician is to play in the patient's care. Additionally, a clear understanding of any current co-morbid psychiatric symptoms or disorders, including anxiety, depression, mania, psychosis, or cognitive disorders such as dementia and delirium, is central to accurate diagnosis. Such co-morbid symptoms and disorders are quite common among those with BPD. Approximately half of these patients also have a history of major depression,[31] one-fifth have a history of anxiety disorders,[32] and two-thirds have a history of substance abuse.[33] In addition to the assessment of current and lifetime substance use, the interview should attempt to identify any self-destructive potential of the patient.

In the initial interview with the house staff, nursing staff, primary physician, and head nurse, the psychiatrist or psychologist should clarify the emotional reactions of the staff and get a history of the patient's behavior and emotional responses to treatment requirements, ward routine, and caretaking during this, and any previous, hospital admission.[8] From the chart, the clinician should focus on tracing the notes that record the patient's reactions to treatment, and should compare medications actually received to those ordered. The clinician should elicit as much psychiatric history as possible from any available family members, paying special attention to any history of trauma.

Through this multi-perspective approach, the psychiatric clinician will gain valuable information concerning the patient's coping processes. Among the most important are the primary defenses used by the patient and the extent to which he or she imposes rigid relationship expectations on staff.

Symptom Control for BPD Patients

The management of treatment–limiting behaviors and psychiatric symptoms evidenced by medically ill borderline patients usually encompasses three broad approaches: psychotherapeutic, psychopharmacological, and staff liaison. All approaches should work toward helping the patient maintain behavioral control, treating co-morbid psychiatric symptoms, maximizing treatment outcomes, and allowing for the adequate functioning of the staff. Reduction of harm to the patient, staff, and treatment caused by regressive, provocative, or impulsive behavior, rather than dramatic personality change, is often a realistic, periodically attainable goal.

Psychotherapeutic management

Problem–centered strategies should set priorities for the patient's treatment, comfort, and safety. Symptom control is generally best provided in a consistent environment that supports frequent re-evaluation. Psychotherapy should focus on providing this environment and helping the patient be as available as possible for palliative care. It is important to soothe patients and help them gain insight into conflicts with staff, such as their role in deskilling.

The psychiatric clinician's attitude and demeanor is critical in approaching these patients. He or she should approach the patient from a position that reflects both a desire to understand and the need to avoid unwitting collusion with the patient's distortions. For instance, the clinician might approach the patient from a "one down" position,[34] which involves taking a genuinely respectful and receptive attitude towards the patient's view of his or her situation, and stating clearly how the clinician might help in addressing problems. This may defuse patient aggression and encourage a collaborative working relationship.[6] It is also important to avoid confronting and interpreting the patient's rage or entitlement, because this can lead to renewed attacks or emotional escalation. Emotional language, and punishments, should categorically be avoided.[35] At the same time, the clinician must avoid overidentification with the patient's distorted view of the disease, treatment, or medical staff, and must be ready to hold to, and sometimes clarify, reality for the patient.

The psychiatrist or psychologist should begin by setting priorities for the patient's agenda. He or she can help the patient clarify questions or requests, and disentangle emotional from physical needs. The therapist can be extremely helpful in modeling effective, nonabusive ways to elicit staff attention, and can teach the patient to communicate distress politely, frankly, and with well-modulated emotion, a technique we refer to as "speaking hospital." Providing effective ways for patients to get their needs met can be valuable in dissipating borderline patients' sense of panic over perceived abandonment. It also bolsters their sense of self-control.

Borderline patients benefit from techniques aimed at increasing their sense of control over, and predictability of, their environments.[5,6,8,10,11] For those with problems adhering to aspects of their treatment regimen, the implementation of a contract that addresses patient responsibilities, such as keeping appointments and complying with medication regimens is helpful. These contracts should have clear information about the repercussions that will ensue from failure to adhere to the guidelines.

Medication should be kept as consistent as possible. Any changes will generally be met with more equanimity if the doctor requests the patient's cooperation in advance of treatment shifts. Avoiding abrupt medication changes will enhance patients' sense of control.

Setting firm limits is required when patients show a real potential to harm themselves, sabotage their medical treatment, disrupt other patients, or interfere with the workings of the staff. Each member of the treatment team should be aware of the limits and be willing to cooperate to enforce them. The responses to unacceptable behaviors should be concrete, and may involve neuroleptics, one-to-one observation, restraints, or psychiatric admission; responses should remain focused on steps required to protect the patient, rather than retribution. Limits should be conveyed calmly. A patient's emotional outburst should be met with verbal recognition of the patient's anger, as well as a request for appropriate behavior. Immediate positive feedback should be given when the patient's behavior improves.

Borderline patients with a history of traumatic childhood abuse may require specific interventions to help them deal with their illness. Such individuals may become highly anxious, panicked, or avoidant in the face of painful or frightening medical procedures. Additionally, they have a greater likelihood of developing symptoms of post-traumatic stress disorder, such as dissociation or sudden flashbacks, after being exposed to sudden or intrusive care, or situations that harken back to the initial trauma. Recent work[14] has elucidated the reciprocal nature of borderline pathology and trauma; borderline patients are more susceptible to developing traumatic reactions, just as a traumatic childhood history can lead to a BPD diagnosis. Therefore, borderline patients may require specific interventions to help them deal with procedures, such as hypnosis, cognitive rehearsing, or the constant presence of a trusted therapist throughout the difficult situation. Additional measures should be taken to enhance a sense of boundaries before entering a room, such as encouraging knocking, or providing the patient a private room if available and desired by the patient.

Psychopharmacological management

There is evidence that personality disorders per se do not respond to drug treatment because of their predominantly psychosocial etiology.[36] Yet, the pan-symptomatic picture often presented by the severely character disordered patient often requires psychotropic intervention,[37] especially in the medical setting. Borderline symptoms can be broken down into treatable clusters and targeted for psychopharmacologic intervention.[38] The identification of target symptoms, including depressive affect, anxiety, behavioral dyscontrol, or distorted thinking, will determine an initial pharmacological intervention.

Depression, anxiety, and delirium
Cognitive symptoms of depression, such as sad mood, helplessness, and pessimism, are very common among those with BPD. However, these patients do not generally manifest the corresponding physical symptoms of depression, such as sleep disturbance, reduced energy, or reduced appetite. Because antidepressants are more efficacious when patients present with both cognitive and physical aspects, borderline patients are sometimes refractory to these drugs.[39,40] In patients who evince both cognitive and physical symptoms, tricyclic antidepressants

(TCAs) may be helpful in managing insomnia, encouraging appetite, and improving mood. Care must be taken, however, in evaluating the suicide potential of such patients, because TCAs may be lethal in overdose. Selective serotonin reuptake inhibitors (SSRIs), such as flouxetine, may be helpful in depressed, relatively healthy patients with few additional physical complaints. Additionally, SSRIs are relatively safe in overdose.

Anxiety is a common complaint among borderline patients. When they must tolerate painful or frightening procedures, or medical confinement, their anxiety may become overwhelming. Benzodiazepines are often quite useful in treating both acute anxiety during procedures and more chronic anxiety associated with hospitalizations or long-term medical illness.[37] The use of longer-acting agents, such as clonazepam, can prevent rebound anxiety, which often inflames characterological defensive maneuvers. It is also important to assess the patient's use of other drugs and alcohol, because benzodiazepines can act synergistically with other drugs to cause oversedation. Although benzodiazepines may be very useful in treating anxiety, it must be recognized that borderline patients may be particularly susceptible to benzodiazepine abuse and addiction. Sedating neuroleptics such as thioridazine can be used for anxiety when benzodiazepines need to be avoided. The newer atypical neuroleptics will likely also play an important role in the management of anxiety in character disordered patients.[38]

Neuroleptics may also be used when patients' behavior is severely disruptive or impulsive, or when distorted thinking such as paranoia becomes an important impediment to treatment. Such symptoms are often controlled with low-dose neuroleptics. These doses pose little risk of serious side effects, such as extrapyramidal symptoms.[6,11]

The diagnosis of delirium may be missed in BPD patients. Once the patient has "declared" himself or herself as peculiar, overly emotional, bizarre, or capable of sudden shifts in behavior, staff can miss early signs of delirium. This can occur if staff become less observant, more avoidant, deskilled, or adopt a sense that virtually anything is possible in terms of the patient's behavioral repertoire. From this perspective, behaviors may be interpreted as volitional rather than organic. In those with BPD and advanced disease or multiple medical complications, the palliative care specialist must be careful not to miss the early signs of delirium or other organic mental disorders.

Pain and symptom management
The borderline patient with pain may present the staff with specific quandaries. Inadequate analgesia can lead to regressive behavior, manipulation, or other forms of acting out.[6] These behaviors, combined with staff knowledge that a patient is a "borderline," may lead to a skeptical attitude toward continued complaints. Problems can be lessened by limiting prescribing to one physician who assumes sole responsibility for analgesics. This physician should frequently reevaluate dosage requirements and, if appropriate, prescribe a fixed scheduled regimen, rather than an "as needed" regimen.

Substance Abuse in BPD Patients

Many patients with BPD periodically abuse illicit substances, alcohol, or pre-scribed and over-the-counter medications. At times, this behavior represents a diagnosable co-morbid substance abuse disorder that complicates all aspects of treatment, particularly pain and symptom management. Such disorders require separate treatment strategies and detailed assessment.[41] Measures such as con-tracts, spot urine toxicology screens, frequent clinic visits with renewal of small quantities of medications, and preference given to longer-acting compounds, are among those preferred to help in the management of these patients. The team can insist that the patient participate in 12-step meetings and document their attendance. Detailed assessments of drug-taking behaviors should be repeated and carefully documented.

A larger subset of BPD patients may have more sporadic patterns of drug abuse. These patterns are suggestive of impulsive or desperate attempts to use the "self-regulating" effects of drugs in an effort to modulate emotional distress, anger with staff or others, self-destructiveness, or feelings of emptiness and boredom. Such self-medication is often haphazard and does not differ significantly from the chaotic and desperate attempts these patients make in using the self-regulating effects of interpersonal contacts, food, exercise, or other means. While behavioral limits similar to those described above for addicts are helpful, separate consideration of the distinct psychodynamics of these situations will govern ultimate treatment decisions, especially after extreme "acting out" has occurred.

Case Example.

A 40-year-old borderline woman with thymoma, chronic pain, and anxiety disorder was angry at her therapist for his prolonged vacation. Her anxiety greatly increased during his time away. While her use of oxycodone had always been difficult to control, her use of alprazolam had been nonconflictual for a period of years (as long as she was provided a few days extra on each prescription so that she would not become panicked at the possibility of running out prior to her scheduled visits). Her physician gave her a prescription for eighty alprazolam tablets on the Friday before the return of her therapist on Monday. The patient impulsively forged a "1" before the "80," more than doubling the number of tablets. The change was detected by a pharmacist who reported it back to her medical team. In consultation with the therapist, the team decided that the behavior represented primarily an expression of the psychodynamics of abandonment and self-defeating expressions of rage, and was dealt with in some detail in her psychotherapy. Nonetheless, for the team's and patient's protection in the face of the illegal nature of the behavior, the patient was placed on a schedule of gradually loosening restrictions (limited prescriptions, pill counts, spot urine checks), until she demonstrated compliance and was returned to her standard management.

Staff Issues

It is generally impossible to manage the hospitalized borderline patient without involving the medical staff. Indeed, Groves[7] considers alliance and support of staff to be the primary approach to managing the hospitalized borderline patient; direct work with the patient is much less critical. The main goals of staff liaison involve addressing the powerful process of deskilling iniated by severely character disordered patients. Through the pull to reenact the dynamics of the patient's childhood world, staff develop intense feelings toward these patients—whether intense sympathy, hatefulness, anger, or rejection. As these patients dismantle doctors' and nurses' normally exceptional caretaking abilities, anger and resentment can increase. Staff liaison that seeks to educate, support, and organize cooperation will go a long way in addressing borderline patients' symptoms, as well as combating staff resentment and burnout.

It is critical that psychiatrists and psychologists educate medical staff about the fact that borderline pathology is a psychiatric disorder. They should understand that these patients are extremely sensitive to feeling out of control or abandoned, and that they have severe problems with personal relationships. Psychiatric clinicians can help staff interpret the patient's alienating behavior within this model; this understanding can help them curb their emotional reactions and maintain consistent care. Psychiatric clinicians can be helpful in modeling a neutral, non-punitive approach to the borderline patient.

In concert with education, it is critical that staff members feel supported in their caretaking of borderline patients. In group meetings, staff should be encouraged to articulate their strong feelings, and to understand that these feelings are useful data about their patients, rather than something to hide or ignore. Indeed, it is more likely that staff will act on negative feelings if they do *not* articulate them.[42] In a group setting, staff members feel supported in their common perceptions. It is the clinician's role to provide a forum for staff to ventilate feelings, and to validate strong negative feelings that are elicited consistently when professionals work with borderline patients.

Education and support must be joined by positive cooperation among staff. The psychiatrist or psychologist should organize a meeting that will ideally be attended by all who treat the patient, including doctors, nurses, and consultants. Limits and consistency of care should be decided through unanimous agreement. Such cooperation will make it more difficult for the patient to engage in staff-splitting maneuvers, and will discourage patient attempts at manipulation or undermining of contracts or limits. Finally, staff can be encouraged to minimize changes both in nursing coverage and in the number of doctors and nurses providing feedback to the patient on a daily basis.

References

1. Massie MJ, Holland JC. Overview of normal reactions and prevalence of psychiatric disorders. In: Holland JC, Rolland JH, eds. *Handbook of Psycho-oncology: Psychological Care of the Patient with Cancer.* New York:Oxford University Press, 1989:273–290.

2. Derogatis LR, Morrow GR, Fetting J, et al. The prevalence of psychiatric disorders among cancer patients. *JAMA* 1983; 249:751–757.

3. Perry S, Veiderman M. Management of emotional reactions to acute medical illness. *Med Clin North Am* 1981; 65:3–14.

4. Crespo VR. The borderline patient with life-threatening illness. In: Klagsbrun SC, Goldberg IK, Rawnsley MM, Kutscher AH, Marcus ER, Siegel M, eds. *Psychiatric Aspects of Terminal Illness.* Philadelphia, Penn.: Charles Press, 1988: 246–256.

5. Fitzgibbon ML, Barbuto J. Approach to the medically-ill borderline patient: A case report. Unpublished manuscript, Memorial Sloan-Kettering Cancer Center.

6. Fogel BS, Martin C. Personality disorders in the medical setting. In: Stoudemire A, Fogel BS, eds. *Principles of Medical Psychiatry.* Orlando, Fla.: Grune & Stratton, 1987:253–270.

7. Groves JE. Management of the borderline patient on a medical or surgical ward: The psychiatric consultant's role. *Int J Psychiatry Med* 1975; 6:337–348.

8. Groves JE. Borderline patients. In: Hackett TP, Cassem NH, eds. *Handbook of General Psychiatry, 2 ed.* Littleton, Mass.: PSG Publishing, 1987:184–207.

9. McDaniel JS, Stoudemire A, Riether AM, Firestone S, Cohen-Cole SA, Cobbs BW. Terminal cardiomyopathy, splitting, and borderline personality organization. *Gen Hosp Psychiatry* 1992; 14:277–284.

10. Sansone RA, Sansone LA. Borderline personality disorder. *Postgrad Med* 1995; 97:169–179.

11. Stoudemire A, Thompson TL. The borderline in the medical setting. *Ann Intern Med* 1982; 96:76–79.

12. Geringer RS, Stern TA. Coping with medical illness: The impact of personality types. *Psychosomatics* 1986; 27:251–261.

13. Sullivan T, Francis AJ. Substance use in borderline personality disorder. *Am J Psychiatry* 1990; 147:1002–1007.

14. Gunderson JG, Sabo AN. The phenomenological and conceptual interface between borderline personality disorder and PTSD. *Am J Psychiatry* 1993; 150:19–27.

15. Waldinger RJ, Guderson JG. *Effective Psychotherapy with Borderline Patients.* New York: Macmillan, 1987.

16. Kernberg O. *Severe Personality Disorders: Psychotherapeutic Strategies.* New Haven, Conn.: Yale University Press, 1984.

17. Stern D. *The Interpersonal World of the Infant.* New York: Basic Books, 1985.

18. American Psychiatric Association. *Diagnostic and Statistical Manual of Mental Disorders,* Fourth Edition. Washington DC: American Psychiatric Association, 1994.

19. Widiger TA, Trull TJ, Hurt SW, Clarkin J, Francis A. A multidimensional scaling of the DSM-III personality disorders. *Arch Gen Psychiatry* 1987; 44:557–563.

20. Kahana RJ, Bebring GL. Personality types in medical management. In: Sinberg NE, ed. *Psychiatry and Medical Practice in a General Hospital.* New York: International Universities Press, 1965:108–123.

21. Kernberg O. *Borderline Conditions and Pathological Narcissism.* New York: Jason Aronson, 1975.

22. Gunderson JG, Singer MT. Defining borderline patients: An overview. *Am J Psychiatry* 1975; 132:1–10.

23. Masterson J. *Treatment of the Borderline Adolescent: A Developmental Approach.* New York: John Wiley, 1972.

24. Vaillant GE. *Empirical Studies of Ego Mechanisms of Defense.* Washington, D.C.: American Psychiatric Association, 1986.

25. Gunderson JG, Zanarini MC, Kisiel CL. Borderline personality disorder: A review of data on DSM-III-R descriptions. *J Personal Disord* 1991; 5:340–352.

26. Sternbach SE, Judd PH, Sabo AN, McGlashan T, Gunderson JG. Cognitive and perceptual distortions in borderline personality disorder and schizotypal personality disorder in a vignette sample. *Compr Psychiatry* 1992; 33:186–189.

27. Gunderson JG, Kerr J, Englund D. The families of borderlines: a comparative study. *Arch Gen Psychiatry* 1980; 37:27–33.

28. Links P. *Family Environment and Borderline Personality Disorder.* Washington, D.C.: American Psychiatric Association, 1990.

29. Herman JL, Perry CC, van der Kolk BA. Childhood trauma in borderline personality disorder. *Am J Psychiatry* 1989; 146:490–495.

30. Torgersen S. Genetic and nosologic aspects of schizotypal and borderline disorders: A twin study. *Arch Gen Psychiatry* 1984; 41:546–554.

31. Pope HG, Jonas JM, Hudson J. The validity of DSM-III borderline personality disorder. *Arch Gen Psychiatry* 1983; 40:23–30.

32. Alnaes R, Torgerson S. *J Nerv Ment Dis* 1990; 178:693–698.

33. Dulit RA, Fyer MR, Hass GL, Sullivan T, Francis AJ. Substance use in borderline personality disorders. *Am J Psychiatry* 1990; 147:1002–1007.

34. Watzlawick P, Beavin JH, Jackson DD. *Pragmatics of Human Communication.* New York: Norton, 1967.

35. Adler G, Buie DH. The misuses of confrontation with borderline patients. *Int J Psychoanal Psychother* 1972; 1:109–120.

36. Searight HR. Borderline personality disorder: diagnosis and management in primary care. *J Fam Pract* 1992; 34:605–612.

37. Berger PA. Pharmacological treatment for borderline personality disorder. *Bull Menninger Clin* 1987; 51:277–284.

38. Joseph S. *Personality Disorders: New Symptom-focused Drug Therapy.* New York: Hawarth Medical Press, 1997.

39. Gunderson JG. Building structure for the borderline construct. *Acta Psychiatr Scand* 1994; 89:12–18.

40. Stone M. *The Fate of Borderline Patients.* New York: Guilford, 1990.

41. Passik S, Portenoy R. Substance Use Disorders In Holland JC, ed. *Psycho-oncology.* New York: Oxford University Press, 1998:576–586.

42. Groves JE. Taking care of the hateful patient. *N Engl J Med* 1978; 298:883–887.

IV

Skin Disorders and Their Management

Introduction

Medical and Psychosocial Implications of Skin Disorders

EDUARDO BRUERA

The majority of terminally ill cancer and AIDS patients suffer from skin abnormalities. The skin may be directly involved by the underlying disease, as in the case of malignancies, or may be affected by a number of associated conditions. These include local and systemic infections, radiation– or chemotherapy–induced dermatitis or mucositis, lymphedema, local or systemic bleeding disorders, and pressure ulcers.

Underlying conditions common to terminally ill patients, such as immobility, malnutrition, delirium, severe pain, immunosuppression, and dehydration, are all risk factors for skin disorders. Skin abnormalities cause numerous physical symptoms and other complications, including incidental and continuous pain, hyperalgesia, pruritus, decreased mobility, odor, and bleeding.

As a consequence of skin disorders, patients and families also suffer from severe psychosocial distress. Changes in body image or odor associated with severe lymphedema or necrotic ulcers may result in the patient's avoidance of contact with friends and relatives or in severe mood changes. In some cases, patients may require hospitalization until death because of the complexity of the physical and psychosocial problems associated with skin complications.

A multidisciplinary approach includes a careful assessment of the etiology and consequences (both physical and psychosocial) of skin disorders. Management requires the consideration of systemic and topical drugs, rehabilitation techniques (physiotherapy and occupational therapy), nursing interventions including mobilization, dressings, and management of odor, planning of interventions in the case of catastrophic hemorrhage, cosmetic interventions, and counseling of both patients and families.

Because of the frequency of these complications in palliative care patients, physicians and nurses treating terminally ill patients should have defined treatment guidelines and access to consulting disciplines. Unfortunately, assessment and management are limited by the scarcity of clinical research on skin disorders in palliative care. The following three chapters address both the importance of a careful clinical approach and recent developments in the management of frequent and devastating complications, such as lymphedema and pressure ulcers. Hopefully, these chapters will encourage researchers from a number of disciplines to focus their interest on the palliative management of the skin complications of terminal illness.

10

Palliative Care and the Clinical Approach to Disorders of the Skin

LLOYD R. HALE AND TERENCE J. RYAN

In the context of palliative care, several new concepts guide the management of skin disease. First, the disease processes that contribute to skin failure in the severely ill result in functional impairment of the skin and consequent handicap. Management may focus on attempting to cure or diminish the causes of skin failure, or it may address the specific impairments. Mostly, it attempts to relieve handicap.

Second, one of the principal functions of the skin is communication. Isolation, loss of confidence, and the feeling of being unwelcome are perhaps the worst handicaps.[1] Remedies include touch, camouflage, the prescription of a prosthesis (after mastectomy, for example) or a wig, and the teaching of communication skills. The "look good, feel good" factor is an important component of well-being, and hence, of health. It is a neglected factor in most "Health for All" documents,[2,3] although it is quite well recognized in the cancer management literature.

Third, the skin is not simply an immobile sleeve. It functions best when it is constantly on the move.

Finally, local cultures and traditions must be considered in the management of skin disease. These disorders occur worldwide. Particularly in the developing world, where palliative care is in its infancy, diseases are diagnosed late and the costs of care are prohibitive. It is necessary to understand local cultures to eliminate some aspects of Western behavior which, for some cultures, can cause great distress. Those who care for the skin must balance the need to communicate with the skin and to feel confident in displaying it with the concurrent need for privacy and the right not to be exposed unnecessarily.

Functions of the Skin

Protective role

Normal healthy skin turns over at a steady rate, allowing the epidermal cells to be replaced, to lose their nuclei as they come to the surface, and to knit together in a surface that is resilient, elastic, supple, and close-knit. It is a surface layer of cells that lies on and is firmly attached to an equally resilient dermis. The dermis consists of a ground substance, which has the capacity to absorb water and other macromolecules. This capacity causes pressure within connective tissue fibers, which are of varying length and resilience (Fig. 10.1). These fibers are attached to cells, such as fibroblasts and the epidermis itself. The blood supply provides the fluid. A controlling factor in maintaining the quality of the dermis is the removal of excess water and macromolecules by the lymphatics, which function primarily by responding to local movement. Movement thus becomes an essential part of the function of the skin. The connective tissue is resilient because of its capacity to maintain the composition and water content of the ground substance in its fibrous environment.[4]

The dermis overlies a layer of adipose tissue. The adipose tissue is an essential organ and has its own functions, including contribution to body shape, insulation,

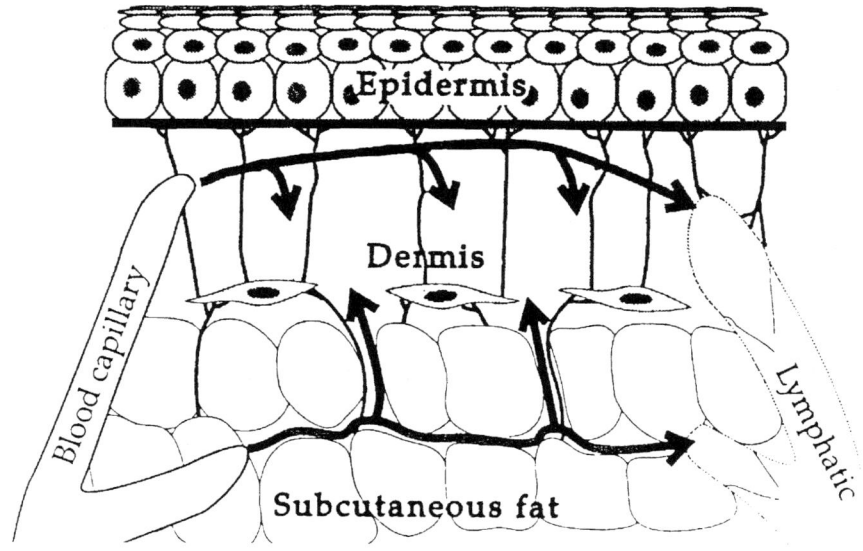

Figure 10.1. Water and macromolecules cause swelling of the ground substance, inducing tractional forces on cell membranes. The lymphatics remove excess fluid in response to local movement. (Reproduced with permission from Ryan TJ, Curri SB. *Genesis of Adipocytes. Clinics in Dermatology.* New York: Elsevier Science Inc., 1989;7:9–24.)

and thermoregulation. It has an innervation that contributes to its capacity to burn fat, to regulate body temperature and to feel pressure, and hence, pain. Because of this innervation, however, discomfort in the fat sometimes results from misinterpretation of signals induced by pressure, cold, or other demands.

An essential function of adipose tissue is the distribution of forces. This is seen best in the soles of the feet, the palms of the hands, and the buttocks. Excessive fat can become a nuisance when attempting to apply forces such as massage or bandages, because it so effectively disperses forces aimed at accumulations of fluid and macromolecules. By contrast, absence of fat, and hence, the loss of the ability to disperse forces, contributes to vulnerability of the skin in the terminally ill, especially over "pressure points."

Fluid balance in the dermis is essential for function. Drying out causes a characteristic loss of elasticity, as seen in dehydrated patients. Excessive accumulation of water and macromolecules leads to changes in the turgor of the skin and also adds to its vulnerability. This is particularly a feature of the immobile, and of dependent tissue subject to the forces of gravity.

Healthy skin normally responds to the frequent stresses, strains, and invasions of its surface with repair processes. An increased blood supply and an acceleration of the turnover of the epidermis is the end result. With respect to the blood supply, it is important to understand that the skin at rest is very undemanding of oxygen. Healthy, resting skin can withstand ischemia for up to 18 hours. Skin that needs to repair itself requires a much more generous blood supply, which can be evoked temporarily through the triple response axon reflex, and the release of chemical agents such as histamine from mast cells. Dermographism is one consequence. However, for most more serious wounds, the skin has to grow a granulation tissue to provide the kind of blood supply that will support adequate healing. Granulation tissue has none of the qualities of normal skin and has no protective role in terms of barrier function or resilience. It has to be removed if health is to be restored.

Thermoregulation

Thermoregulation requires that the skin retain heat. This is primarily a result of vasoconstriction and the use of clothing. Adipose tissue is the most significant endogenous insulation. Loss of heat is one of the most common terminal events. Its extent has not been adequately measured, but worldwide, body cooling—particularly at night and particularly in the neonate or the very old—may be a significant terminal event. Protection of the body against overheating is usually accomplished by insensible perspiration and by sweating. The thermoregulatory role of sweating requires evaporation, which usually requires some movement, either of the body or of the surrounding air. Without the use of a fan, the immobile or dying patient may not be able to take advantage of the capacity to sweat. The interaction of vasodilatation with sweating to achieve thermoregulation is most important in the upper body, particularly the head and hands.

Perception

The skin's sensory role allows it to perceive its environment, and in particular, to sense pain, which is a warning sign of a threatening environment. Pain perception requires alertness, as well as a fully functioning peripheral and central nervous system. Without the sensation of pain, tissues are easily damaged. Pain is usually manageable and bearable. Itch, on the other hand, may be neither manageable nor bearable, and the degree of distress that itch can produce is poorly recognized.

Endocrine function

For many decades, it has been understood that skin produces Vitamin D, but only one decade has passed since the realization that the skin is a major site of manufacture of significant cytokines, including the interleukins, tumor necrosis factor alpha, and interferon gamma. The local production of agents, such as 5-alpha reductase, also has been shown to be important in the metabolism of the sex hormones, and, in part, explains acne and hirsutism. Inflammation of the skin may produce huge metabolic demands. Many terminal events such as weight loss, fever, and heart failure can be a direct consequence of loss of control of skin function.

Immune function

The skin is at the interface with the environment and is in constant interaction with foreign material. It has a well-adapted system for recognizing such foreign material and presenting it to the immune system. These mechanisms include special cells within the skin, such as Langerhans cells, and pathways from the epidermis through the lymphatics to lymph nodes. These systems require both chemical (cytokine) and mechanical forces (skin movement) to perform effectively. The immune defense system may be depressed by skin failure, for example, after severe sun exposure or in any widespread disease.

Sociosexual communication and display

In many ways this is the most important function of the skin. The basis of human communication is determined first by sight, and only second by speech. Animal behavior includes smell and touch, but humans form opinions based initially on sight and then through conversation. It is the first sight which may be the most important in palliative care. Disfigurement can be extremely distressing. The "look good, feel good" factor is one of the strongest components of well-being and only the newborn and the completely demented make no effort to communicate effectively in this way. Grooming is important in the provision of caring and those who are not well groomed may well find themselves receiving less care. There is, thus, a vicious circle in which those who receive the least grooming become the most isolated. The co-components of sociosexual communication include "love at first sight," color prejudice, body scents, and the closest communication, touch.

Those who are disfigured often have less contact and are separated from other people by greater distance. This aspect of management, which includes touch, is important for well-being.

Cutaneous Manifestations of Malignancy

Malignancy may be manifested in the skin by direct or secondary spread of internal malignancies, primary skin malignancies, paraneoplastic phenomena, genodermatoses, or carcinogenic agents. Indirect manifestations may be due to mucocutaneous side effects of treatment or to immunosuppression associated with the disease or treatment.

Spread of internal malignancies

In a retrospective review of tumor registry data on 7316 patients with cancer, skin involvement by internal carcinoma occurred at an overall rate of 5%.[5] As the authors acknowledge, this is probably an underestimate. The highest rates of skin metastasis were for carcinomas of the breast (23.9%), nasal sinuses (10%), oral cavity (5.3%), larynx (3.9%), ovary (3.0%), kidney (2.6%), colon/rectum (2.3%), and lung (1.7%).

In another study of 724 patients with cutaneous metastases, the most frequent primary tumors in men were lung carcinoma (24%), colorectal carcinoma (19%), melanoma (13%), and oral squamous cell carcinoma (12%). In women, the most frequent primary tumors were breast carcinoma (69%), colorectal carcinoma (9%), melanoma (5%), and ovarian carcinoma (4%).[6]

Direct malignant invasion of the skin usually presents as ulceration or inflammation. Carcinoma of the breast may cause fungating ulceration, Paget's disease of the nipple, carcinoma erysipelatoides, or carcinoma en cuirasse. Extra-mammary Paget's disease may, not invariably, be associated with carcinoma in adjacent organs, such as the rectum or uterus.[7]

The subject of cutaneous metastases has been extensively reviewed by Rosen.[8] Metastasis from a distant tumor usually presents as one or more, firm to rubbery, skin-colored, reddish or bluish, rapidly growing papules or nodules presenting anywhere on the skin surface. The scalp is commonly involved by metastases from lung, kidney, and breast tumors.[9] On the scalp, the clinical appearance may be of a scleroderma-like plaque with associated alopecia, rather than a papule or nodule.[10]

Primary skin tumors

New primary tumors may develop in the skin during the course of a terminal illness. Basal cell carcinoma and squamous cell carcinoma are the most common skin malignancies, but a patient with pre-existing metastatic melanoma is at an increased risk of developing a new primary melanoma. Angiosarcoma, a rare and highly malignant neoplasm, may develop in a lymphedematous extremity. Usually, this occurs after mastectomy for breast carcinoma (Stewart-Treves syndrome); it rarely complicates other malignancies.[11] In Africa, albinos, who are particularly common (170,000 being recorded in Tanzania), have an early death from skin tumors and often present for treatment late in their disease.[12]

Genodermatoses and acquired paraneoplastic phenomena

Inherited and acquired skin conditions that may be associated with underlying malignancy have been the subject of recent reviews.[13-16] While some are relatively specific for a given malignancy, others may be associated with a large range of malignancies (Table 10.1). In some, the association with malignancy is rare or disputed.

Carcinogens

Various carcinogens may cause skin changes. Smoking may cause nicotine staining of the skin and oral cavity and is linked to bronchial carcinoma, accelerated aging, reduced nitric oxide effects, and the consequences of atherosclerosis.

Radiation effects on the skin, such as atrophy, pallor, telangiectasia, and chronic radiodermatitis, may be associated with thyroid, hematological, and skin malignancies.[7] Vinyl chloride has been linked with angiosarcoma of the liver.[17] It may also cause acrosclerosis, acro-osteolysis, and papular skin changes.[18]

Arsenic ingestion may result in pigmentary change, keratoses, Bowen's disease (intraepithelial carcinoma), superficial basal cell carcinomas, and multiple sebaceous tumors. This agent has been linked to an increased risk of internal malignancy, especially bronchial.[18]

Immunosuppression–related problems

Internal malignancy may cause a reduction in immunocompetence through indirect mechanisms, such as nutritional deficiency. Lymphoproliferative and hematological malignancies may directly predispose to infection.

Clinical assessment and selective microbiological culture are important in the diagnosis of skin infections. However, a culture of skin biopsy tissue in the immunocompromised patient with cancer and a rash has been shown to have low diagnostic value.[19]

Skin Impairment in Patients with Progressive Systemic Illness: Common Clinical Phenomena

The skin of patients with terminal illness may be subject to a large number of adverse factors. These include immobility, gravitational effects, environmental

Table 10.1. Inherited and acquired dermatological conditions associated with internal malignancy

Dermatological condition	Associated internal malignancy
Genodermatoses	
Adult progeria	Mesenchymal tumors, skin cancer
Ataxia-telangiectasia syndrome	Lymphoreticular malignancy
Bloom syndrome	Leukemia, lymphoma, gastrointestinal
Bruton's X-linked agammaglobulinemia	Lymphoma, leukemia
Chédiak-Higashi syndrome	Lymphoma
Cowden syndrome	Breast, thyroid, uterine
Dyskeratosis congenita	Squamous cell carcinoma (oral, nasal, esophageal, cervical)
Fanconi's anemia	Leukemia, squamous cell carcinoma (oral, esophageal)
Gardner's syndrome	Gastrointestinal (colon, duodenal)
Hemochromatosis	Hepatoma
Howel-Evans' syndrome	Esophageal
Muir-Torre syndrome	Gastrointestinal (colon), genitourinary
Multiple endocrine neoplasia III	Medullary thyroid carcinoma, pheochromocytoma
Nevoid basal cell carcinoma (Gorlin's syndrome)	Central nervous system tumors (medulloblastoma), various
Neurofibromatosis	Neurofibrosarcomas, various
Peutz-Jeghers syndrome	Gastrointestinal, pancreatic, breast, lung, genitourinary
Primary immunodeficiency disorders	Leukemia, lymphoma
Wiskott-Aldrich syndrome	Lymphoreticular malignancy
Acquired Paraneoplastic Dermatoses	
Acanthosis nigricans	Gastrointestinal (stomach), liver, lung, breast
Acanthosis palmaris	Gastrointestinal (stomach), lung
Amyloidosis	Multiple myeloma
Bazex's syndrome	Squamous cell carcinoma (upper respiratory and gastrointestinal)
Carcinoid syndrome	Carcinoid tumor
Cronkhite-Canada syndrome	Gastrointestinal (colon)
Cryoglobulinemia	Waldenström's macroglobulinemia, myeloma
Cushing's syndrome secondary to ectopic corticotropin	Lung (small cell), carcinoid tumor
Dermatomyositis	Various
Digital clubbing	Intrathoracic neoplasms
Erythema gyratum repens	Lung, breast

(continued)

Table 10.1. Inherited and acquired dermatological conditions associated with internal malignancy (*Continued*)

Dermatological condition	Associated internal malignancy
Hypertrichosis lanuginosa	Gastrointestinal (colon), lung
Icthyosis—acquired	Lymphoma (Hodgkin's), Kaposi's sarcoma
Leser-Trélat sign	Gastrointestinal (stomach), leukemia, lymphoma, breast
Multicentric reticulohistiocytosis	Various
Necrolytic migratory erythema	Glucagonoma
Paraneoplastic pemphigus	Lymphoma, leukemia, thymoma, sarcoma
Sweet's syndrome	Myeloproliferative (leukemia)
Trousseau's syndrome	Pancreas, lung, stomach, colon
Less Common Associations	
Dermatitis herpetiformis	Lymphoma
Erythema annulare centrifugum	Various
Erythema elevatum diutinum	Myeloma
Erythema multiforme	Various
Erythema nodosum	Lymphoma, leukemia
Erythroderma	Lymphoma, leukemia
Porphyria cutanea tarda	Hepatoma
Pruritus	Hodgkin's disease, cutaneous T-cell lymphoma
Pyoderma gangrenosum	Lymphoma, leukemia
Raynaud's phenomenon	Various
Scleroderma-like changes	Lung, various
Scleromyxedema	Myeloma
Urticaria	Lymphoma, leukemia
Xanthomas	Myeloma

Source: Adapted with permission from Poole and Fenske.[14]

factors, and poor nutrition. Various skin diseases become more troublesome as the patient's general condition deteriorates.

Poor Mobility

With advancing illness and incapacity for movement, patients are likely to spend an increasing proportion of their time in a sitting, semirecumbent, or recumbent position. Unrelieved pressure on the skin covering bony prominences (such as ischial tuberosities, sacrum, hips, or heels) will cause changes in lymphatic and blood flow and extracellular fluid distribution. Edema and changes in the turgor of the skin cause it to be more vulnerable to associated stretching and shearing forces, which result in damaged cells of the epidermis, dermis, and adipose tissue, and damage to dermal connective tissue and vessels.[4] These changes result in skin inflammation and ultimately necrosis, which is clinically recognized as pressure sores or decubitus ulcers.

Movement of the patient, either active or passive, should be encouraged from the onset of the illness. As incapacity increases, a regular regimen for turning the patient should be implemented.

Family involvement in terminal care is a feature of the developing world, while in the developed world there is a greater dependence on the night nurse. Factors such as the position of a television may determine the degree of stress and the direction of forces on the skin. Massage may be helpful by providing touch, relaxing the body, and activating the lymphatic system. The increasing interest of the nursing profession in aromatherapy, with its associated massage, is an example of the role of complementary medicine in the field of palliative care.

Poor nutrition

The skin is the largest organ of the body and undergoes constant regeneration as the surface keratinocytes are shed. If minimum requirements for energy and protein intake are not met, the skin's regenerative and repair capacity will be impaired, along with its structural and functional integrity. Additionally, essential fatty acid, vitamin, and mineral deficiencies may be manifest in a variety of dermatoses (Table 10.2). Nutritional supplements may be required when eating is no longer a pleasure or when there is inadequate absorption or excessive use by cancer or exfoliative dermatitis.

Poor hydration

Reduced skin turgor and dry oral mucosa are classic clinical signs of dehydration. Reduced water content of the skin will impair skin function. In particular, dehydration reduces skin resilience and pressure dispersal, which are important in the prevention of pressure sores. Dryness of the oral mucosa is an unpleasant symptom in itself and increases susceptibility to many other oral conditions, such as halitosis, dental caries, periodontal disease, mucosal ulceration, and oral infections. When oral intake is diminished, alternative provision of fluids may be indicated.

Environmental factors and dry skin

Dry skin is extremely common and may be related to chronic illness, malnutrition, poor hygiene, or immunologic deficit.[21] The ill or dying patient is often cared for in an environment that is warm in temperature and low in humidity, which may result in dry, itchy skin. Regimens of skin care such as frequent bathing, reduced clothing, the liberal use of soap, and vigorous toweling often unintentionally

Table 10.2. Skin manifestations and their related nutritional deficiences in palliative care

Dermatitis
  Seborrhea-like: Riboflavin, pyridoxine
  Xerotic: Essential fatty acids
  Scrotal: Riboflavin
  Intertriginous and periorificial: Biotin
  Acral and periorificial pustulobullous: Zinc (acrodermatitis
    enteropathica)
  Intertriginous erosions: Essential fatty acid
  Perirectal sores: Niacin
  Pellagra-like: Niacin (pellagra), pyridoxine

Xerosis: Vitamin A, biotin, calories, protein

Skin hemorrhage: Vitamin C (perifollicular), vitamin K

Poor wound healing: Vitamin C, zinc

Peripheral edema: Protein

Pigmentary changes
  Hypopigmentation: Protein
  Hyperpigmentation: Niacin ("Casal's necklace"), vitamin B_{12}

Hair/follicular changes
  Follicular hyperkeratosis: Vitamin A (phrynoderma), vitamin C
  Alopecia: Energy, biotin, zinc, essential fatty acids, iron
  "Corkscrew hairs": Vitamin C
  Poliosis: Vitamin B_{12}

Oral lesions
  Angular stomatitis: Riboflavin, pyridoxine, niacin, zinc, iron
  Cheilosis: Riboflavin, pyridoxine, niacin, folate
  Glossitis: Vitamin B_{12}, folate, pyridoxine, zinc, riboflavin
  Swollen, friable gums: Vitamin C
  Erosions: Pyridoxine

Source: Adpated from Miller SJ. Nutritional deficiency and the skin. *J Am Acad Dermatol* 1989; 21:1–30, by permission of Mosby-Year Book, Inc.

exacerbate these drying influences. Certain sites, such as the extensor surfaces of the forearms or lower legs, often show the first effects. The dried surface cracks (Fig. 10.2); irritants such as soap easily penetrate and cause dermatitis.

The factors can be easily corrected. Any heating can be reduced to a comfortable temperature of 18–20°C. A humidifying device, even a bowl of water in the room, may be beneficial. Less frequent bathing using a soap substitute, such as a bath oil, aqueous cream, or emulsifying ointment, and patting the skin dry gently with a soft towel, help to preserve the natural barrier effect of the epidermis. Regular application of a moisturizer, after bathing and as often as required, is beneficial. Table 10.3 lists some simple moisturizers in descending order of effectiveness. In general, the effectiveness of a moisturizer is proportional to its greasiness, but this may limit patient acceptability. In the desert-like atmosphere

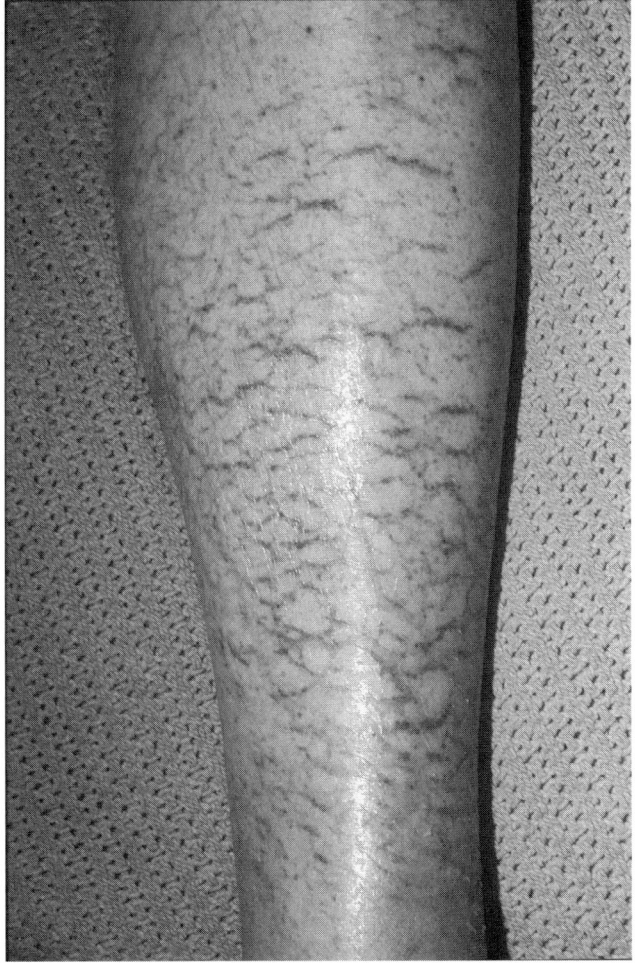

Figure 10.2. Dry, cracked skin. The legs are a common site for this phenomenon.

of some hospitals, the fully dressed patient maintains a microclimate which is less drying than flimsy nightwear.

For very dry skin and associated itch, *wet wrapping* is helpful. It consists of a generous application of a moisturizer (such as 50% liquid paraffin/50% white soft paraffin) covered by a wet cloth or clothing (vest or pajamas or netting) from which excess water has been wrung. This in turn is covered by a dry cloth or clothing to hold it in place. It is not always necessary to remove more than the outer layer to maintain moisture; water may be sprayed onto the under garment and the outer layer reapplied.

Table 10.3. Simple moisturizing applications (in descending order of effectiveness)

50% liquid paraffin/50% white soft paraffin
  greasy but relatively easy to apply to large areas of very dry skin

10%–20% white soft paraffin in aqueous cream
  mildly greasy
  suitable for moderately dry skin

Aqueous cream BP
  least greasy
  suitable for minimally dry skin
  also useful as a soap substitute

Seborrheic dermatitis

Scaling and erythema in a seborrheic distribution, i.e., eyebrows, nasolabial folds, beard and mustache area, scalp, retroauricular, chest, and pubic areas, are usually asymptomatic, but when treatment is required for cosmetic reasons, it is relatively easy to control with standard therapies.[21] This dermatitis is especially found in AIDS and some neurological conditions such as parkinsonism. It responds to low potency topical steroids (e.g., 1% hydrocortisone acetate to the face or 0.025% betamethasone valerate to the trunk). The role of *Pityrosporum* yeast infection has been controversial, but the density of the *P. ovale* has been found to correlate with the clinical severity of seborrheic dermatitis.[22] Topical azoles, in particular ketoconazole, are often effective.[23] Anti-dandruff shampoos containing tar, zinc pyrithione, selenium sulfide, or ketoconazole may be useful for scalp involvement.

Excessive sweating

Excessive sweating may be due to the underlying disease or its complications, or to environmental factors such as excessive temperature and humidity or the use of impermeable mattress covers. It may result in skin irritation, pruritus, maceration, occlusion of sweat ducts (miliaria), and secondary bacterial or fungal infections (e.g., *C. albicans, P. aeruginosa*). Overhydration of the skin increases the shearing stresses between skin and bed clothes, and this may play a part in the development of pressure sores.

Simple measures, such as cooling fans and air conditioning, are useful. Cool, wet compresses may be distressingly uncomfortable if the patient is suffering from fever, and should be used only if tolerated. Clothing should be light and changed frequently. A moisture–absorbent layer under the patient may help to disperse excessive perspiration. Positioning of the patient so as to expose the largest possible surface area will contribute to the effectiveness of evaporative cooling. Overheating is reduced by extending the limbs and frequent movement.

Incontinence

Prolonged exposure of the skin to urine and feces will initially cause an irritant dermatitis. Ultimately, ulceration and secondary infection with bowel flora may occur. Suitable nursing care, possibly with the use of a urine collection device, is important. A barrier-type application such as zinc oxide, silicone, or white soft paraffin, will help to protect the skin.

Pruritus

There are many possible causes or aggravating factors for pruritus (Table 10.4). Management involves the elimination of the cause, if possible. Dryness of the skin is frequently a precipitating or exacerbating factor, and therefore, moisturizers are essential. Wet wrapping techniques in which moisturizers are placed on the skin under a wet dressing, covered by a dry dressing, are often the most effective way of moisturizing the skin. Topical steroid applications reduce the itch associated with skin inflammation. These may be best applied in ointment rather than cream formulations to alleviate dryness. Menthol in aqueous cream, 0.5%–2% applied to the skin as required is a mild antipruritic, acting partially as a counter-irritant or anesthetic. Antihistamines may be helpful in relieving itch which is clearly associated with histamine release, such as urticarial eruptions. H_1 antihistamines, sometimes with H_2 antihistamines, may be used in this situation.[24] H_1 antihistamines and topical corticosteroids should not be used in the absence of visible inflammatory changes in the skin.[25] Tricyclic antidepressants may be useful for intractable itch.[26] Treatments for the relief of itch associated with chronic cholestasis have been reviewed recently.[27]

Oral problems

The principal mouth problems encountered in terminal care are dryness, dirty mouth, coated tongue, infection, halitosis, pain, and alteration in taste.[28] Dry-

Table 10.4. Causes of pruritus

Metabolic: Hepatic impairment, renal impairment, hypothyroidism, hyperthyroidism

Hemotological: Iron deficiency, polycythemia

Malignancy: Leukemia, lymphoma, myeloma, internal malignancy

Drugs: Opioids, aspirin, drug reactions

Dermatological: Dryness (xerosis), wetness, irritation, skin disease (e.g., eczema, psoriasis)

Infestation: Scabies, lice, bed-bugs, insects

Infection: Candida, dermatophyte

Allergy: Urticaria, contact allergic dermatitis

Psychogenic: Parasitophobia, psychogenic itch

ness may be due to drug effects (e.g., tricyclic antidepressants, antihistamines, phenothiazines, antispasmodics, or opioids), dehydration (systemic and local, e.g., as a result of mouth breathing or oxygen therapy), reduced salivary flow (e.g., secondary to malignant involvement, radiotherapy, surgery), widespread erosion of the buccal cavity (e.g., stomatitis or infections) or depression or anxiety.[28,29]

Measures to reduce xerostomia include stimulation of salivary flow (by sucking or chewing ice cubes, sweets, small pieces of fruit or chewing gum); frequent mouth washes (preferably tap water); frequent sips of cold, clear drinks; the use of a saliva substitute; and possibly drug treatments. Medications that may aggravate xerostomia should be avoided or reduced in dosage if possible.

Cleaning of the oral cavity may be ideally effected with a toothbrush with a soft, small head.[30] Other available tools include a foam stick, gauze swabs, and cotton buds. When the patient is unable to use a toothbrush, or has a bleeding tendency, a foam stick may be the treatment of choice, although this may not be as effective in plaque reduction.[31,32] Oral care may be required every two hours or more often. Although tap water and toothpaste are the simplest agents, a heavily coated tongue may require the use of Vitamin C (one-quarter of a 1 g effervescent tablet dissolved on the tongue four times a day) or small pieces of fresh pineapple (containing the enzyme ananase); other treatments include sodium bicarbonate, hydrogen peroxide, and sodium perborate, but each may have unpleasant or undesirable effects.[28] The osmotic properties of food and medicines should be taken into account. Some medicines are less irritating when diluted. Foods that leave multiple small particles in the mouth may collect in oral crevices; soft diets should be prepared with this in mind.

Infection with *Candida albicans* is a common problem in the terminally ill. Treatment with nystatin suspension 100,000 units/ml, 1 ml 4 times a day (up to every 4 hr) is indicated if Candidal infection is present or suspected. Dentures should be removed and cleaned with nystatin.[28] Ice cubes of nystatin diluted with water can be used to increase the contact time with oral mucosa.[29] Other topical alternatives include miconazole gel and amphoteracin lozenges. When systemic treatment is required, the newer triazole derivatives, fluconazole and itraconazole, may be preferable to ketoconazole because they have a lower incidence of side effects.

Wound care

Malignant ulceration and fungating tumors require careful assessment of possible palliative measures, such as surgical debulking, radiotherapy, chemotherapy, or hormonal therapy. These may improve the quality of life for the terminally ill patient. Exudate, malodor, infection, and bleeding may require specific attention in the planning of rational wound care.[20,33,34] An algorithm for wound care of fungating and malignant ulcers is reproduced in Figure 10.3.

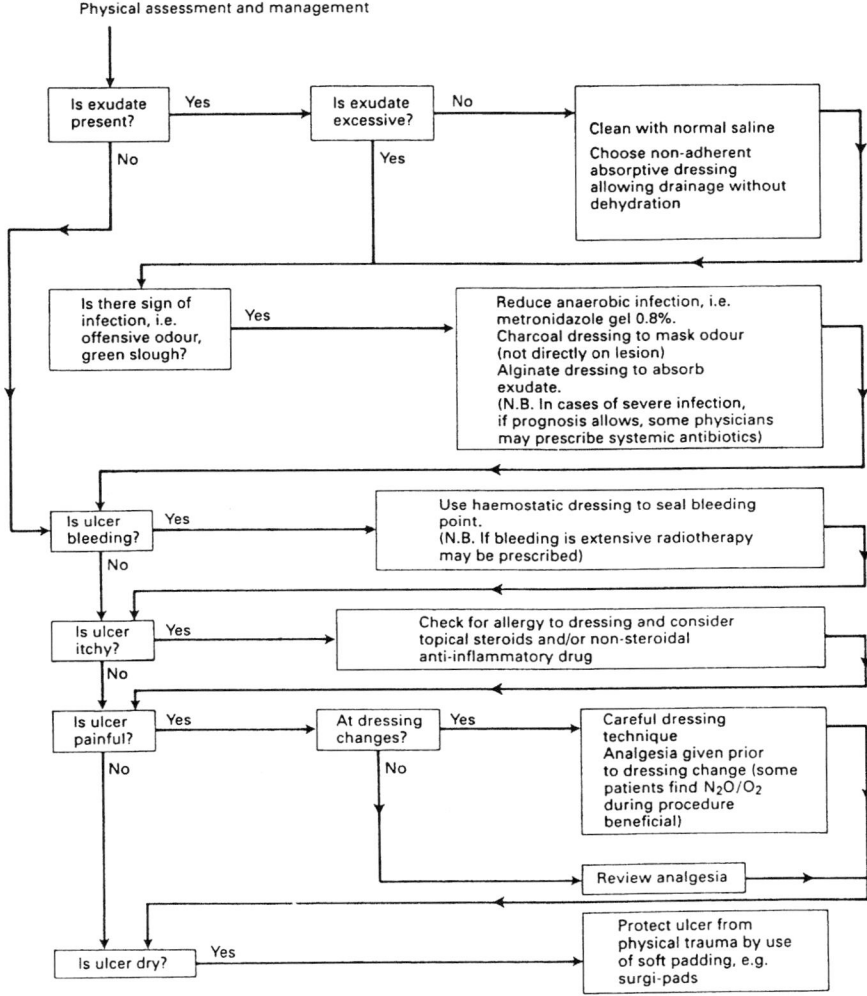

Figure 10.3. An algorithm for managing fungating and malignant ulcers. (Reproduced with permission from Miller CM, O'Neill A, Mortimer PS.[20])

Malodor

Malodor may result from incontinence, fungating wounds, poor hygiene, bacterial contamination of the skin, or certain skin diseases that have a characteristic odor. Removing debris and necrotic tissue, counteracting bacteria, and occluding the odorous area are some of the ways in which this can be managed. Some dressings, e.g., hydrocolloid, are made of gelatin and can themselves be malodorous.

Larval therapy has recently been re-introduced as an adjunct to modern wound therapy. It is a low-cost, easily established treatment useful in the debridement of open wounds and ulcers and in the control of infection, including that of antibiotic-resistant organisms. It is also an effective way of managing odor.[35-38]

Perfumes and airing of the room, or placing the patient in the most easily ventilated space, can be helpful. Meeting visitors in the open space of a garden may be a possibility.

Acquired immunodeficiency syndrome

AIDS is commonly associated with dermatological conditions, and the reader is referred to reviews of the cutaneous,[23,39-41] oral,[42-44] and pediatric cutaneous[45] manifestations of HIV infection. A comprehensive list of the dermatological manifestations of HIV infection is reproduced in Table 10.5.

Smith et al. observed the frequency of cutaneous disease in 912 HIV-1-positive patients in all stages of disease progression over a period of 42 months.[46] Dry skin and seborrheic dermatitis were common and tended to increase in severity with disease progression. Tinea infections, verrucae, and condyloma acuminata became more diffuse and resistant to treatment, while herpes simplex infections, oral candidiasis, molluscum contagiosum, S. aureus infections, and oral hairy leukoplakia showed a marked increase in occurrence with advanced disease.

Assessment of the skin is an important part of the management of the HIV-infected patient. When the CD4 lymphocyte count falls below 200, the clinical picture may be complex. Skin biopsy is often necessary for histology and microbiological culture (for bacteria, mycobacteria, fungi, yeasts, and viruses).[23]

Conclusion

The provision of palliative care involving the skin places special demand on the skills of the nursing profession. In elite units, more is known than ever before about the mechanisms underlying disease; health service organization, however, is usually unable to meet demand outside of these elite units. In the field of dermatology, there are increasing attempts to improve skills by enhancing the knowledge and availability of the dermatological nurse. Armed with training required to give comfort to a patient who has a skin problem, nurses are often better than doctors at relieving soreness, and they are best at providing detailed instructions about skin care. Such nurses trained in specialist skin units should be available to visit the home or hospice of a patient and share their expertise with caretakers at all levels. Patients should be protected from "rejection episodes." Ideally, those who have odor or shed skin or exudate should not be exposed to an open general ward where other patients, visitors, or cleaners might complain. A balance between privacy and display needs sensitive handling. Boosting confidence in appearance and encouraging contact with others is not the same as

Table 10.5. Cutaneous manifestations associated with HIV infection

Neoplastic
  Kaposi's sarcoma
  Lymphoma (usually B-cell)
  Squamous cell carcinoma
  Basal cell carcinoma
  Melanoma

Viral infections
  Herpes simplex
  Herpes zoster
  Chickenpox
  Molluscum contagiosum
  Oral hairy leukoplakia
  Common warts
  Condyloma acuminatum
  Epstein-Barr virus exanthem

Bacterial infections
  Abscesses
  Folliculitis
  Impetigo
  Ecthyma
  Cellulitis
  Ulcers (*Pseudomonas* and polymicrobial)
  Mycobacterial
  Actinomycosis
  Atypical syphilis
  Scalded skin syndrome

Fungal and yeast infections
  Candidiasis
  Dermatophytosis
  Tinea versicolor
  Alternariosis
  Cryptococcosis
  Histoplasmosis
  Sporotrichosis
  Scopulariopsis

Mixed Infections
  Viral, bacterial, and fungal

Protozoal infections
  Amebiasis cutis

Arthropod infection
  Scabies
  Crusted scabies

Vascular lesions
  Vasculitis
  Telangiectasia
  Splinter hemorrhages
  Thrombocytopenic purpura
  Hyperalgesic pseudothrombophlebitis
    syndrome
  Cutis marmorata

Papulosquamous
  Seborrheic dermatitis
  Psoriasis
  Pityriasis rosea

Oral
  Angular stomatitis
  Aphthosis
  Gingivitis (simple and necrotizing)

Hair and nails
  Thinning of hair
  Premature graying
  Alopecia areata
  Telogen effluvium
  Nail deformities
  Nail color changes

Exaggeration of
  Infections (e.g., syphilis)
  Infestations (e.g., scabies)
  Dermatoses (e.g., psoriasis)

Miscellaneous
  Exanthemas and erythroderma
  Xerosis and ichthyosis
  Atopic dermatitis
  Nurtritional deficiencies
  Eosinophilic pustular folliculitis
  Papular and lichenoid eruptions (some with
    atypical infiltrate)
  Pseudolymphoma cutis
  Granuloma annulare
  Drug eruptions
  Pruritus
  Pyoderma gangrenosum
  Focal acantholytic dyskeratosis (Grover's)
  Bullous pemphigoid
  Erythema elevatum diutinum
  Urticaria
  Premature aging

Source: Reproduced from Fisher BK, Warner LC[39], by permission of Blackwell Science Ltd.

exposing the shy. An understanding of the views of different cultures is especially required. The management of diseased skin requires that affected areas be exposed transiently to the caretaker. There is no need for prolonged exposure and the caretaker need be no other than the well-trained patient or the nurse. Nevertheless, for complete and effective care, a careful examination of the whole skin surface is necessary. Cultural sensitivity should not lead the examiner to neglect sanctuary sites, possibly overlooking development of skin disease.

In conclusion, an understanding of the principles of management for patients suffering from disorders of the skin in palliative care is helpful. While disability cannot be remedied, handicap often can be so. It should always be remembered that the skin is an organ of communication. Sensitive management of privacy and display, an understanding of the "look good, feel good" factor, and remedying isolation through touch are important. In the past, except in the management of pressure sores, the role of mobility has been under-emphasized. The skin normally is on the move and this is an important part of its long-term function. Patients should be helped to maintain mobility, and alternative therapies, which include massage, may be helpful.

References

1. Ryan TJ. Disability in dermatology. *Br J Hosp Med* 1991; 46:33–36.
2. Ryan TJ. Healthy skin for all. *Int J Dermatol* 1994; 33:829–835.
3. Finlay AY, Ryan TJ. Disability and handicap in dermatology. *Int J Dermatol* 1996; 35:305–311.
4. Ryan TJ. Exchange and the mechanical properties of the skin: Oncotic and hydrostatic forces control by blood supply and lymphatic drainage. *Wound Rep Reg* 1995; 3:258–264.
5. Lookingbill DP, Spangler N, Sexton FM. Skin involvement as the presenting sign of internal carcinoma. *J Am Acad Dermatol* 1990; 22:19–26.
6. Browstein MH, Helwig EB. Patterns of cutaneous metastasis. *Arch Dermatol* 1972; 105:862–868.
7. Mortimer PS. Skin problems in palliative care: medical aspects. In Doyle D, Hanks G, MacDonald N, eds. *Oxford Textbook of Palliative Medicine*. Oxford: Oxford University Press, 1993:384–395.
8. Rosen T. Cutaneous metastases. *Med Clin North Am* 1980; 64:885–900.
9. McLean DI, Haynes HA. Cutaneous manifestations of internal malignant disease. In: Fitzpatrick TB, Eisen AZ, Wolff K, et al., eds. *Dermatology in General Medicine* 4th ed. New York: McGraw Hill, 1993:2229–2249.
10. Browstein MH, Helwig EB. Spread of tumours to the skin. *Arch Dermatol* 1973; 107:80–86.
11. Kirchmann TT, Smoller BR, McGuire J. Cutaneous angiosarcoma as a second malignancy in a lymphedematous leg in a Hodgkin's disease survivor. *J Am Acad Dermatol* 1994; 31:861–866.
12. Ryan TJ. The African albino. *Radiological Protection Bulletin* 1996; 183:34–37.

13. Poole S, Fenske NA. Cutaneous markers of internal malignancy. I. Malignant involvement of the skin and the genodermatoses. *J Am Acad Dermatol* 1993; 28:1–13.
14. Poole S, Fenske NA. Cutaneous markers of internal malignancy. II. Paraneoplastic dermatoses and environmental carcinogens. *J Am Acad Dermatol* 1993; 28:147–164.
15. Loucas E, Russo G, Millikan LE. Genetic and acquired cutaneous disorders associated with internal malignancy. *Int J Dermatol* 1995; 34:749–758.
16. Higgins EM, du Vivier AWP. Cutaneous manifestations of malignant disease. *Br J Hosp Med* 1992; 48:552–561.
17. Hodgsons ES. Occupational and environmental health and safety: gastrointestinal tract. In: Weatherall DJ, Ledingham JGG, Warrell DA, eds. *Oxford Textbook of Medicine*, 3rd ed. Oxford: Oxford University Press, 1996:1171–1172.
18. Weismann K, Graham RM. Systemic disease and the skin. In: Champion RH, Burton JL, Ebling FJG, eds. *Textbook of Dermatology*, 5th ed. Oxford: Blackwell Scientific Publications, 1992:2407–2453.
19. Chren M-M, Lazarus HM, Salata RA, et al. Cultures of skin biopsy tissue from immunocompromised patients with cancer and rashes. *Arch Dermatol* 1995; 131:552–555.
20. Miller CM, O'Neill A, Mortimer PS. Skin problems in palliative care: nursing aspects. In: Doyle D, Hanks G, MacDonald N, eds. *Oxford Textbook of Palliative Medicine*. Oxford: Oxford University Press, 1993:395–406.
21. Johnson RA, Dover JS. Cutaneous manifestations of human immunodeficiency virus disease. In: Fitzpatrick TB, Eisen AZ, Wolff K, et al., eds. *Dermatology in General Medicine*, 4th ed. New York: McGraw Hill, 1993:2637–2689.
22. Heng MCY, Henderson CL, Barker DC, et al. Correlation of Pityrosporum ovale density with clinical severity of seborrheic dermatitis as assessed by a simplified technique. *J Am Acad Dermatol* 1990; 23:82–86.
23. Wong D, Shumack S. HIV and skin disease. *Med J Aust* 1996; 164:352–356.
24. Champion RH. Urticaria. In: Champion RH, Burton JL, Ebling FJG, eds. *Textbook of Dermatology*. Oxford: Blackwell Scientific Publications, 1992:1865–1880.
25. Greaves MW. Pruritus. In: Champion RH, Burton JL, Ebling FJG, eds. *Textbook of Dermatology*. Oxford: Blackwell Scientific Publications, 1992:527–535.
26. Newbold PCH. Antidepressants and skin disease. *BMJ* 1988; 296:379.
27. Raiford DS. Pruritus of chronic cholestasis. *QJM* 1995; 88:603–607.
28. Lethem W. Mouth and skin problems. In Saunders C, Sykes N, et al. *The Management of Terminal Malignant Disease*, 3rd ed. London: Edward Arnold, 1993:139–148.
29. Ventafridda V, Ripamonti C, Sbanotto A, De Conno F. Mouth Care. In Doyle D, Hanks G, MacDonald N, eds. *Oxford Textbook of Palliative Medicine*. Oxford: Oxford University Press, 1993:434–447.
30. Barnett J. A reassessment of oral health care. *Prof Nurse* 1991; 6:703–708.
31. Porter H. Mouth care in cancer. *Nurs Times* 1994; 90:27–29.
32. Holmes S. The oral complications of specific anticancer therapy. *Int J Nurs Stud* 1991; 28:343–360.
33. Hallett A. Fungating wounds. *Nurs Times* 1995; 91:81–85.
34. Clark L. Care for fungating tumours. *Nurs Times* 1992; 88:66–70.
35. Church JCT. ETRS working party consensus paper on wound debridement. *Surgery* 1995; 13:228.

36. Sherman RA, Wyle F, Vulpe M, et al. The utility of maggot therapy for treating chronic wounds. *Am J Trop Med Hyg* 1993; 49(Suppl 3):266
37. Sherman RA, Wyle F, Vulpe M. Maggot therapy for treating pressure ulcers in spinal cord injury patients. *J Spinal Cord Med* 1995; 18:71–74.
38. Thomas S. Using larvae in modern wound management. *J Wound Care* 1996; 5:60–69.
39. Fisher BK, Warner LC. Cutaneous manifestations of the acquired immunodeficiency syndrome. *Int J Dermatol* 1987; 26:615–630.
40. Dover JS, Johnson RA. Cutaneous manifestations of human immunodeficiency virus infection. Parts I and II. *Arch Dermatol* 1991; 127:1383–1391 & 1549–1558.
41. Zalla MJ, Su WPD, Fransway AF. Dermatologic manifestations of human immunodeficiency virus infection. *Mayo Clin Proc* 1992; 67:1089–1108.
42. Itin PH, Lautenshlager S, Fluckiger R, Rufli T. Oral manifestations in HIV-infected patients: Diagnosis and management. *J Am Acad Dermatol* 1993; 29:749–760.
43. Scully C, McCarthy G. Management of oral health in persons with HIV infection. *Oral Surg Oral Med Oral Pathol* 1992; 732:215–225.
44. Foltyn P, Marriott D. HIV and oral disease. *Med J Aust* 1996; 164:357–359.
45. Prose NS. Mucocutaneous disease in pediatric human immunodeficiency virus infection. *Pediatric Clin North Am* 1991; 38:977–990.
46. Smith KJ, Skelton HG, Yeager J, et al. Cutaneous findings in HIV-1 positive patients: A 42 month prospective study. *J Am Acad Dermatol* 1994; 31:746–754.

11

The Pathophysiology and Management of Pressure Ulcers

PAUL WALKER

Pressure ulcer, pressure sore, decubitus ulcer, and *bed sore* are the terms used to describe a universally recognized and age-old problem of humankind.

Many similar definitions for these lesions can be found in the literature. The Agency for Health Care Policy and Research states: "A pressure ulcer is any lesion caused by unrelieved pressure resulting in damage of underlying tissue."[1] Implicit in this statement is the compression of tissue between a bony prominence and an external surface, resulting in necrosis. Localized pressure is a key factor, reflected in the preferred term of *pressure ulcer*. The older term, decubitus ulcer, is less desirable in that it implies that a lying position is required to sustain an injury of this type. In fact, some of the worse pressure ulcers occur in spinal cord injury patients because of prolonged sitting in a wheelchair.[2]

History

Written records of pressure ulcers can be found dating back to Biblical times.[3] Egyptian mummies at necropsy have demonstrated these lesions.[4] In the late 19th and early 20th centuries, pressure ulcers occurred mainly in young persons with chronic wasting diseases such as tuberculosis, osteomyelitis, and chronic renal disease.[5] Today, pressure ulcers are seen in elderly, debilitated, or spinal cord injury patients.[5,6] Advanced cancer patients may be in one or more of these groups and are therefore at high risk for developing these lesions.

Incidence and Prevalence

It is estimated that 1.5 to 3 million patients in the United States have pressure ulcers.[7] In acute care facilities the incidence ranges from 2.7%[8] to 29.5%,[9] and prevalence varies between 3.5%[10] and 29.5%.[11] In long-term care facilities, prevalence rates range from 2.4%[12] to 23%.[13,14] Incidence studies in nursing home residents have indicated that the longer the patient stays, the greater the likelihood of ulcer development.[7] One study indicated that 13.2% of nursing home residents had an ulcer within one year and 21.6% had an ulcer at two years.[15] It is estimated that 100,000 nursing home residents in the United States have a pressure ulcer.[15]

Age is a risk factor for pressure ulcers; 50% to 70% of these lesions develop in patients older than 70 years.[16] For elderly patients with femoral fractures, the incidence is 66%;[17] there is a high perioperative mortality rate of 27% in these patients.[18] Other populations at high risk include hospitalized quadriplegic patients, who exhibit a 60% prevalence,[19] and intensive care patients, who have an incidence of 33%[20] and a prevalence of 41%.[21]

Between 1975 and 1984, 19% of 7000 patients at St. Christopher's Hospice were found to have pressure ulcers during the terminal phases of their illnesses, despite preventive measures.[22] Kaasa et al. studied 87 consecutive admissions to our palliative care unit and found an incidence of 33%.[23] This was reduced to 7% following the implementation of an interdisciplinary wound management committee.

Costs

Estimates of the economic burden of treatment for pressure ulcers vary greatly: One estimate exceeds $1.3 billion annually in the United States,[24] and others place this in excess of $5 billion.[25–27] The increased duration of hospitalization required to treat these lesions is an important cost factor.[28] In addition, the psychological burden to the patient and family of dealing with this problem can be extremely high.

Nurses have played a vital role in the research and management of pressure ulcers. Other disciplines that have become involved include family medicine, plastic surgery, rehabilitation medicine, dermatology, critical care, physiotherapy, occupational therapy, nutrition science, geriatrics, and palliative care.

Etiology and Pathophysiology

Central to the development of pressure ulcers is the loss of a protective mechanism. This has been explained by Chicarilli.[3] "The key factors that provide for avoidance of pressure ulcerations include the sensory input of discomfort followed by voluntary motor execution to alter one's position and alleviate the noxious stimulus. These actions are such an integral part of our daily living that we accept them as second nature. We continually alter compressive weight bearing forces by shifting our weight while standing or sitting and adjusting our position when lying down, mitigating their injurious nature. It is only when these conscious and subconscious safeguards become impaired that the destructive consequences of unmitigated pressure become evident." Many conditions can affect this protective mechanism by limiting spontaneous movement (Table 11.1).

Intrinsic and extrinsic factors

The classic factors *intrinsic* to the patient, which increase the risk for developing pressure ulcers,[16] include those listed in Table 11.1, as well as conditions that reduce tissue oxygenation (Table 11.2).

Increasing age causes changes in the skin such as decreased numbers of elastic fibers, fewer dermal blood vessels, and reduced epidermal proliferation.[7,29] Thinner, less resilient skin, which has a decreased rate of healing, occurs as a result of aging. Malnutrition is also an important intrinsic factor.[26,30,31]

The *extrinsic* physical factors of friction, maceration, and shear add to the risk of injury.[7,16] Friction occurs when the patient's skin is dragged across the bed sheets. Shearing forces occur most commonly when the head of the bed is elevated, causing the patient to slide downward while the tissue remains in a relatively fixed position.[6] This causes deformation of the vasculature of the skin, impeding perfusion. Maceration is largely due to urinary and fecal incontinence, but profuse sweating can also contribute to this problem. Chemical irritants in

Table 11.1. Conditions affecting spontaneous movement

Pain
Paralysis or weakness secondary to:
Spinal cord compression
Brain metastasis
Cerebrovascular accident
Spinal cord trauma
Other neurological injuries
Sedation from medications (opioids, benzodiazepines, etc.)
Massive ascites or edema
Joint contractures
Fractures
Dementia, delirium, or severe depression
Coma

Source: Adapted from Miller CM, O'Neill A, Mortimer PS.[104]

Table 11.2. Conditions reducing tissue oxygenation

Dehydration

Surgical interventions

Radiation fibrosis

Fever

Peripheral vascular disease

Diabetes

Massive ascites or edema

Anemia

Heart failure

Respiratory disease

Smoking

Source: Adapted from Miller CM, O'Neill A, Mortimer PS.[104]

urine and feces have been implicated in direct injury to epithelial cells. Bacterial ureases in feces have been reported to degrade to ammonia and cause an increased pH of the skin, which results in increased permeability; further investigation of this mechanism is required to confirm its importance.[16,32] Of all the extrinsic risk factors, pressure remains the critical factor in development of a pressure ulcer.[1,3,5,33]

The tissue damage that occurs in the formation of pressure ulcers is due to ischemia. Normal tissue has tolerance for ischemia of short duration. When this is exceeded, normal capillary filling pressure has been surpassed. A cascade of adverse events occurs, beginning with capillary collapse and cessation of perfusion.[3,5,6,28] Hypoxia ensues with acidosis, vessel leakage, hemorrhage, and accumulation of toxic cellular wastes.[33] The final result is tissue necrosis, which can then become a locus for infection. Necrosis begins closest to bone, where pressure is the highest and resulting tissue deformation the most severe. The result is a cone of tissue destruction that is greatest adjacent to the bone and extends outward to a smaller area superficially.[3,5] It is often not appreciated that tissue damage occurs deep in muscle and subcutaneous tissue before extending to the skin. What is seen at physical examination is the "tip of the iceberg,"[3] as a larger area of injury lies deep under the skin. This explains the undermining that occurs in advanced pressure ulcers.

Pressure ulcers occur predominant in the pelvic region because of the bony prominence of the sacrum (23% of ulcers), ischium (24% of ulcers), and greater trochanters (15% of ulcers).[3] Other common areas of ulceration include the heels, malleoli, knees, elbows, spinous processes, scapula, fibular head, ears (secondary to immobility of the head or the pressure of oxygen tubing), and nares (secondary to nasal cannulae).

The diagnosis of a pressure ulcer is usually straightforward. The lesion is usually over a dependent bony prominence, under sustained pressure, in a patient who has incurred some loss of the protective mechanism of spontaneous movement. Differential diagnoses worth considering include stasis or ischemic ulcers, vasculitides, neoplastic ulcers, radiation injury, and pyoderma gangrenosum.[33]

Staging

Pressure ulcers are clinically staged from I to IV, according to the degree of tissue destruction. This clinical tool, which is used to direct management, is based on the level of tissue destruction from the "outside looking in," (i.e., the level of tissue destruction evident to observation). It is important to remember that tissue necrosis occurs from the "inside out." As a result, the staging of pressure ulcers has the potential to confuse caregivers about the mechanism or extent of injury, and this may lead to under-management.

Two points are worth remembering in dealing with this staging system. First, it is not possible to stage a pressure ulcer until the eschar has been removed.[1] Second, diagnosis of Stage I pressure ulcers may be difficult in darkly pigmented skin.[1] With these caveats, the staging is as follows:

Stage I: Non-blanchable erythema of intact skin, the heralding lesion of skin ulceration.

Stage II: Partial thickness skin loss involving epidermis, dermis, or both. The ulcer is superficial and presents as an abrasion, shallow crater, or blister.

Stage III: Full thickness skin loss involving damage to or necrosis of subcutaneous tissue that may extend down to, but not through, underlying fascia. The ulcer presents clinically as a deep crater with or without undermining of adjacent tissue.

Stage IV: Full thickness skin loss with extensive destruction, tissue necrosis, or damage to muscle, bone, or supporting structures (e.g., tendon, joint capsule). Undermining and sinus tracts also may be associated with Stage IV pressure ulcers.

Ulcer staging should be part of a comprehensive assessment of the entire person, which includes a complete history and physical examination and a full delineation of the clinical problems. An assessment of the patient's nutritional status is essential. The psychosocial dynamics that may be relevant include the patient's comprehension of the problem, his or her motivation and plans, and the goals and needs expressed.[1]

Prevention

Avoidance of pressure ulcer formation represents the best level of care achievable for those at risk for such lesions. To help recognize vulnerable patients who may require preventive interventions, bed- or chair-bound individuals may be given a *risk assessment tool*, such as the Norton[34] or Braden scales.[20,35] The Braden Scale assesses six domains: sensory perception, moisture, activity, mobility, nutrition, and friction/shear. The total score indicates the level of risk. Our experience with advanced cancer patients has been that, almost without exception, they score as being at high risk. Palliative care units may therefore find limited application for this structured assessment, whereas earlier in the course of cancer treatment, such as in the oncology center, this type of assessment may be helpful.

Attention to *skin care* is necessary in those patients deemed to be at risk for tissue breakdown. Avoidance of undue trauma, harsh chemicals, or excessive drying is recommended when cleaning the skin.[1] Avoiding maceration of the skin is also important. To encourage this, incontinent patients should wear garments that absorb moisture. The use of ointments or protective dressings that act as moisture barriers is helpful. Massage over bony prominences should be avoided.[36] There is no evidence that massage stimulates blood flow and there is preliminary evidence to suggest that deep tissue trauma may result.[37,38] Friction forces on the skin can be avoided by using a lift sheet or trapeze to move patients. This avoids dragging the dependent area of skin across the bed linen.

Patients at high risk should be considered for a *pressure reducing support surface* (Table 11.3). Attention to positioning is important and it is recommended that the patient not be placed in the lateral decubitus position with the trochanters bearing weight.[1,36,39,40] Because elevating the head of the bed can result in increased friction or shear forces, it should be kept at the lowest degree of elevation consistent with care, and be elevated for short periods only.[1,41] The use of a donut or ring-type device is contraindicated as these impair circulation, causing venous congestion and edema, and are likely to cause new pressure points and contribute to pressure ulceration.[1,42] Alteration of weight-bearing surfaces (repositioning or turning) is a time-honored nursing tradition. This simulation of normal spontaneous movement allows different skin surfaces to carry the brunt

Table 11.3 Support surfaces recommended for pressure reduction

DYNAMIC

Air–fluidized bed: A high rate of air flow is used to fluidize fine particulate material (such as sand) to produce a support medium that has characteristics similar to a liquid (e.g., Clinatron, Fluid–Air).

Low–air–loss bed: A series of interconnected woven fabric air pillows that allow some air to escape through the support surface. The pillows can be variably inflated to adjust the level of pressure relief (e.g., Flexicair, KinAir).

Alternating–air mattress: A mattress or overlay with interconnecting air cells that cyclically inflate and deflate to produce alternating high and low pressure intervals. Cells with larger depth and diameter produce greater pressure relief over the body (e.g., Dyna–Care, Sof–Care).

STATIC

Static air or water mattress: A vinyl mattress or overlay composed of interconnected compartments filled with air or water to distribute pressure uniformly over the support surface to create a flotation effect (e.g., Roho).

Foam mattress overlay: Thick foam slab with a textured surface designed to be placed on top of the standard hospital mattress to reduce pressure by enveloping the body. Its effectiveness is influenced by its thickness, density, and stiffness (e.g., Geo–Matt, Clinizert, Ultra–Foam).

Source: Adapted from Bergstrom et al.[1]

of the body's pressure, as would occur in the healthy individual. It is recommended that the patient be turned at least every two hours if feasible.[1,36] Often, in the terminally ill patient, pain and other symptom control issues may preclude a vigorous turning schedule.

Treatment

When a pressure ulcer is discovered, the areas of concern outlined for prevention require increased attention. Ulcer management, concerns regarding bacterial infection, the option of surgical repair, and nutritional support must also be addressed. To facilitate healing, complete relief of pressure from the injured area is advised.[1,7,16] This requires great attention to positioning techniques. Several pillows and foam wedges may be useful in making frequent small adjustments to the patient's position.[1] Although the position causing the pressure ulcer should be avoided completely if possible, this is often impossible in the symptomatic cancer patient (Fig. 11.1). Specialized mattresses and beds have been developed to lessen the pressure exerted over the bony prominences. This is done primarily by increasing the surface area of weight dispersion. Added benefits of these support surfaces include low moisture retention, decreased heat accumulation, and shear force reduction. These devices come in two major categories, static or dynamic (Table 11.3).

Ulcer care

Ulcer care comprises debridement, wound cleansing, dressings, and adjuvant therapies. *Debridement* of necrotic tissue is vital to reduce the risk of infection and improve wound healing. This may be achieved by one of four methods:[1]

1. *Sharp* or *surgical debridement* is the most rapid treatment and is recommended, especially for infection, large necrotic areas, or thick eschar.
2. *Mechanical debridement* includes hydrotherapy, wound irrigation, dextranomers and the archaic technique of wet–to–dry dressing changes. A simple method of providing the correct pressure for ulcer irrigation is to inject fluid from a 35 ml syringe through a 19 gauge needle or angiocatheter. The pressure produced by this combination is effective for removing necrotic tissue, but does not increase the risk of infection by driving bacteria into the wound.
3. *Enzymatic debridement* with collagenase or other enzymes may be indicated if sharp debridement is not tolerated and the ulcer is not infected; this is a slower form of debridement.
4. *Autolytic debridement* allows digestion of the necrotic tissues through enzymes normally present in wound fluid. This is an especially slow process and is not indicated for infected ulcers.

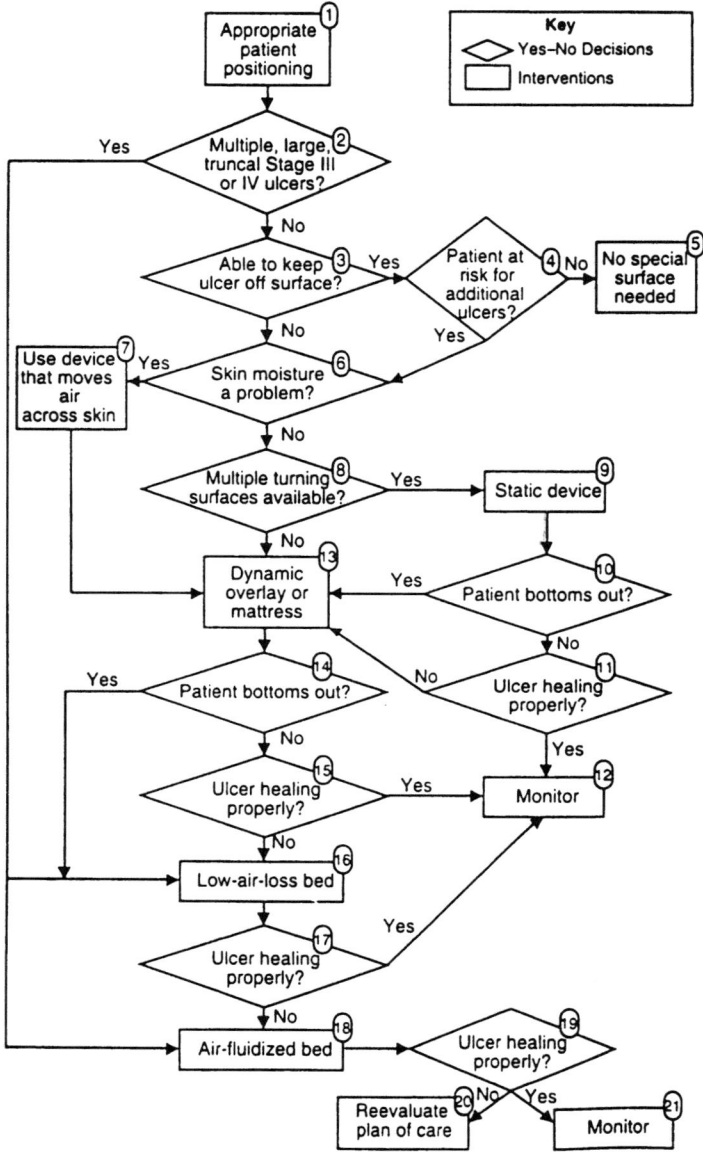

"Bottoming out" refers to an inadequate mattress overlay determined by placing the hand (palm up) under the mattress and detecting a <1 inch thickness under the involved area.

Figure 11.1. Mangement of tissue loads. (Reproduced with permission from Bergstrom et al.[1])

Once the wound has been cleaned of necrotic tissue, *irrigation of the ulcer* is recommended at each dressing change, using a 35 ml syringe and a 19 gauge angiocatheter. Saline is advised for this irrigation, as other skin cleansers and antiseptic agents have been found to exhibit various degrees of cytotoxicity to fibroblasts and leukocytes.[43-49]

The goal of *wound dressings* is to keep the ulcer tissue moist and the surrounding skin dry and intact.[50-54] A moist wound environment promotes migration of fibroblasts and epithelial cells. In addition, the presence of growth factors in the serous exudate may speed healing. In five controlled trials comparing various types of moist wound dressings, no differences were noted in pressure ulcer healing.[55-59] The clinician may therefore choose the most appropriate moist wound dressing for the situation. Moist saline gauze dressings are inexpensive but require frequent changes and therefore more nursing care. More expensive alternatives that require less frequent dressing changes include hydrocolloids, foams, hydrogels, and alginates. Semi-permeable film dressings may be suitable for Stage I ulcers.[7]

Hydrocolloid dressings are self-adhesive and promote autolysis, angiogenesis, and granulation. They may remain in place for 5–7 days, but one study revealed an average duration of 3½ days.[60] Both film and hydrocolloid dressings are difficult to use over ulcers near the anus, and many investigators report that they fail to remain intact.[61-64] Dobrzanski et al. reported that the edges of hydrocolloid dressings placed at the sacral area often roll because of position changes of the patient.[62] Taping the edges of the dressing may help prevent this.[1] Hydrocolloid dressings may not adhere to highly exudative wounds, and in these cases, dressings with a greater ability to absorb wound exudate, such as foams, hydrogels, or alginates, may be more appropriate. It is important that wound exudate not macerate the surrounding skin, thereby creating further susceptibility to injury. Alternatively, caution must be taken with highly absorbent alginate dressings so that wound desiccation does not occur.

A panel of the Agency for Health Care Policy and Research (AHCPR) reviewed the multitude of *adjunctive therapies*.[1] Recommendation for the use of electrotherapy for Stage III and IV pressure ulcers that have not responded to conventional therapy, and recalcitrant Stage II ulcers, was given based on enhanced healing rates documented in clinical trials.[65-69] Adverse reactions to this therapy were mild, with 15% of patients in one study reporting tingling sensations. Presently this treatment appears to be limited to a small number of research centers. Treatment with infrared, ultraviolet, and low-energy laser were not supported by the AHCPR because of the lack of controlled clinical trials and adequate data relating to pressure ulcers. Current studies with new cytokine growth factors, such as recombinant platelet-derived growth factor-BB[70,71] and basic fibroblast growth factor[72] show encouraging results, but with only limited data on the treatment of pressure ulcers, the AHCPR did not recommend their use, pending further study.

Bacterial colonization and infection

High levels of bacterial colonization have been linked to failure of pressure ulcers to heal.[73–76] Lesions in the pelvic region are at particular risk, as fecal incontinence has been linked to slower ulcer healing, and fecal exposure to the ulcer area has resulted in increased levels of bacterial colonization.[77] Even without fecal contamination, all pressure ulcers are colonized by bacteria. If infection is suspected, then swabbing the area for culture will not be helpful, as all ulcers, both colonized and infected, will grow organisms. To obtain a meaningful culture, the Centers for Disease Control and Prevention (CDC) in the United States recommend a simple injection of sterile fluid subcutaneously at the margin of the ulcer, followed by aspiration.[78] This procedure is less traumatic than the alternative of tissue biopsy.

An algorithm for managing infection related to pressure ulcers helps to provide a rational approach (Fig. 11.2). Local ulcer infections are commonly caused by polymicrobial infections, with gram negative, gram positive, and anaerobic organisms. Two studies support the use of topical antibiotics[73,79] and, therefore, topical broad spectrum agents such as silver sulfadiazine are appropriate. When evidence of spreading infection is present (advancing cellulitis, bacteremia, sepsis, or osteomyelitis) systemic antibiotics are recommended. Staph aureus, gram negative bacilli, and *Bacteroides fragilis* are the organisms commonly found in bacteremia and sepsis associated with pressure ulcers. Empiric systemic antiobiotic coverage is required until blood culture results are available.[80–83] Mortality in this situation is high, approaching 50% or more.[80,82] Osteomyelitis is difficult to diagnose, and is associated with 26% of non-healing pressure ulcers.[84]

Surgical repair

Surgical repair for non-infected Stage III and IV pressure ulcers that do not respond to optimal treatment may be considered.[1] Musculocutaneous flaps are usually the best treatment for paraplegic patients. Alternative procedures include skin grafting and skin flaps. Musculocutaneous flaps can aid in the treatment of osteomyelitis by improving blood flow and providing a barrier to infection.[85–87] A surgical procedure of this type can require anesthesia for 1–3 hr and result in blood loss of up to 1500 mL.[1] Therefore, patients must be carefully selected. They must be medically stable, have good nutritional status, express appropriate goals and preferences, and have a reasonable expectation of a good rehabilitative outcome and a lowered risk of pressure ulcer recurrence.

Advanced cancer patients frequently are debilitated and nutritionally compromised secondary to their disease. Our team has found it exceedingly rare that surgery of this type is desirable in this setting. Earlier in the management of cancer, or when complications are due to spinal cord compression with otherwise acceptable medical status, surgery may be a viable option.

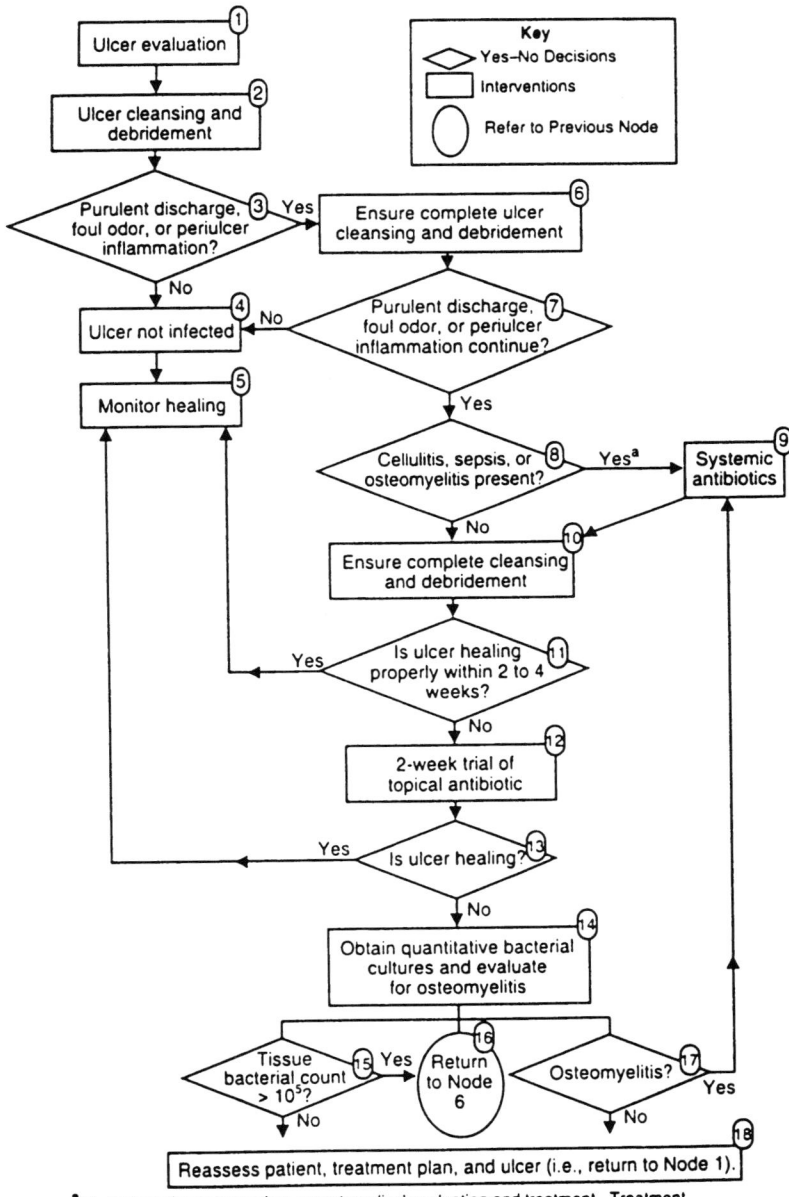

Figure 11.2. Managing bacterial colonization and infection. (Reproduced with permission from Bergstrom et al.[1])

Nutrition

Poor nutrition is a known risk factor for pressure ulcers. The severity of malnutrition correlates with the stage of the pressure ulcer.[26,30,88–93] In a non-randomized trial, Breslow et al. found that high protein and calorie intake (up to 40 kcal per kg of body weight per day) speeded pressure ulcer healing in poorly nourished nursing home patients.[94]

Nutritional support is more complicated in patients with advanced disease. The use of tube feeding or total parenteral nutrition is unlikely to benefit cancer patients suffering from the cachexia–anorexia syndrome. This common complication of cancer occurs in 85% of cancer patients.[95] In controlled clinical studies, total parenteral nutrition (TPN) has been shown not to improve survival, enhance tumor response to antineoplastic treatment, or decrease toxicity of treatment.[96] There are no data on whether quality of life is improved by TPN[95] and it is controversial whether surgical complications are decreased.[97] Megestrol acetate has been shown to provide weight gain through increased fat deposition and to increase appetite in cancer patients with the cachexia–anorexia syndrome.[98–100] It is unclear, however, whether megestrol acetate would enhance pressure ulcer healing through improved nutrition in cancer patients. This is an area requiring further research.

Presently, there is scant evidence regarding the use of vitamin and mineral supplements. In a small controlled study, Taylor et al. found that patients receiving 500 mg of vitamin C twice daily exhibited improved pressure ulcer healing.[101] If vitamin or mineral deficiencies are suspected, then high potency vitamin and mineral supplements containing vitamin C and zinc are recommended.[101,102] In the advanced cancer patient, optimizing oral nutrition, and possible use of megestrol acetate and vitamin and mineral supplementation, may improve pressure ulcer healing.

Conclusion

The development of skin care teams that educate patients, families, and caregivers about the means to prevent and treat pressure ulcers is recommended.[1] In patients with advanced disease, considerations in the management of pressure ulcers include the goals of treatment, the patient's preferences, expected outcomes, and both the benefits and burdens of treatment.[36,103] The dogma that all patients should have treatment directed at healing these lesions has been challenged,[103] and it must be acknowledged that repositioning, surgical debridement, dressing changes, and nutritional interventions can cause significant discomfort in some cases, with no resulting benefit.[36,103] For some patients, the goal of providing comfort through the use of analgesic drugs[1] and the selection of appropriate support surfaces and dressings, may be deemed the most desirable approach to management.[36,103] Pressure ulcer formation must not always be viewed as a quality-of-care issue.[103] Although most pressure ulcers can be prevented, it must be remembered that even the most exemplary care may not prevent the development of these lesions in high risk patients.[36,103]

References

1 Bergstrom M, Bennett MA, Carlson CE, et al. *Treatment of Pressure Ulcers. Clinical Practice Guideline*, No. 15. Publication No. 95-0652. Rockville, Md: Agency for Health Care Policy and Research, Public Health Service, U.S. Department of Health and Human Services, AHCPR 1994.

2. Preventing pressure sores (editorial). *Lancet*, 1990; 54:409.

3. Chicarilli AN. Pressure sores in the elderly. In: Katlic MR, ed. *Geriatric Surgery, Comprehensive Care of the Elderly Patient*. Baltimore: Urban & Schawarzenberg, 1990:549–87.

4. Thompson S, Rowling J. Pathological changes in mummies. *Proc R Soc Med* 1961; 54:409.

5. Reuler JB, Cooney TG. The pressure sore: pathophysiology and principles of management. *Ann Int Med* 1981; 94:661–666.

6. Bar CA, Pathy MSJ. Pressure sores. In: Pathy MSI, ed. *Principles and Practice of Geriatric Medicine*, 2nd ed. New York: John Wiley and Sons Ltd., 1991:1037–1060.

7. Evans JM, Andrews KL, Chutka DS, Fleming KC, Garness SL. Pressure ulcers: Prevention and management. *Mayo Clin Proc* 1995; 70:789–799.

8. Gerson LW. The incidence of pressure sores in active treatment hospitals. *Int J Nurs Stud* 1975; 12(4):201–204.

9. Clarke M, Kadhom HM. The nursing prevention of pressure sores in hospital and community patients. *J Adv Nurs* 1988; 13(3):365–373.

10. Shannon ML, Skorga R. Pressure ulcer prevalence in two general hospitals. *Decubitus* 1989; 2(4):38–43.

11. Oot-Guromini B, Bidwell FC, Heller NB, Parks ML, Prebish EM, Wicks P, et al. Pressure ulcer prevention versus treatment, comparative product cost study. *Decubitus* 1989; (3):52–54.

12. Petersen NC, Bittinann S. The epidemiology of pressure sores. *Scand J Plast Reconstr Surg* 1971; 5(1):62–66.

13. Langemo DK, Olson B, Hunter S, Bund C, Hansen D, Cathcart-Silkenberg T. Incidence of pressure sores in acute care, rehabilitation, extended care, home health, and hospice in one locale *Decubitus* 1989; 2(2):42.

14. Young L. Pressure ulcer prevalence and associated patient characteristics in one long term care facility. *Decubitus* 1989; 2(2):52.

15. Brandeis GH, Morris JN, Nash PJ, Lipsitz LA. The epidemiology and natural history of pressure ulcers in elderly nursing home residents. *JAMA* 1990; 264:2905–2909.

16. Patterson JA, Bennett RG. Prevention and treatment of pressure sores. *J Am Geriatr Soc* 1995; 43:919–927.

17. Versluyson M. How elderly patients with femoral fractures develop pressure sores in hospital. *Br Med J (Clin Res Ed)* 1986; 292(6531):1311–1313.

18. Versluyson M. Pressure sores in elderly patients: the epidemiology related to hip operations. *J Bone Joint Surg Br* 1985; 67:10–13.

19. Richardson PR, Meyer PR Jr. Prevalence and incidence of pressure sores in acute spinal cord injuries. *Paraplegia* 1981; 19(4):235–247.

20. Bergstrom N, Demuth PJ, Braden BJ. A clinical trial of the Braden Scale for predicting pressure sore risk. *Nurs Clin North Am* 1987; 22(2):417–428.

21. Robnett MK. The incidence of skin breakdown in a surgical intensive care unit. *J Nurs Qual Assur* 1986; 1(1):77–81.

22. Guggisberg E, Terumalui K, Carron JM, Rapin CH. New perspectives in the treatment of decubitus ulcers. *J Palliat Care* 1992; 8(2):5–10.

23. Kaasa T, MacMillan K, Bruera E. Reducing the incidence of skin breakdown in the palliative care setting (Abstract). *J Palliat Care* 1995; 11(3):65–66.

24. Miller H, Delozier J. *Cost Implications of the Pressure Ulcer Treatment Guideline.* Contract No. 282-91-0070. Sponsored by the Agency for Health Care Policy and Research. Columbia, Md: Center for Health Policy Studies, 1994.

25. Eckman KL. The prevalence of dermal ulcers among persons in the U.S. who have died. *Decubitus* 1989; 2:36–40.

26. Pinchcofsky-Devin GD, Kaminski MV Jr. Correlation of pressure sores and nutritional status. *J Am Geriatr Soc* 1986; 34(6):435–440.

27. Moss RJ, La Pumer J. Pressure sores: more than meets the eye. *J Clin Ethics* 1990; 1:304–305.

28. Donovan WH, Garber SL, Hamilton SM, Krouskop TA, Rodriguez GP, Stal S. Pressure ulcers. In: Delisa JA, ed. *Rehabilitation Medicine Principles and Practice.* Philadelphia: J.B. Lippincott, 1986:476–491.

29. Carier DM, Balin AK. Dermatological aspects of aging. *Med Clin North Am* 1993; 67:531–543.

30. Berlowitz DR, Wilking SVB. Risk factors for pressure sores: a comparison of cross-sectional and cohort-derived data. *J Am Geriatr Soc* 1989; 37(11):1043–1050.

31. Breslow RA, Hallfrisch J, Guy DG, et al. The importance of dietary protein in healing pressure ulcers. *J Am Geriatr Soc* 1993; 42:357–362.

32. Berg RW, Milligan MC, Scarbaugh PC. Association of skin wetness and pH with diaper dermatitis. *Pediatr Dermatol* 1994; 11:18–20.

33. Goode PS, Allman RM. The prevention and management of pressure ulcers. *Med Clin North Am* 1989; 73(6):1511–1124.

34. Norton D, McLaren R, Exton-Smith AN. *An Investigation of Geriatric Nursing Problems in Hospitals*, London: Corporation for the Care of Old People, 1962.

35. Braden BJ, Bergstrom N. Clinical utility of the Braden Scale for predicting pressure sore risk. *Decubitus* 1989; 2:44–51.

36. Bergstrom N, Allman RM, Carlson CE, et al. *Pressure Ulcers in Adults: Prediction and Prevention. Clinical Practice Guideline*, No. 3. AHCPR Publication No. 92-0047. Rockville, Md.: Agency for Health Care Policy and Research, Public Health Service, U.S. Department of Health and Human Services, 1992.

37. Ek AC, Gustavsson G, Lewis DH. The local skin blood flow in areas at risk for pressure sores treated with massage. *Scand J Rehabil Med* 1985; 17(2):81–86.

38. Dyson R. Bed sores—the injuries hospital staff inflict on patients. *Nurs Mirror* 1978; 146(24):30–32.

39. Garber SL, Campion LJ, Krouskip KA. Trochanteric pressure in spinal cord injury. *Arch Phys Med Rehabil* 1982; 63(11):549–552.

40. Seiler WO, Allen S, Stahelin HB. Influence of the 30 degrees laterally inclined position and the 'super-soft' 3-piece mattress on skin oxygen tension on areas of maximum

pressure—implications for pressure sore prevention. *Gerontology* 1986; 32(3):158–166.

41. Reichel SM. Shearing force as a factor in decubitus ulcers in paraplegics. *JAMA* 1958; 166(7):762–763.

42. Crewe RA. Problems of rubber ring nursing cushions and a clinical survey of alternative cushions for ill patients. *Care Sci Pract* 1987; 5(2):9–11.

43. Custer J, Edlich RF, Prusak M, Madden J, Panek P, Wangensteen OH. Studies in the management of the contaminated wound: V. An assessment of the effectiveness of pHisoHex and Betadine surgical scrub solutions. *Am J Surg* 1971; 121:572–575.

44. Johnson AR, White AC, McAnalley B. Comparison of common topical agents for wound treatment: cytotoxicity for human fibroblasts in culture. *Wounds* 1989; 1(3):186–192.

45. Rodeheaver GT, Pettry D, Thacker JG, Edgerton MT, Edlich RF. Wound cleansing by high pressure irrigation. *Surg Gynecol Obstet* 1975; 141(3):357–362.

46. Rydberg B, Zederfeldt B. Influence of cationic detergents on tensile strength of healing skin wounds in the rat. *Acta Chir Scand* 1968; 134(5):317–320.

47. Burkey JL, Weinberg C, Brenden RA. Differential methodologies for the evaluation of skin and would cleansers. *Wounds* 1993; 5(6):284–291.

48. Foresman PA, Payne DS, Becker D, Lewis D, Rodeheaver GT. A relative toxicity index for would cleansers. *Wounds* 1993; 5(5):226–231.

49. Bryant CA, Rodeheaver GT, Reem EM, Nichter LS, Kenney JG, Edlich RF. Search for a nontoxic surgical scrub solution for periorbital lacerations. *Ann Emerg Med* 1984; 13(5):317–321.

50. Kurzuk-Howard G, Simpson L, Palmieri A. Decubitus ulcer care: a comparative study. *West J Nurs Res* 1985; 7(1):58–79.

51. Saydak SJ. A pilot test of two methods for the treatment of pressure ulcers. *J Enterostomal Ther* 1990; 17(3):139–142.

52. Fowler E, Goupil DL. Comparison of the wet–to–dry dressing and a copolymer starch in the management of debrided pressure sores. *J Enterostomal Ther* 1984; 11(1):22–25.

53. Gorse GJ, Messner RL. Improved pressure sore healing with hydrocolloid dressings. *Arch Dermatol* 1987; 123(6):766–771.

54. Sebern M. Home-team strategies for treating pressure sores. *Nursing* 1987; 17(4):50–53.

55. Alm A, Hornmark AM, Fall PA, Linder L, Bergstrand B, Ehrnebo M, Madsen SM, Setterberg G. Care of pressure sores: a controlled study of the use of a hydrocolloid dressing compared with wet saline gauze compresses. *Acta Derm Venereol* (Stockh) 1989; 149(suppl):1–10.

56. Colwell JC, Foreman MD, Trotter JP. A comparison of the efficacy and cost-effectiveness of two methods of managing pressure ulcers. *Decubitus* 1992; 6(4):28–36.

57. Neill KM, Conforti C, Kedas A, Burris JF. Pressure sore response to a new hydrocolloid dressing. *Wounds* 1989; 1(3):173–185.

58. Oleske DM, Smith XP, White P, Pottage J, Donovan MI. A randomized clinical trial of two dressing methods for the treatment of low-grade pressure ulcers. *J Enterostomal Ther* 1986; 13(3):90–98.

59. Xakellis GC, Chrischilles EA. Hydrocolloid versus saline gauze dressings in treating pressure ulcers: a cost–effectiveness analysis. *Arch Phys Med Rehabil* 1992; 73:463–469.

60. Yarkony GM, Kramer E, King R, LuKanc C, Carle TV. Pressure sore management: efficacy of a moisture reactive occlusive dressing. *Arch Phys Med Rehabil* 1984; 65:597–600.

61. Ahmed MC. Op-site for decubitus care. *Am J Nurs* 1982; 82(1):61–64.

62. Dobrzanski S, Kelly CM, Gray JI, Gregg AJ, Cosgrove CA. Granuflex dressings in treatment of full thickness pressure sores. *Prof Nurse* 1990; 5(11):594–599.

63. Goren D. Use of Omiderm in treatment of low-degree pressure sores in terminally ill cancer patients. *Cancer Nurs* 1989; 12(3):165–169.

64. Lingner C, Rolstad BS, Wetherill K, Danielson S. Clinical trial of a moisture vaporpermeable dressing on superficial pressure sores. *J Enterostomal Ther* 1984; 11(4):147–149.

65. Carley PJ, Wainapel SF. Electrotherapy for acceleration of wound healing: low intensity direct current. *Arch Phys Med Rehabil* 1985; 66(6):443–446.

66. Feedar JA, Kloth LC, Gentzkow GD. Chronic dermal ulcer healing enhanced with monophasic pulsed electrical stimulation. *Phys Ther* 1991; 71(9):639–649.

67. Gentzkow GD, Pollack SV, Kloth LC, Stubbs HA. Improved healing of pressure ulcers using dermapulse, a new electrical stimulation device. *Wounds* 1991; 3(5):158–170.

68. Griffin JW, Tooms RE, Medius RA, Clifft JK, Vander Zwaag R, El-Zeky F. Efficacy of high voltage pulsed current for healing of pressure ulcers in patients with spinal cord injury. *Phys Ther* 1991; 71(6):433–442.

69. Kloth LC, Feedar JA. Acceleration of wound healing with high voltage, monophasic, pulsed current. *Phys Ther* 1988; 68(4):503–508.

70. Robson M, Phillips LG, Tomason A, Robson LF, Pierce GF. Recombinant human growth factor-BB for the treatment of chronic pressure ulcers. *Ann Plast Surg* 1992a; 29:193–201.

71. Robson M, Phillips LG, Thomason A, Robson LF, Pierce GF. Platelet-derived factors BB for treatment of chronic pressure ulcers. *Lancet* 1992b; 339:23–25.

72. Robson MC, Phillips LG, Lawrence WT, Bishop JB, Youngerman JS, Hayward PG, Broemeling LD, Heggers JP. The safety and effect of topically applied recombinant basic fibroblast growth factor on the healing of chronic pressure sores. *Ann Surg* 1992; 216(4):401–408.

73. Bendy RH Jr, Nuccio PA, Wolfe E, Collins B, Tamburro C, Glass W, Martin CM. Relationship of quantitative wound bacterial counts to healing of decubiti: effect of topical gentamicin. *Antimicrob Agents Chemother* 1964; 4:147–155.

74. Daltrey DC, Rhodes B, Chattwood JG. Investigation into the microbial flora of healing and non-healing decubitus ulcers. *J Clin Pathol* 1981; 34(7)701–705.

75. Lyman IR, Tenery JH, Basson RP. Correlation between decrease in bacterial load and rate of wound healing. *Surg Gynecol Obstet* 1970; 130(4):616–621.

76. Sapico FL, Ginunas VJ, Thornhill-Joynes M, Canawati HN, Capen DA, Klein NE, Khawam S, Montogomerie JZ. Quantitative microbiology of pressure sores in different stages of healing. *Diagn Microbiol Infect Dis* 1986; 5(1):31–38.

77. Ferrell BA, Osterweil D, Christenson P. A randomized trial of low–air–loss beds for treatment of pressure ulcers. *JAMA* 1993; 269(4):494–497.

78. Garner JS, Jarvis WR, Emori TG, Horan TC, Hughes JM. CDC definitions for nosocomial infections, 1988. *Am J Infec Control* 1988; 16(3):128–140.

79. Kucan JO, Robson MC, Heggers JP, Ko F. Comparison of silver sulfadiazine, povidone-iodine and physiologic saline in the treatment of chronic pressure ulcers. *J Am Geriatr Soc* 1981; 29(5):232–235.

80. Bryan CS, Dew CE, Reynolds KL. Baceremia associated with decubitus ulcers. *Arch Intern Med* 1983; 143(11):2093–2095.

81. Chow AW, Galpin JE, Guze LB. Clindamycin for treatment of sepsis caused by decubitus ulcers. *J Infec Dis* 1977; 135(suppl):S65–S68.

82. Galpin JE, Chow AW, Bayer AS, Guze LB. Sepsis associated with decubitus ulcers. *Am J Med* 1976; 61(3):346–350.

83. Lewis VL Jr, Bailey MH, Pulawski G, Kind G, Bashioum RW, Hendrix RW. The diagnosis of osteomyelitis in patients with pressure sores. *Plast Reconstr Surg* 1988; 81(2):229–232.

84. Surgarman B. Pressure sores and underlying bone infection. *Arch Intern Med* 1987; 147(3):553–555.

85. Anthony JP, Huntsman WT, Mathes SJ. Changing trends in the management of pelvic pressure ulcers: a 12-year review. *Decubitus* 1992; 5(3):44–47, 50–51.

86. Becker H. The distally-based gluteus maximus flap. *Plast Reconstr Surg* 1979; 63(5):653–656.

87. Bruck JC, Buttermeyer R, Grabosch A, Gruhl L. More arguments in favor of myocutaneous flaps for the treatment of pelvic pressure sores. *Ann Plast Surg* 1991; 26(1):85–88.

88. Allman RM, Laprade CA, Noel LB, Walker JM, Moorer CA, Dear MR, Smith CR. Pressure sores among hospitalized patients. *Ann Intern Med* 1986; 105(3):337–342.

89. Bergstrom N, Braden B. A prospective study of pressure sore risk among institutionalized elderly. *J Am Geriatr Soc* 1992; 40(8):747–758.

90. Breslow RA, Hallfrisch J, Goldberg AP. Malnutrition in tubefed nursing home patients with pressure sores. *JPEN J Parenter Enteral Nutr* 1991; 15(6):663–668.

91. Ek AC, Unosson M, Bjurulf P. The modified Norton Scale and the nutritional state. *Scand J Caring Sci* 1989; 3(4):183–187.

92. Hanan K, Scheele L. Albumin vs. weight as a predictor of nutritional status and pressure ulcer development. *Ostomy Wound Manage* 1991; 33(2):22–27.

93. Holmes R, Macchiano K, Jhangiani SS, Agarwal NR, Savino JA. Nutrition know-how: combating pressure sores—nutritionally. *Am J Nurs* 1987; 87(10):1301–1303.

94. Breslow RA, Hallfrisch J, Guy DG, Crawley B, Goldberg AP. The importance of dietary protein in healing pressure ulcers. *J Am Geriatr Soc* 1993; 41(4):357–362.

95. Bruera E, Fainsinger R. Clinical management of cachexia and anorexia. In: Doyle D, Hanks G, MacDonald N, eds. *Oxford Textbook of Palliative Medicine*. London: Oxford Medical Publications, 1993:330–337.

96. Koretz R. Parenteral nutrition: is it oncologically logical? *J Clin Oncol* 1984; 2:534–538.

97. Detsky AS, Baker JP, O'Rourke K, Goel V. Perioperative parenteral nutrition: a meta-analysis. *Ann Int Med* 1987; 107:195–203.

98. Bruera E, Macmillan K, Hanson J, Kuehn N, MacDonald RN. A controlled trial of megestrol acetate on appetite, caloric intake, nutritional status, and other symptoms in patients with advanced cancer. *Cancer* 1990; 66:1279–1282.

99. Loprinzi CL, Ellison NM, Schaid DJ, et al. Controlled trial of megestrol acetate for the treatment of cancer, anorexia and cachexia. *J Natl Cancer Inst* 1990; 82:1127–1132.

100. Tchekmedyian S, Hakman M, Siau J, et al. Megestrol acetate in cancer anorexia and weight loss. *Cancer* 1992; 69:1268–1274.

101. Taylor TV, Rimmer S, Day B, Butcher J, Dymock IW. Ascorbic acid supplementation in the treatment of pressure sores. *Lancet* 1974; 2(7880):544–546.
102. Burr RG. Blood zinc in the spinal patient. *J Clin Pathol* 1973; 26(10):773–775.
103. Darovich SL. When is no treatment the right treatment? *Nursing 96* 1996; 26(7):47.
104. Miller CM, O'Neill A, Mortimer PS. Skin problems in palliative care: nursing aspects. In: Doyle D, Hanks G, MacDonald N, eds. *Oxford Textbook of Palliative Medicine*. London: Oxford Medical Publications, 1993:395–407.

Lymphedema: Current Treatments and Controversies

RICHARD S. TUNKEL
AND PHYLLIS RAMPULLA

Lymphedema is characterized by the regional accumulation of large amounts of interstitial fluid, especially in the subcutaneous tissues of the affected area. *Primary lymphedema* or *lymphedema praecox* is an uncommon form usually affecting the lower limbs. *Hereditary lymphedema*, which can first be seen at birth or puberty, is rare. In the palliative care setting, *secondary lymphedema* is the form most frequently encountered. It usually arises from focal lymphatic obstruction caused by neoplastic infiltration, en bloc resection, or irradiation of regional lymph nodes.[1]

The effect of lymphedema on the patient's quality of life may be quite profound. There is increased risk of infection in the affected limb, and there may be impaired limb function, pain, and significant alteration of the patient's body image. Therapeutic interventions are available to patients with this condition and should be offered when appropriate.

Structure and Function of the Lymphatic System

The lymphatic drainage system plays an important role in the management of interstitial fluid. Net transendothelial pressure at the capillary wall causes production of interstitial fluid. The escape of some macromolecules, especially proteins, maintains interstitial oncotic pressure. These large molecules resist reuptake into the capillary lumen. If proteins are broken down by macrophages, the resulting polypeptides and amino acids can return directly to the bloodstream. This process, however, may be insufficient to maintain a homeostatic pressure gradient.

An intact lymphatic network drains excess proteinaceous fluid from the interstitium, eventually returning it to the blood.[2] Interstitial fluid is brought into the "terminal" lymphangioles when gaps form between the endothelial cells.[3] This presumably occurs with movement of the individual endothelial cell relative to the surrounding tissue to which it is tethered by anchoring filaments.[4] This may occur by intrinsic tissue movement caused by skeletal muscle contraction or arterial pulsation, or by extrinsic tissue motion, such as with gentle, intermittent massage. The endothelial cells themselves may bring in fluid and particles by active vesicular transport.[3]

The lymphatic system is also integral to the function of the immune system. Lymphatics pick up antigenic material from the tissues they drain, including viral and bacterial debris. These antigens are carried in the afferent lymph to the regional lymph nodes into which the lymphatics drain. Although some of this material is taken up by lymphatic endothelium, most is presented to lymphocytes within the lymph nodes, thereby initiating the immune response.[5]

The superficial lymphatic system of the skin begins at the initial lymphatics found below the epidermis. These valveless "capillaries" drain into the deeper reticular layer of lymphatics, where valves prevent backflow.[6] These "precollectors," in turn, conduct the lymph fluid into subcutaneous collectors which have both valves and smooth muscle, providing a means of actively propelling the fluid proximally.[7] Some precollectors drain directly into deep periarterial lymphatics that follow the course of the neurovascular bundle. These collectors drain into four major lymph node groups situated at the base of each limb. For example, the lymphatics of the upper limb, ipsilateral upper torso, and ipsilateral head and neck drain into the axillary lymph nodes. There are rather superficial collateral channels on the torso that connect the drainage areas of these four major lymph node groups.[8,9] Eventually, the lymph fluid is carried to the thoracic duct and returned to the blood.

Presentation of Lymphedema

Lymphatic drainage may be disrupted by regional lymph node dissection, irradiation, or other types of local injury. Acute, transient edema which may arise after surgery usually resolves within about two months.[10] Its appearance does not foretell the onset of chronic lymphedema. Chronic lymphedema may first appear months or years after surgery or irradiation.[11]

After radical mastectomy, the reported incidence of upper limb lymphedema has varied greatly.[2,12] The literature reports decreasing incidence as more conservative surgical management for breast cancer is employed. This probably is related to decreasing the extent of lymphadenectomy.[13-15] There also is some evidence, however, that lymphedema may be more prevalent with less extensive surgery for breast carcinoma; scatter radiation from the breast field may be absorbed in the area of the axilla, increasing the risk of lymphedema by its synergistic effect.[16] At least some of the apparent differences in reported incidence of lymphedema result from different measuring techniques and definitions of lymphedema.

In patients who have focal obstruction of regional lymphatic drainage, the onset or exacerbation of chronic lymphedema of the affected limb may be provoked by any of several etiologies. Perhaps the most commonly recognized is infection.[17] Sluggish lymphatic drainage, the presence of increased amounts of interstitial fluid (even if not clinically apparent), and impairment of regional lymph nodes into which afferent lymph drains may all predispose to infection. The usual pathogen is either *Staphylococcus* or *Streptococcus* skin flora. The resulting cellulitis or erysipelas can cause a macular or maculopapular erythematous rash with increased warmth and swelling. There may be a red macular line, which represents lymphangitis. In some cases, infection may occur with little erythema, mild warmth, and induration of the affected area. Indeed, a chronic, low grade infection may exist without clinical evidence of inflammation.[18] Some patients have reported increased warmth, swelling, and redness that spontaneously resolved. Some of these patients even have constitutional symptoms.[19] A local portal of entry for infection is not always apparent.

Appropriate treatment for a local infection that may be inciting lymphedema includes an oral antibiotic with adequate skin penetration and good coverage of gram positive cocci. An example would be dicloxacillin 500 mg taken 4 times a day for approximately 2 weeks, or longer if needed. If there are accompanying constitutional symptoms or signs such as fever, chills, or sweats, or if local infection is severe, intravenous antibiotics may be necessary. The very real potential of local infection to further interfere with the superficial lymph system justifies prompt treatment. The majority of those who develop an infection are at increased risk for its recurrence.[20]

Irradiation of the lymphadenectomized region is generally believed to predispose the corresponding limb to lymphedema.[10,14,21-25] Obesity, persistent seroma, and delayed wound healing also have been associated with an increased incidence of lymphedema.[12,25,26] Overuse of the affected limb, which fatigues its musculature, may exacerbate edema. Some patients report increased swelling when exposed to heat or to decreased atmospheric pressure, such as during a commercial airline flight.

Chronic lymphedema may present in a generalized pattern throughout the limb or be focally apparent. Common presentations in the upper limb include edema limited to the elbow and forearm, the upper arm, or the hand and digits. If affected, only a portion of the dorsum of the hand may be edematous, often the radial aspect. Similarly, edema may first appear in the proximal or distal aspect of the lower limb. The patient often complains of heaviness or fullness of the limb and a significant number experience a generalized ache caused by stretching of the local soft tissues.[27] The report of pain is not directly related to the degree of swelling.

Initial onset of limb swelling necessitates evaluation. Evidence of infection, even if equivocal, usually requires initiation of antibiotic therapy. Neurologic examination demonstrating new focal deficit may require further studies to rule out cancer recurrence. Concurrent limb pain may result from recurrence or post-radiation plexopathy, though the latter is less common, or from painfully stretched soft tissues of the limb.[28] Studies may be needed to rule out deep venous thrombosis, which can also cause limb swelling. A finding of venous edema does not exclude the possibility of coexisting obstructive lymphedema. When the diagnosis is uncertain, imaging with lymphoscintigraphy is usually preferred over lymphangiography.[29,30] Magnetic resonance imaging can also visualize subcutaneous fluid collections.[31]

Initially, lymphedema is soft and pitting in quality. Pitting is usually more pronounced in the more dependent portions of the limb, for example, over the ulna when the elbow and forearm are involved. The skin of the affected limb may become dry and scaly. Over time, the volume of lymphedema increases and becomes less pitting and more fibrous and firm to palpation. This may be the result of fibroblasts converting excess interstitial proteins into fibrous tissue. As more fibrous subcutaneous tissue forms, the edema becomes brawny and non-pitting.[1] With this severe lymphedema, there is restriction of range of motion because of thicker, less compliant tissues and excessive bulk. The skin may become hyperkeratotic. Verrucous and vesicular lesions containing lymph fluid may occur, giving rise to elephantiasis.[2] Although rare, chronic lymphedema may give rise to lymphangiosarcoma (Stewart-Treves syndrome), a malignant tumor with a very poor prognosis.[32]

Lymphedema, especially of the upper limb, may give rise to significant psychological sequelae. For example, physical changes arising from surgical or radiotherapeutic intervention for breast cancer are usually easily concealed by the patient. Upper limb lymphedema, especially when affecting the hand, is often readily apparent, at least to the patient. Compression garments attract further attention to the swollen limb, also serving as a reminder to the patient of the malignancy. This may undermine previously successful psychological strategies for coping with the condition. Significant related psychosocial and sexual difficulties may also appear.[33]

Preventive Measures with Lymphedema

Even with significant lymphedema, some lymph production and functional lymphatic drainage from the limb continues. It is prudent for the patient to avoid circumstances that promote interstitial fluid production (Table 12.1). Because of the effects of gravity, back pressure in the lymphatic vessels, like venous pressure, increases when the limb is maintained in a dependent position. When possible, prolonged dependency should be avoided. Activity in the affected limb sufficient to fatigue its musculature may cause reflex shunting of blood to the area (to provide oxygen and nutrients and remove excess lactic acid), which can increase production of interstitial fluid. Not only heavy work, but also light, sustained

Table 12.1. Circumstances and activities that may exacerbate lymphedema

Heavy lifting or sustained activity of the limb

Maintaining the limb in a gravity-dependent position for prolonged periods

Focal limb constriction
  Tight jewelry or clothing
  Blood pressure cuff

Inflammation of the integument of the limb
  Closed trauma
  Thermal injury
  Infection
      Open trauma
      Needle sticks
      Wounds or cuts (even trivial)
    Insect bites
    Breaks in the skin
      Tinea unguium
      Dry, scaly skin requiring moisturizer

Decreased atmospheric pressure
  Commercial airline flights
  High-altitude environment

Heat and humidity

activity may produce fatigue. Tight or constrictive clothing or jewelry may act like a tourniquet and provoke swelling, usually distal to the constriction. For this reason, blood pressure cuffs are avoided on the affected limb. Heat may increase lymph fluid production and therefore local heat applications to the affected limb are best avoided. Static compression over the affected limb may be advisable with any exposure to decreasing atmospheric pressures, including airplane flights.

Anything that may induce an inflammatory response, such as trauma or thermal injury, may cause swelling. Infection is most problematic. The natural barrier of the integumentary system needs to be maintained. Trivial injuries such as a crack in dry skin, a paper cut, a tear of the cuticle around the nail, or an insect bite, may become a portal of entry for skin bacteria. An interdigital or subungual tinea infection does not cause cellulitis but may breach the integumentary barrier. Breaks in the skin should be cleaned, treated with topical antibiotic, and covered. Patients must be instructed to tell the physician about any evidence of infection in the affected limb.

Management of Lymphedema

The specific treatment of lymphedema depends upon the nature and degree of edema and the patient's abilities and compliance with the treatment plan (Table 12.2). The natural history of lymphedema is one of gradual increase over time.

Table 12.2 Therapeutic interventions available for lymphedema treatment

Limb elevation

Therapeutic exercise

Static limb compression
  Gradient pressure garment
  Limb wrapping or bandaging
  Legging orthosis

Self-massage by patient and/or caregiver

Pneumatic compression pumping

Combination of physical therapies (CPT)
  Manual lymphedema treatment (MLT)
  Limb wrapping or bandaging
  Therapeutic exercise
  Appropriate skin care

Pharmacologic measures

Surgical intervention

This is especially true of secondary arm lymphedema, particularly in older patients.[34] Limb elevation should be encouraged when possible, especially when pitting edema is present. Periods of time throughout each day may be set aside toward this end. However, arm elevation after axillary lymph node dissection may cause very little reduction when edema is not pitting in nature.[35] Non-fatiguing therapeutic exercise is designed to encourage the action of the "muscle pump" in the affected limb. The intermittent compression against the local vasculature displaces fluid within lymphatics and veins. This fluid is directed proximally by intraluminal valves, facilitating its return to the bloodstream.

Static compression applied over the affected limb is routinely used in treatment. The net relative pressure pushing fluids out through capillary walls is slightly lessened by external compression, discouraging interstitial fluid production.[36] This is especially important when the limb will be in a gravity-dependent position or it is exposed to decreased atmospheric pressure, such as occurs at high altitudes or during airline flights in partially pressurized cabins. External compression may also facilitate the action of the "muscle pump."

Gradient pressure garments are most commonly employed to accomplish external compression. In the upper limb, a sleeve extending from wrist to axilla may be sufficient if there is no distal lymphedema and none is provoked. Otherwise, a hand piece, as part of or separate from the sleeve, may be needed.[37] If the arm is excessively large or unusually proportioned, a custom-made garment will be needed. In some cases, shoulder straps are used instead of an elastic band at the axilla. In the lower limb, the stocking almost always has an attached foot piece. When possible, it should extend above the upper limit of the edema; this sometimes requires a waist-high garment. A legging orthosis using a series of Velcro inelastic straps has been used with some success, especially for edema distal to the knee.[38] Wrapping or bandaging the limb with relatively inelastic materials is also used, especially during active hands-on treatment. Both this and the legging orthosis conform automatically when applied to a limb with fluctuating edema.[39]

Pneumatic compression pumping of the affected limb has been widely used throughout the United States in the treatment of lymphedema. A gradient pressure garment is usually applied throughout the day between pumping sessions. Pneumatic compression involves intermittent inflation of a plastic sleeve by a pneumatic pump to which it is connected by one or more hoses. The first devices had only a single chamber throughout the length of the plastic sleeve. Later units had multiple chambers, each with its own hose attached to the pump. Sequential inflation applies centripetal compression to the limb, which "milks" edematous fluid from the limb. Currently, many sequential pumps use an adjustable pressure gradient, which is greater in the distal aspect of the limb. The pressures applied to the limb are adjustable in all units. The duty cycle of some pumps is also adjustable; this may increase patient comfort and compliance.

Pneumatic pumps have been used at a wide range of pressures in lymphedema, and the ideal pressure is controversial. This applies to all varieties of pneumatic pumps including single chamber models and sequential, multichambered units.[10,23,37,40–50] Some have suggested that pressures greater than 50 mmHg or 60 mmHg may be injurious to lymphatic vessels.[51] There is also no consensus on the optimal period of pumping or frequency of pumping. An example would be one- to two-hour pumping sessions once daily.

Although some patients report perceived benefit from pneumatic pumping at home, this does not appear to be true for many others. To many patients, pumping on a daily basis represents a drawback and is, therefore, an impediment to patient compliance. Some patients report that edema reduction is only temporary, even with application of a gradient pressure garment immediately after pumping. Others report a buildup of fluid at the base of the limb or at the adjacent trunk after pumping, sometimes transiently but occasionally without complete resolution. This can sometimes be addressed with post-pumping local massage by the patient or helper.

Specialized medical massage treatments have been used for many years in Europe for the treatment of lymphedema. These treatments, which are sometimes termed *manual lymphedema treatment* (MLT), are used in combination with multilayer bandaging, therapeutic exercise, and meticulous skin care to help reduce limb swelling. As such, these may together be termed a *combination of physical therapies* (CPT).[52] Several different forms of MLT exist, although the general principles and treatment schema are similar.

Manual deformation of the skin during MLT is believed to facilitate opening of the gap junctions of the terminal, superficial lymphatic channels by dynamically changing the position of the lymphangiole in relation to a small portion of its wall which is attached to a static anchoring filament.[53] This, in turn, allows entrance of interstitial fluids and macromolecules into the vessel lumen. This stimulation may have the additional benefit of encouraging an increased rate of contractility of the superficial lymph vessels, thus increasing centripetal flow of lymph fluid.[54] To accomplish these responses, relatively light massage techniques are employed. More forceful pressure would, theoretically, collapse the superficial lymphangioles, actually impeding lymph flow. Indeed, it has been suggested that excessively forceful or improperly sequenced MLT may damage superficial lymphatics or cause pooling of edema around scars where superficial lymphatics have insufficiently regenerated.[53] Most forms of MLT emphasize the importance of massage applied to the torso. Here, the goal is to "open" the collateral channels connecting the different major drainage areas at the bases of the limbs. For example, if the right axillary lymph nodes have been dissected, significant time would be spent in an effort to facilitate flow through the collateral channels connecting this drainage area with that on the left.[55] Massage techniques would be applied across the front and back of the torso.

The application of multilayer bandaging is believed to encourage the distal to proximal flow of the fluids within the lymphatic channels and maintain adequate external compression, which may create an optimal pressure gradient for lymphatic channel function.[55] Gentle therapeutic exercise is, therefore, done with bandaging in place, in an effort to encourage the effect of the local muscle pumping action. Typically, bandaging materials have little compliance. This is possible since it is wrapped onto the limb, not pulled over the limb like a sleeve or stocking. A further advantage over a gradient pressure garment is that the bandaging is form-fitted with each application, thereby accommodating small reductions after each MLT session. The bandaging is to be worn between MLT sessions, both day and night. Patients with advanced breast cancer occasionally respond favorably to multilayer bandaging with therapeutic exercise as the sole treatment intervention. Inappropriate application of bandages may result in unacceptable areas of fluid collection, especially distally, if proper technique is not achieved.

There are no specific studies indicating the optimal frequency for MLT treatments. Some patients only are able to get these treatments once or twice a week and seem to achieve lesser results than those receiving MLT treatments as often as every day. Some clinics administer MLT treatments twice a day. CPT is usually not done ad infinitum. In milder cases, two or three weeks may be recommended, whereas severe lymphedema may require four or more weeks, or more than one treatment period. Some advocate periodic maintenance MLT sessions on a long-term basis.

Results of CPT are generally favorable.[56–58] Some patients may achieve more than a 50% reduction in swelling. The long-term effects of treatment are variable, with results lasting weeks, months, or longer. For some, swelling may slowly return over time, at least in part. Occasionally a further decrease of edema is recorded at follow-up. Further improvement may be the result of continued collateral flow. Variability in outcome with CPT may be related to individual pathophysiological differences or the degree of skill and expertise of the treating therapist. However, at least in part, differences appear to be the result of degrees of patient compliance. This could also be said of the other available treatment modalities.

There is a paucity of scientific studies comparing the efficacy of different CPT approaches or pneumatic pumping. Almost all reports in the literature, even those with large numbers of participants, are not controlled and are essentially outcome surveys, often pooled from different clinics. In spite of this, it seems that many clinicians have "chosen sides." Those advocating CPT will frequently balk at the idea of using pneumatic pumping, concerned about the untoward effects it may provoke. Those using pneumatic pumping obviously do not feel that there are any long-term side effects of pumping and point out the labor-intensive nature of CPT. In our experience, a significantly greater number of patients seem to have done well with CPT than with pneumatic pumping, and over a significantly shorter period of time. A very small number seem to have benefited from the combination of approaches. For example, if fluid collects in the proximal limb or adjacent torso, massage may be applied to the area at the completion of pumping.

There may be contraindications for MLT/CPT and even pneumatic pumping when active malignancy is present.[52] Massage over irradiated tissue may also be relatively contraindicated. Significant congestive heart failure may contraindicate these treatments, as may acute thrombophlebitis. When present, cellulitis or other significant pathology on the affected limb may contraindicate any therapeutic intervention except, perhaps, elevation and gentle exercise.

Dietary modifications have not been reported to play a major role in lymphedema management. Restricted sodium intake may have a modest effect in a small number of cases. Diuretics may be helpful in acute exacerbations, but are of limited benefit in chronic lymphedema.[23,55] Benzopyrones, particularly coumarin, have been used, especially outside of the United States. They appear to cause macrophage aggregation, which, in turn, causes breakdown of interstitial proteins into amino acids and small polypeptides which can traverse the capillary walls.[59,60] Decreased edema and incidence of infection usually require many months of continued use.[61] Few side effects have been reported in patients; these include a chemical hepatitis.[62]

Surgical intervention has also been reported. These procedures are considered when physical interventions fail. Conservative treatment is usually continued after surgery. Recreating lymphatic drainage from the severely lymphedematous limb has been attempted using pedicle grafts or lymphovenous anastomoses.[63–67] Debulking of the limb may be necessary in severely refractory cases.[68–70] If the limb loses function and interferes with remaining function, amputation is rarely considered.

Conclusion

With an increasing incidence of new cases of cancer and increasing life expectancies of patients with cancer, chronic lymphedema will remain a highly prevalent condition. The natural history of lymphedema is that it increases over time when not treated. This fact, combined with its adverse effects on physical and psychological functioning, mandate intervention even in mild cases. It is unfortunate that few studies address optimal treatment plans and virtually none successfully compare different treatment modalities. Logic dictates that the rational approach would be to employ the modality that most benefits the patient. Equally important is to design an intervention that optimizes patient compliance. Biases for or against certain interventions continue, but it is in the patient's best interest to keep an open mind as to the most effective interventions available for each individual patient.

References

1. Brennan MJ. Lymphedema following the surgical treatment of breast cancer: a review of pathophysiology and treatment. *J Pain Symptom Manage* 1992; 7(2):110–116.
2. Mortimer P, Regnard C. Lymphostatic disorders. *Br Med J* 1986; 293:347–348.
3. Huth F, Bernhardt D. The anatomy of lymph vessels in relation to function. *Lymphology* 1977; 10:54–61.
4. Ryan TJ. The endothelial cell. In: Cluzan RV, Pecking AP, Lokiec FM, eds. *Progress in Lymphology-XIII*. Amsterdam: Elsevier Science Publishers B.V., 1992:147–148.
5. Castenholz A. The histochemical role of the lymphatic endothelium for lymph formation and lymph transport. In: Cluzan RV, Pecking AP, Lokiec FM, eds. *Progress in Lymphology-XIII*. Amsterdam: Elsevier Science Publishers B.V., 1992:125–129.
6. Kubik S. Lymphatics of the skin. In: Cluzan RV, Pecking AP, Lokiec FM, eds. *Progress in Lymphology-XIII*. Amsterdam: Elsevier Science Publishers B.V., 1992:11–14.
7. Olszewski WL, Engeset A. Intrinsic contractility of leg lymphatics in man—preliminary communication. *Lymphology* 1979; 12:81–84.
8. Leduc A, Caplan I, Leduc O. Lymphatic drainage of the upper limb. Substitution lymphatic pathways. *Eur J Lymphology* 1993; 4:11–18.
9. Bruna J. Types of collateral lymphatic circulation. *Lymphology* 1974; 7:61–68.
10. Leis HP, Bowers WF, Dursi J. Postmastectomy edema of arm. *NY State J Med* 1966; 66:618–624.
11. Brennan MJ, Weitz J. Lymphedema 30 years after radical mastectomy. *Am J Phys Med Rehabil* 1992; 71:12–14.
12. Markowski J, Wilcox JP, Helm PA. Lymphedema incidence after specific postmastectomy therapy. *Arch Phys Med Rehabil* 1981; 62:449–452.
13. Getz DH. The primary, secondary and tertiary nursing interventions of lymphedema. *Cancer Nurs* 1985; 8(3):177–184.
14. Kissin MW, Querci della Rovere G, Easton D, Westbury G. Risk of lymphoedema following the treatment of breast cancer. *Br J Surg* 1986; 73:580–584.
15. Heytmanek G, Kubista E. Therapie des post-operativen lymphodems beim mammakarzinom: die lymphdrainage. *Geburtshilfe Frauenheilkd* 1988; 48:433–435.
16. Petrek JA, Blackwood MM. Axillary dissection: current practice and technique. *Curr Probl Surg* 1995; 32:262–323.
17. Mozes M, Papa MZ, Karasik A, Reshef A, Adar R. The role of infection in post-mastectomy lymphedema. *Surg Ann* 1982; 14:73–83.

18. Britton RC, Nelson PA. Causes and treatment of postmastectomy lymphedema of the arm. Report of 114 cases. *JAMA* 1962; 180:95–102.

19. Ohkuma M. Trial treatment dispensing antibiotics for acute cellulitis in lymphedema. In: Witte MH, Witte CL, eds. *Progress in Lymphology-XIV*. Zurich: International Society of Lymphology, 1994:539–542.

20. Benda K, Svestkova S. Incidence rate of recurrent erysipelas in our lymphedema patients. In: Witte MH, Witte CL, eds. *Progress in Lymphology-XIV*. Zurich: International Society of Lymphology, 1994:519–522.

21. Tsyb AT, Bardychev MS, Guseva LI. Secondary limb edemas following irradiation. *Lymphology* 1981; 14:127–132.

22. Durand JC, Poljicak M, Lefranc P, Pilleron JP. Wide excision of the tumor, axillary dissection and postoperative radiotherapy as treatment of small breast cancers. *Cancer* 1984; 53:2439–2443.

23. Tish Knobf MK. Primary breast cancer: physical consequences and rehabilitation. *Semin Oncol Nurs* 1985; 1(3):214–224.

24. Robinson DS, Senofsky GM, Ketcham AS. Role and extent of lymphadenectomy for early breast cancer. *Semin Surg Oncol* 1992; 8:78–82.

25. Segerström K, Bjerle P, Graffman S, Nyström Å. Factors that influence the incidence of brachial oedema after treatment of breast cancer. *Scand J Plast Reconstr Surg Hand Surg* 1992; 26:223–227.

26. Pezner RD, Patterson MP, Hill LR, et al. Arm lymphedema in patients treated conservatively for breast cancer: relationship to patient age and axillary node dissection technique. *Int J Radiat Oncol Biol Phys* 1986; 12(12):2079–2083.

27. McGuire WL, Foley KM, Levy MH, Osborne CK. Pain control in breast cancer. *Breast Cancer Res Treat* 1989; 13:5–15.

28. Kori SH, Foley KM, Posner JB. Brachial plexus lesions in patients with cancer: 100 cases. *Neurology* 1981; 31:45–50.

29. McNeill GC, Witte MH, Witte CL, et al. Whole-body lymphangioscintigraphy: preferred method for initial assessment of the peripheral lymphatic system. *Radiology* 1989; 172:495–502.

30. Bruna J, Brunova J. Complications and side-effects after lymphography. In: Witte MH, Witte CL, eds. *Progress in Lymphology-XIV*. Zurich: International Society of Lymphology, 1994:321–324.

31. Unger EC, Baker MR. Role of magnetic resonance imaging in evaluation of lymphedema and diseases of the lymphatics. In: Witte MH, Witte CL, eds. *Progress in Lymphology-XIV*. Zurich: International Society of Lymphology, 1994:249–252.

32. Stewart FW, Treves N. Lymphangiosarcoma in postmastectomy lymphedema: a report of 6 cases in elephantiasis chirurgica. *Cancer* 1948; 1:64–81.

33. Passik S, Newman M, Brennan M, Holland J. Psychiatric consultation for women undergoing rehabilitation for upper-extremity lymphedema following breast cancer treatment. *J Pain Symptom Manage* 1993; 8(4):226–233.

34. Casley-Smith JR. Alterations of untreated lymphedema and its grades over time. *Lymphology* 1995; 28:174–185.

35. Swedborg I, Norrefalk JR, Piller NB, Åsard C. Lymphoedema post-mastectomy: is elevation alone an effective treatment? *Scand J Rehabil Med* 1993; 25:79–82.

36. Gray B. Management of limb oedema in advanced cancer. *Nurs Times* 1987; 83(49):39–41.

37. Swedborg I. Effects of treatment with an elastic sleeve and intermittent pneumatic compression in post-mastectomy patients with lymphoedema of the arm. *Scand J Rehabil Med* 1984; 16:35–41.

38. Vernick SH, Shapiro D, Shaw FD. Leg orthosis for venous and lymphatic insufficiency. *Arch Phys Med Rehabil* 1987; 68:459–461.

39. Casley-Smith JR. Modern treatment of lymphedema. *Modern Med Aust* 1992; 32:70–83.

40. Ziessler RH, Rose GB, Nelson PA. Postmastectomy lymphedema: late results of treatment in 385 patients. *Arch Phys Med Rehabil* 1972; 53:159–166.

41. Wood C, Gerber LH. Rehabilitation of the patient with breast cancer. In: Lippman ME, Lichter AS, Danforth DN, eds. *Diagnosis and Management of Breast Cancer*. Philadelphia: WB Saunders, 1988:457–467.

42. Zanolla R, Monzeglio C, Balzarini A, Martino G. Evaluation of the results of three different methods of postmastectomy lymphedema treatment. *J Surg Oncol* 1984; 26:210–213.

43. McNair TJ, Martin IJ, Orr JD. Intermittent compression for lymphoedema of arm. *Clin Oncol* 1976; 2:339–342.

44. Yamazaki Z, Idezuki Y, Nemoto T, Togawa T. Clinical experiences using pneumatic massage therapy for edematous limbs over the last 10 years. *Angiol J Vasc Dis* 1988; 39:154–163.

45. Pappas CJ, O'Donnell TF. Long-term results of compression treatment for lymphedema. *J Vasc Surg* 1992; 16(4):555–562.

46. Zelikovski A, Manoach M, Giler SH, Urca I. Lympha–Press: A new pneumatic device for the treatment of lymphedema of the limbs. *Lymphology* 1980; 13:68–73.

47. Zelikovski A, Haddad M, Reiss R. The "Lympha-Press" intermittent sequential pneumatic device for the treatment of lymphoedema: five years of clinical experience. *J Cardiovasc Surg* 1986; 27:288–290.

48. Alexander MA, Wright ES, Wright JB, Bikowski JB. Lymphedema treated with linear pump: pediatric case report. *Arch Phys Med Rehabil* 1983; 64:132–133.

49. Kim-Sing C, Basco VE. Postmastectomy lymphedema treated with the Wright linear pump. *Can J Surg* 1987; 30(5):368–370.

50. Klein MJ, Alexander MA, Wright JM, Redmond CK, LeGasse AA. Treatment of adult lower extremity lymphedema with Wright linear pump: statistical analysis of a clinical trail. *Arch Phys Med Rehabil* 1988; 69:202–206.

51. Eliska O, Eliskova M. Lymphedema—morphology of the lymphatics after manual massage. In: Witte MH, Witte CL, eds. *Progress in Lymphology-XIV*. Zurich: International Society of Lymphology, 1994:132–135.

52. International Society of Lymphology Executive Committee. The diagnosis and treatment of peripheral lymphedema. *Lymphology* 1995; 28:113–117.

53. Eliskova O, Eliskova M. Are peripheral lymphatics damaged by high pressure manual massage? *Lymphology* 1985; 28:21–30.

54. Foldi E, Foldi M, Weissleder H. Conservative treatment of lymphoedema of the limbs. *Angiol J Vasc Dis* 1985; 36:171–180.

55. Foldi E, Foldi M, Clodius L. The lymphedema chaos: a lancet. *Ann Plast Surg* 1989; 22(6):505–515.

56. Bunce IH, Mirolo BR, Hennessy JM, Ward LC, Jones LC. Post mastectomy lymphoedema treatment and measurement. *Med J Aust* 1994; 161:125–128.

57. Hutzschenreuter PO, Wittlinger H, Wittlinger G, Kurz I. Post-mastectomy arm lymphedema: treated by manual lymph drainage and compression bandage therapy. *Eur J Phys Med Rehabil* 1991; 1:166–170.
58. Casley-Smith JR, Casley-Smith JR. Lymphoedema therapy in Australia; complex physical therapy, exercises and benzopyrones, on over 600 limbs. In: Witte MH, Witte CL, eds. *Progress in Lymphology-XIV*. Zurich: International Society of Lymphology, 1994:622–626.
59. Casley-Smith JR, Casley-Smith JR. Modern treatment of lymphoedema II. The benzopyrones. *Aust J Dermatol* 1992; 3:69–74.
60. Casley-Smith JR, Morgan RG, Piller NB. Treatment of lymphedema of the arms and legs with 5,6-Benzo-[1]-pyrone. *N Engl J Med* 1993; 329:1158–1163.
61. Casley-Smith JR, Casley-Smith JR. The pathophysiology of lymphedema and the action of benzo-pyrones in reducing it. *Lymphology* 1988; 21:190–194.
62. Cox D, O'Kennedy R, Thornes RD. The rarity of liver toxicity in patients treated with coumarin (1,2-Benzopyrone). *Hum Toxicol* 1989; 8:501–506.
63. Degni M. Surgical management of selected patients with lymphedema of the extremities. *J Cardiovasc Surg* 1984; 25:481–488.
64. Campisi C. A rational approach to the management of lymphedema. *Lymphology* 1991; 24:48–53.
65. Egorov YS, Avalmasov KG, Ivanov VV, Abramov YA, Gainulin RM, Chatterjee SS, Khussainov BE. Autotransplantation of the greater omentum in the treatment of chronic lymphedema. *Lymphology* 1994; 27:137–143.
66. Rada IO, Rada FC, Cristodor P, Hancu M. Upper limb late postoperative secondary lymphoedema. In: Cluzan RV, Pecking AP, Lokiec FM, eds. *Progress in Lymphology-XIII*. Amsterdam: Elsevier Science Publishers B.V., 1992:451–452.
67. Campisi C. Lymphatic microsurgery: a potent weapon in the war on lymphedema. *Lymphology* 1995; 28:110–112.
68. Louton RB, Terranova WA. The use of suction currettage as adjunct to the management of lymphedema. *Ann Plast Surg* 1989; 22:354–357.
69. O'Brien B McC, Khazanchi RK, Kumar PAV, Dvir E, Pederson WC. Liposuction in the treatment of lymphoedema: a preliminary report. *Br J Plast Surg* 1989; 42:530–533.
70. Talarico F, Brunetto D, Scialabba M, et al. Fibrosclerotic lymphedema: pathophysiology and therapy. *Lymphology* 1991; 24:11–15.

Index

abscesses, in HIV patients, 249

abstinence syndrome, from opioid withdrawal, 23

abuse, in childhood, as factor in borderline personality disorder, 217

acantholytic dyskeratosis, in HIV patients, 249

acanthosis nigricans, internal malignancies associated with, 239

acanthosis palmaris, internal malignancies associated with, 239

acetabular lesions, classification of, 142

acetaminophen
   antipyretic effect of, 13
   for bone pain, 87, 119
   for cancer pain in children, 12, 13
   opioid use with, 14, 20, 87, 206
   pediatric dosages of, 13

acidemias, nausea and vomiting from, 55

acne, 5-alpha reductase role in, 236

acrodermatitis enteropathica, nutritional deficiency in, 242

acro-osteolysis and acrosclerosis, vinyl chloride-induced, 238

actinomycosis, in HIV patients, 249

acute lymphocytic leukemia
   depression in, 193
   methylphenidate for, 64

acyclovir (Zovirax), depression induced by, 196
   for oral herpes, 53

adenocarcinoma, bone resorption inhibitors for, 92

adhesions, bowel obstruction by, 54

adipose tissue
   damage to, 240
   function of, 235
   of skin, 234

adjustment disorders, in terminal patients, 168, 182–183

adjuvant analgesics
   for bone pain, 75, 86–91
   for cancer pain in children, 12, 21–23
   for neuropathic pain, 167

adolescents
   AIDS in, antidepressant for, 62
   cancer pain in, 9
   desipramine for hyperactivity in, 62
   methylphenidate use as psychostimulant in, 64
   patient-controlled analgesia use by, 18
   role in pediatric palliative care, 44

Adriamycin, 205

affective disorders, in cancer patients, 182, 183

affect tolerance, in borderline personality disorder, 215

Africa, skin tumors in albinos of, 238

Agency for Health Care Policy and Research (AHCPR), 253, 261

aggression
   in borderline personality disorder, 218
   pediatric treatment of, 61–62

aging
   accelerated, from smoking, 238
   premature, in HIV patients, 249

AIDS
   in adolescents, antidepressant for, 62
   diaper dermatitis in, 65
   diarrhea in, 57
   dyspnea in, 60
   encephalopathies from, 63
   in pediatric patients, 53, 60, 248
   psychiatric disorders in, 166
   seborrheic dermatitis in, 244
   skin disorders in, 231, 248
   Sting lyrics based on death from, 165
   wasting in, treatment of, 54

air-fluidized bed, for pressure reduction, 258

air pillows, for pressure reduction, 258

airplane flights, exacerbated lymphedema from, 273, 275, 276

akatheisia, drug-induced, 206

alcohol abuse
   bone pain management and, 86
   in borderline personality disorder, 223
   depression induced by, 183, 195, 196
   NSAID use and, 90
   role in cancer development, 178